HANDBOOK OF

OVARIAN STIMULATION

HANDBOOK OF OVARIAN STIMULATION

Series Editors

Juan A García-Velasco MD PhD
Director
IVI Madrid
Madrid, Spain
IVI Director
Nova IVI Fertility, India and
GCC, Abu Dhabi, UAE
Professor
Obstetrics and Gynecology
Rey Juan Carlos University
Madrid, Spain

Manish Banker MD DGO
Director
NOVA IVI Fertility and Pulse Women's Hospital
Ahmedabad, Gujarat, India
Past President
Indian Society for Assisted Reproduction (ISAR)

Editor

Sulbha Arora MD DNB
Clinical Director
Consultant Reproductive Medicine
Nova IVI Fertility
Mumbai, Maharashtra, India

Foreword

Nozer Sheriar MD DNBE FICOG FCPS DGO

JAYPEE The Health Sciences Publisher
New Delhi | London | Panama

JAYPEE Jaypee Brothers Medical Publishers (P) Ltd

Headquarters
Jaypee Brothers Medical Publishers (P) Ltd.
4838/24, Ansari Road, Daryaganj
New Delhi 110 002, India
Phone: +91-11-43574357
Fax: +91-11-43574314
E-mail: jaypee@jaypeebrothers.com

Overseas Offices
J.P. Medical Ltd.
83, Victoria Street, London
SW1H 0HW (UK)
Phone: +44-20 3170 8910
Fax: +44(0)20 3008 6180
E-mail: info@jpmedpub.com

Jaypee-Highlights Medical Publishers Inc.
City of Knowledge, Bld. 237, Clayton
Panama City, Panama
Phone: +1 507-301-0496
Fax: +1 507-301-0499
E-mail: cservice@jphmedical.com

Jaypee Brothers Medical Publishers (P) Ltd.
17/1-B, Babar Road, Block-B, Shaymali
Mohammadpur, Dhaka-1207
Bangladesh
Mobile: +08801912003485
E-mail: jaypeedhaka@gmail.com

Jaypee Brothers Medical Publishers (P) Ltd.
Bhotahity, Kathmandu, Nepal
Phone: +977-9741283608
E-mail: kathmandu@jaypeebrothers.com

Website: www.jaypeebrothers.com
Website: www.jaypeedigital.com

Inquiries for bulk sales may be solicited at: jaypee@jaypeebrothers.com

Handbook of Ovarian Stimulation

First Edition: 2018

ISBN: 978-93-5270-060-8

Printed at:

Dedicated

This book is dedicated to our patients whose dreams and hopes inspire us to constantly search for solutions and strive to scale newer heights of success.

Juan A García-Velasco
Manish Banker
Sulbha Arora

CONTRIBUTORS

Carlo Alviggi MD PhD
Assistant Professor
University of Naples
Federico II
Naples, Italy

Sulbha Arora MD DNB
Clinical Director
Consultant Reproductive
Medicine
Nova IVI Fertility
Mumbai, Maharashtra, India

Puneet R Arora MBBS MS (O&G) MRCOG MSc
Senior Consultant and Clinical
Director
Nova IVI Fertility
New Delhi, India

Manish Banker MD DGO
Director
NOVA IVI Fertility and Pulse
Women's Hospital
Ahmedabad, Gujarat, India
Past President
Indian Society for Assisted
Reproduction (ISAR)

Natalia Basile MSc PhD
Embryologist
IVI Madrid
Madrid, Spain

Julia K Bosdou MD MSc PhD
Obstetrics and Gynecology Resident
Unit for Home Reproduction
First Department of Obstetrics
and Gynecology, Papageorgiou
Hospital, Aristotle University of
Thessaloniki Medical School
Thessaloniki, Greece

Carlos Dosouto Capel MD
Physician/Doctor
Hospital Universitario Dexeus
Reproductive Medicine Service
Barcelona, Spain

Alessandro Conforti MD
Professor of Gyne and Obs
Department of Neurosciences
Reproductive Sciences and
Odontostomatology
University of Naples Federico II
Naples, Italy

Giuseppe De Placido MD
Professor
Department of Neurosciences
Reproductive Sciences and
Odontostomatology
University of Naples Federico II
Naples, Italy

Ashvini Deshmukh MBBS MS (Obs & Gyn)
Associatc Gynecologist
Nova IVI Fertility
Mumbai, Maharashtra, India

Sandro C Esteves PhD MD
Medical and Scientific Director
ANDROFERT
Andrology and Human Reproduction Clinic
Center for Male Reproduction
Sao Paulo, Brazil

Human M Fatemi MD PhD
Director
Middle-East Operations
IVI Middle-East Fertility Clinic
Abu Dhabi, UAE

Pilar Alamá Faubel MD PhD
Gynecologist
Oocyte Donation Program
Coordinator, Instituto Valenciano de Infertilidad (IVI)
Valencia, Spain

Juan Antonio García-Velasco MD PhD
Director, IVI Madrid
Madrid, Spain
IVI Director
Nova IVI Fertility
India and GCC, Abu Dhabi, UAE
Professor
Obstetrics and Gynecology
Rey Juan Carlos University
Madrid, Spain

Korula George MD MRACOG
Professor and Head
Reproductive Medicine Unit
Bangalore Baptist Hospital
Bengaluru, Karnataka, India

Alfredo Guillén MD
Gynecologist
Vice Director, IVI Madrid
Madrid, Spain

Reena Gupta MBBS MS FNB
Obstetrician and Gynecologist
Fellowship in Reproductive Medicine
Nova IVI Fertility
Ahmedabad, Gujarat, India

Ritu Hinduja MD DRM (Germany)
Fellowship in Reproductive Medicine
Consultant
Nova IVI Fertility
Mumbai, Maharashtra, India

Peter Humaidan DMSc
Professor
Skive Regional Hospital and Faculty of Health
Aarhus University
Aarhus, Denmark

Krithika Devi J MBBS MD (OG)
Consultant
Fellowship in Andrology and Reproductive Medicine
Nova IVI Fertility
Chennai, Tamil Nadu, India

Mohan S Kamath MS DNB PGDMLS
Fellow (Reproductive Medicine)
Christian Medical College
Vellore, Tamil Nadu, India
Commonwealth Fellow (Reproductive Medicine)
United Kingdom
Professor
Reproductive Medicine Unit
Christian Medical College
Vellore, Tamil Nadu, India

Stratis Kolibianakis MD MSc PhD
Associate Professor
Obstetrics, Gynecology and
Assisted Reproduction Unit for
Human Reproduction
Medical School
Aristotle University
Thessaloniki, Greece

Barbara Lawrenz MD PhD
Consultant Obstetrician and
Gynecologist
Fakih IVF
Abu Dhabi, UAE

Diana Collado Muñoz MD PhD
Oocyte Donation Program
Gynecologist, IVI Madrid
Madrid, Spain

Javier Martínez-Salazar Romero MD
Gynecologist
Assisted Reproduction Unit
IVI Madrid
Madrid, Spain

Israel Ortega Sanchez MD
Gynecologist
IVI Madrid
Madrid, Spain

Kalyani Shrimali DNB MNAMS DRM (Germany)
Fellowship in Reproductive
Medicine
Indian College of Obstetricians &
Gynaecologists (ICOG)
Mumbai, Maharashtra, India
Consultant
Nova IVI Fertility
Indore, Madhya Pradesh, India

Haahr T MD PhD
Clinical Assistant
The Fertility Clinic Skive
Skive Regional Hospital and Skive
Department of Clinical Medicine
Aarhus University,
Aarhus, Denmark

FOREWORD

"There was never a night or a problem that could defeat sunrise or hope."
—Bernard Williams

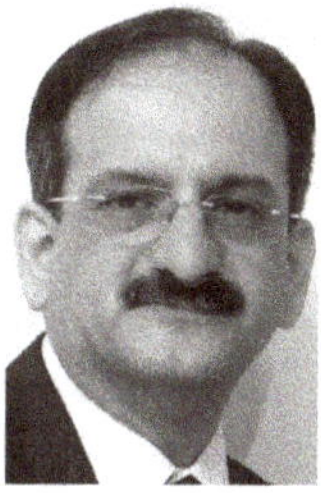

Addressing the cause of reproductive health and rights championed by gynecologists, the primary care givers for women would be incomplete, unfair and unjust, if the difficulty in conception faced by about a tenth of couples each year is not acknowledged, cared for and supported. This makes the treatment of infertility not just an essential part of care of women and the practice of gynecology but also a major public health issue.

Ovarian function fascinates me since the story of all human life begins with gonads and with gametes. The study, assessment, manipulation and stimulation of the ovaries thus allow us a glimpse into and give us a privileged role in the processes at the very start of life. This makes it necessary to keep abreast with the scientific advances and therapies related to ovarian function, its related problems and solutions. Broad principles have to be understood and yet individualization has to be ensured to create a predictable response in an often unpredictable situation. Exciting advances in our knowledge and capacity to influence ovarian function make it necessary for us to periodically update ourselves on the subject of ovarian stimulation.

It is hence an honor for me to write this foreword for this important *Handbook of Ovarian Stimulation* edited by Dr Sulbha Arora and Dr Manish Banker both of whom I have long known and respected for their professional sincerity and capability, along with Dr Juan A García-Velasco a renowned specialist and much published academician. This book is a thoughtful compilation of topics ranging from the basics of ovarian stimulation to protocols for tailored solutions for different situations in clinical practice to strategies to promote safety and preempt complications. This challenging task has been achieved by bringing together between its covers, the work, experience and expertise of an exceptional panel of internationally renowned contributors.

For me the editors of a book are its heart and its guiding light. I have known Sulbha Arora for over a decade in both organizational and professional roles. This polite charming young doctor is not only a successful fertility specialist, but is also passionate about sharing knowledge through conferences, chapters and books. Manish Banker has been a friend and colleague for twice as long. He is a polite and soft spoken individual and a nationally acclaimed fertility specialist. In his many organizational roles he has worked hard to promote reproductive medicine in India and document practice through a decade long involvement with the National ART Registry. Juan A García-Velasco brings the book a truly international perspective along with his acknowledged scholarship in this subject.

I wish the editors and the panel of contributors the very best for this book, their labor of love for addressing and confronting subfertility. I also thank them on behalf of all the couples whose hopes and dreams they will help fulfill, by virtue of this book influencing the care that will be provided to them by their doctors going ahead.

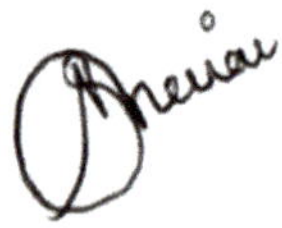

Nozer Sheriar MD DNBE FICOG FCPS DGO
Consultant Obstetrician and Gynecologist
Breach Candy, Hinduja Healthcare and Holy Family Hospitals
Mumbai, Maharashtra, India

PREFACE

The conception of the first in vitro fertilization (IVF) baby, Louise Brown, was the result of a natural or unstimulated cycle. However, it was soon realised that the success rates of natural cycle IVF were low, mainly due to the limited number of oocytes retrieved. To address this problem, urinary gonadotropin preparations were introduced to stimulate the production of multiple follicles by the ovaries. The advent of ovarian stimulation heralded a significant increase both in the number of oocytes retrieved as well as the success rates of IVF. Today, ovulation induction and controlled ovarian stimulation are integral parts of every assisted reproductive program.

Stimulation protocols are currently chosen mainly based on personal preferences and individual experience rather than objective evidence. This book, aimed at physicians whose practices include assisted reproductive techniques (ART), discusses ways in which clinicians might better predict ovarian response to stimulation with gonadotropins, as well as select the ideal stimulation protocol and tailor it to the individual patient. It includes chapters on the different oral ovulogens as well as the different gonadotropins; stimulation protocols for IUI and IVF; for poor and hyper-responders; for egg donors and for oncofertility patients. It also includes information on complications of stimulation, as well as newer drugs and drug delivery systems.

In almost four decades of IVF practice, numerous textbooks discussing reproduction and ART have been published. Is a new textbook actually needed? This question would evidently be answered merely by skimming through the table of contents of this handbook. IVF is not a perfect science and we are constantly faced with the question "what next?". What else can be done to help the most challenging cases? How can we build on existing knowledge and improve our success rates further?

Reproductive medicine is a young science and, as such, all innovations are happening in our lifetime by our seniors, peers and even by young stars in the field. In this comprehensive compilation, we aim to offer an easy approach to Ovarian Stimulation by experts pioneering in reproductive medicine.

Sulbha Arora

ACKNOWLEDGMENTS

I would like to acknowledge the efforts and contribution of all the authors and co-editors in the compilation of this Handbook. I am thankful to Mr Jitendar P Vij (Group Chairman), Mr Ankit Vij (Group President) and Ms Chetna Malhotra Vohra (Associate Director-Content Strategy) for their kind cooperation; and Ms Angima Shree (Senior Development Editor) and the editorial team of M/s Jaypee Brothers Medical Publishers (P) Ltd, for their pivotal role in coordinating the release of this book.

CONTENTS

Chapter 1

Oral Ovulogens

Mohan S Kamath, Korula George

INTRODUCTION

Ovulatory dysfunction is one of the common reasons for infertility and accounts for about 40% of female infertility.[1] According to World Health Organization (WHO) classification ovulatory dysfunctions are mainly categorized into: (1) Class I—consisting of hypothalamic pituitary failure, (2) Class II—being hypothalamic pituitary dysfunction, and (3) Class III—representing ovarian failure. The hypothalamic pituitary failure (5 - 10%) and ovarian failure (5%) are less common groups with majority of the ovulatory dysfunction belonging to the Class II category. Polycystic ovarian syndrome (PCOS), which belongs to WHO Class II, is the most common cause of ovulatory dysfunction.[1] Diagnosis of PCOS can be made using Rotterdam criteria or National Institute of Health (NIH) criteria. Out of the three criteria (oligo- and/or anovulation, clinical and/or biochemical signs of hyperandrogenism, and polycystic ovaries on ultrasound), presence of two are considered essential for diagnosis of PCOS under the Rotterdam criteria.[2] Additionally, other endocrine disorders such as congenital adrenal hyperplasia and androgen secreting tumors should be excluded.

Oral ovulogens are drugs, which are mainly used for inducing ovulation in women with anovulatory dysfunction. They are usually the first line of treatment for patients belonging to WHO Class II. They are also used to achieve super ovulation during intrauterine insemination (IUI) in couples with unexplained infertility.[3] During in vitro fertilization (IVF) treatment, they may also be combined with gonadotropins for controlled ovarian hyperstimulation (COH), commonly known as mild stimulation protocols.[4]

Most common oral ovulogens used in contemporary practice are clomiphene citrate (CC), aromatase inhibitors (e.g. anastrozole), and insulin sensitizers such as metformin.[1,5,6] Less commonly used drugs are tamoxifen, dexamethasone, and thiazolidinediones (e.g. rosiglitazone).[7,8]

ORAL DRUGS FOR OVULATION INDUCTION

Clomiphene Citrate

Clinical Case # 1

"A 23-year-old Mrs X and her husband Mr Y, aged 26 years, presented with complaints of inability to conceive from last 1 year. They have been married for 2 years. Menstrual cycles are irregular (40–45 days). No dysmenorrhea. No obvious clinical signs of excess androgen observed during examination. Body mass index 24 kg/m^2. On ultrasound, polycystic ovaries were seen. Thyroid-stimulating hormone (TSH) and serum prolactin levels were normal. Husband semen analysis reported as normozoospermia. Wife diagnosed as a case of PCOS. No previous treatment for infertility. The first pharmacological line of treatment for treatment naive PCOS woman is..."

Clomiphene citrate is the first-line drug used to induce ovulation in women with PCOS. It consists of two isomeric components: zu-clomiphene and en-clomiphene. Among the two, zu-clomiphene is considered more potent for ovulation induction.[1] The estrogen receptors in hypothalamus are blocked by clomiphene citrate, which prevents a negative feedback of estrogen, causing a release of gonadotropin releasing hormone (GnRH). The release of GnRH results in increase in endogenous gonadotropins—follicle stimulating hormone (FSH) and luteinizing hormone (LH)—from the anterior pituitary, which promotes follicular development in the ovary. The negative impact of estrogen receptor blockade by CC at the endometrial and cervical level is considered to be the reason for lower pregnancy rates (30–40%) even though ovulation is achieved in almost 80% of the PCOS women.[1]

Though the starting dose is 50 mg daily for 5 days and can be initiated from anytime between day 2 to day 5 of menstrual cycle, many clinicians prefer 100 mg daily as the starting dose. The reason for this is higher ovulation rate (67%) with 100 mg compared to 46% following 50 mg dosage, without any apparent increase in multiple pregnancy rate.[9] The follicular development can be documented by an ultrasound by day 12–14 at least in the index cycle. Those with follicular development can be advised timed intercourse for at least 1 week after ultrasound. The routine administration of human chorionic gonadotropin (hCG) as a trigger for follicular rupture during ovulation induction with CC has not been found to be beneficial.[10]

Ultrasound monitoring helps in identifying those women who have responded to a particular dose of CC and the same dose can be adhered to for subsequent treatment cycles. In few cases, hyper-response can be noted and when more than three dominant follicles are noted, it is advisable to cancel the cycle and advise sexual abstinence for next 2 weeks.

In case no follicular development is noted, the daily dose of CC can be increased by 50 mg and a maximum of 150–200 mg per day is advised.

Women who do not respond to the maximum dose of CC are categorized under CC resistance, and those who respond but do not conceive after three to six treatment cycles are known as CC failure. It is advisable to restrict the number of CC cycles to a maximum of 12, due to potential threefold increase in risk of ovarian malignancy in future.[11]

For women with CC resistance which signifies a severe form of PCOS, next treatment options include aromatase inhibitors, gonadotropins, insulin sensitizers and in some cases, laparoscopic ovarian drilling.[1,12] In cases of CC failure, tubal evaluation is warranted to rule out tubal pathologies before moving to alternative options.

Clomiphene citrate may cause side effects such as nausea, hot flushes, and rarely visual disturbances.[1] In case of any visual disturbance following CC is noted, it should be promptly discontinued and alternative ovulation induction agents should be offered.

Some of the less common CC regimens include stair step protocol and using CC for longer duration.

In stair step protocol, starting dose of CC (50 mg) is given for 5 days from day 2 of the menstrual cycle and ultrasound is done on day 11–14.[13] In case no follicle develops, the dose is increased by 50 mg (100 mg for 5 days) and started immediately while the ultrasound is planned 1 week after the first follicular ultrasound. If no response is noted again, then the daily dose is increased to 150 mg for 5 days and repeat ultrasound done 1 week later. In clinical practice, this protocol reduces time to ovulation (23–35 days) compared to standard cyclical protocol (55–88 days). PCOS women with anovulation are more suited for this protocol than oligo-ovulation.

Clomiphene citrate is sometimes used in couples with unexplained infertility. In the Cochrane review, no significant increase in clinical pregnancy rates following CC compared to expectant management after pooling results from two trials (OR 1.03, 95% CI 0.64–1.66).[11] In unexplained infertility, use of CC should be avoided since it has no proven benefit, though it increases risk of multiple pregnancies.

Aromatase Inhibitors

Clinical Case # 2

"A 27-year-old Mrs X and her husband Mr Y, age 36 years, presented with complaints of inability to conceive from last 6 years. They have been married for 7 years. Menstrual cycles are irregular (40–45 days). No dysmenorrhea. No obvious clinical signs of excess androgen observed during examination. Body mass index 26 kg/m². On ultrasound, polycystic ovaries were seen. TSH, serum prolactin, and testosterone levels were normal. Husband semen analysis reported as normozoospermia. Wife diagnosed as a case of PCOS. She gives history of ovulation induction with CC with no response at 200 mg daily dose

(CC resistance). Hysterosalpingography demonstrated patent tubes. Sugar levels are normal. The next possible medical option for such women with CC resistance is..."

Aromatase inhibitors act at the ovarian level and prevent the conversion of androgen to estrogen. The reduced systemic levels of estrogen release the hypothalamo-pituitary axis from the negative feedback exerted by estrogen, thus resulting in increase in FSH levels. The higher androgen levels in the ovary also increases follicular sensitivity to FSH.[14] Unlike CC, aromatase inhibitors do not exert peripheral antiestrogenic action and are cleared from systemic circulation more rapidly due to shorter half-life (48 hours) compared to CC which has a prolonged half-life (2 weeks). Another advantage of aromatase inhibitor is reduced chances of multifollicular development due to intact estrogen negative feedback mechanism, which reduces FSH levels with rising estrogen.[14] With CC, this negative feedback mechanism is interrupted due to blockade of estrogen receptors by CC.

There were initial concerns about teratogenic effect of letrozole, an aromatase inhibitor. Subsequent studies have not shown increased congenital anomaly rate following the drug.[15]

Anastrozole, another aromatase inhibitor, is being used in clinical practice as an alternative oral ovulogen to CC. The recommended dose of anastrozole is 1 mg daily for 5 days from day 2 of menstrual cycle.[16] The ovulation rates following anastrozole are comparable to CC (67% vs. 68%).[5] It may have role in treating CC resistant PCOS women who constitute about 20–25%.[17,18]

Tamoxifen

Tamoxifen, a triphenyl ethylene derivative, is less commonly used drug for ovulation induction purpose. It is sometimes used in women who experience side effects following CC and rarely in CC resistant PCOS cases.[8,19] The dosage is between 20 mg and 40 mg daily from day 2 or day 3 of menstrual cycle for 5 days. Live birth rates following tamoxifen were not significantly different compared to CC.[8]

Dexamethasone

Clinical Case #3

"A 27-year-old Mrs X and her husband Mr Y, aged 36 years, presented with complaints of inability to conceive from last 6 years. They have been married for 7 years. Menstrual cycles are irregular (40–45 days). No dysmenorrhea. No obvious clinical signs of excess androgen observed during examination. Body mass index 26 kg/m². On ultrasound, polycystic ovaries were seen. TSH, serum prolactin, and testosterone levels were normal. Her dehydroepiandrosterone (DHEA) level is elevated. Husband semen analysis reported as normozoospermia. Wife diagnosed as a case of late onset congenital adrenal

hyperplasia. She wants regularization of cycles and wishes to conceive. The recommended medical option for such women with late onset congenital adrenal hyperplasia (CAH) is..."

The role of dexamethasone as an ovulation induction agent is mainly confined to treating endocrinological conditions such as late onset congenital adrenal hyperplasia. However, it has been also offered in CC resistant PCOS case with normal levels of dehydroepiandrosterone sulfate (DHEAS). A randomized trial found significantly higher ovulation rates (75% vs. 15%; $p < 0.01$) with CC and dexamethasone compared to CC with placebo in women with CC resistance.[20] The low dosage of 0.5 mg per day from day 1 to day 14 of menstrual cycles is generally recommended. Earlier study has found better pregnancy rates with higher dose of 2 mg per day instead of low dose.[20]

Insulin Sensitizers

Clinical Case # 4

"A 28-year-old Mrs X and her husband Mr Y, aged 36 years, presented with complaints of inability to conceive from last 4 years. They have been married for 7 years. Menstrual cycles are irregular (40–45 days). No dysmenorrhea. No obvious clinical signs of excess androgen observed during examination. Body mass index 30 kg/m^2. On ultrasound, polycystic ovaries were seen. TSH, serum prolactin, and testosterone levels were normal. Husband semen analysis reported as normozoospermia. Wife diagnosed as a case of PCOS. She gives history of ovulation induction with CC with no response at 200 mg daily dose (CC resistance). Hysterosalpingography demonstrated patent tubes. She is diagnosed with impaired glucose tests. She has been advised weight reduction and given dietary advice. The next possible medical option for such women with CC resistance is.."

Most common insulin sensitizer used in PCOS women is metformin. Though its influence on weight reduction is not clearly established, it is commonly advised in PCOS women with impaired glucose.[2] It is also an option in women with CC resistant PCOS. In a randomized controlled trial (RCT) which included women with CC resistance, intervention arm consisted of metformin for 6 months followed by CC again. In the control arm, ovulation induction with gonadotropin was planned. No significant difference in clinical pregnancy rates was observed in the two groups and lower cost of metformin was an added advantage.[21] Recent update has reported improvement in menstrual cycle regularity and ovulation rate following metformin compared to placebo.[22] Metformin is associated with severe gastrointestinal side effects, which can lead to patient compliance issues. Usual recommended dose is 500–1,500 mg daily though it should be initiated with low dose and gradually titrated after assessing the tolerance.[22]

Since metformin is considered safe in pregnancy, clinicians continue its use during pregnancy once the woman conceives. This is done to help in improving metabolic profile and reduce the risk of gestational diabetes in PCOS women. A recent large trial however did not show any improvement in complication rate during pregnancy by continuing metformin throughout the gestation.[23]

There is paucity of trials evaluating other newer insulin sensitizers such as thiazolidionedines and d-chiro-inositol. Thiazolidionedines are mainly used for treating type 2 diabetes mellitus. Due to their beneficial action in improving insulin resistance, many clinicians have advocated its use in women with PCOS. A study found young PCOS women with pioglitazone had improvement in menstrual symptoms.[24]

However, there are ongoing concerns regarding side effects, weight gain, and safety during pregnancy with these drugs. Though many of these drugs showed initial promise, currently the evidence is insufficient to recommend their use for ovulation induction purpose.[22,25]

Oral Ovulogens for Ovarian Stimulation during Intrauterine Insemination

Commonly, ovarian stimulation is combined with intrauterine insemination (IUI) to achieve super ovulation (more than one follicle) in couples with unexplained infertility, mild male factor, or minimal endometriosis. Various agents are used for ovarian stimulation such as CC, aromatase inhibitors, gonadotropin or combination of oral ovulogens with gonadotropins.

Clomiphene or aromatase inhibitors are combined with gonadotropin to lower total dosage requirement of gonadotropin, which reduces the cost without compromising on IUI outcomes. Clomiphene citrate (100 mg) is started from day 2 of menstrual cycle and continued for 5 days. The gonadotropin (75 IU) is initiated from day 5 and given on alternate days and follicular monitoring is done from day 10. Satisfactory pregnancy rates are achieved using combination of CC and gonadotropin during IUI.[26] Similar combination protocol (CC and gonadotropin) also can be used for achieving ovulation induction instead of gonadotropin alone in CC resistant or CC failure cases as pregnancy rates are comparable.[12]

Use of Oral Ovulogens in Mild Stimulation Protocols

Clinical Case # 5

"A 37-year-old Mrs X and her husband Mr Y, aged 46 years, presented with complaints of inability to conceive from last 6 years. They have been married for 7 years. Menstrual cycles are regular. Body mass index 21 kg/m^2.

On ultrasound, normal ovaries and total antral follicle count of 5 was noted. TSH and serum prolactin levels were normal. Husband semen analysis reported as severe oligoasthenozoospermia. Couple underwent for IVF with conventional stimulation of high gonadotropins. Three oocytes were retrieved and cycle was unsuccessful. The couple wishes to try another autologous IVF. The possible options for controlled ovarian hyperstimulation (COH) include..."

Oral ovulogens such as CC and aromatase inhibitors have been used for mild stimulation protocol during IVF. Use of CC in these protocols is quite common and some of the benefits include lower gonadotropin requirements and less cost during IVF.[27,28] They also are patient-friendly protocols and pregnancy rate for certain subset of patients is comparable to conventional IVF. The milder stimulation has added advantage of higher yield of euploid embryos compared to conventional high dose gonadotropins.[29]

The Cochrane review which included 12 trials and 2,536 participants found comparable live birth rates following CC and gonadotropin compared to gonadotropin alone during IVF (OR 0.93, 95% CI 0.69–1.24). The ovarian hyperstimulation syndrome (OHSS) rates were significantly lower in the CC and gonadotropin group (0.8–1.8%) compared to gonadotropin agonist protocol (3.5%).[4] The mild stimulation protocol has been advocated in women who had poor response or unsuccessful outcome in previous conventional IVF with high dose of gonadotropins. A recent systematic review which included four trials, evaluated CC with gonadotropin versus conventional gonadotropin alone in poor responders. They found no significant differences in live birth rates (OR: 0.71, 95% CI 0.22–2.2) and clinical pregnancy rates (OR: 1.11, 95% CI 0.80–1.55) following CC with gonadotropin compared to gonadotropin alone.[27]

Clomiphene citrate has also been used to prevent premature LH surge during IVF instead of GnRH analogs. In this protocol, CC is initiated from day 2 of the cycle and continued till the day hCG trigger is given. Continuous use of clomiphene citrate blocks estrogen receptors' sites at the hypothalamus and pituitary. Clomiphene used in this fashion mimics the action of a GnRH analog and prevents an LH surge due to rising estrogen levels, a result of follicular development. Low dose gonadotropins 75–150 IU are also added to enhance the response. Hence, conventional GnRH analogs are not required for prevention of premature LH surge.[30] This protocol is quite useful in low cost IVF program since the GnRH analogs are not used, and gonadotropin requirement is less.[28]

KEY SUMMARY POINTS

Lifestyle changes are the first line of therapy for ovulation induction in PCOS.

- Clomiphene citrate is the first choice for inducing ovulation medically in PCOS.
- For CC failure, alternatives are aromatase inhibitors or gonadotropins alone or in combination with CC or aromatase inhibitors.
- If resistant to CC, the next options are aromatase inhibitors, insulin sensitizers, gonadotropins, or surgical intervention for ovarian drilling.
- Metformin is recommended for women with PCOS who have impaired glucose tolerance and CC resistance. Currently other insulin sensitizers are not recommended for routine ovulation induction due to insufficient evidence.
- Tamoxifen is another alternative antiestrogen which can be advised in CC failure.
- Dexamethasone can be offered as an adjuvant along with CC in women with CC resistance.
- Clomiphene citrate and aromatase inhibitors can be combined with gonadotropins in mild stimulation IVF protocols, especially in poor responders.

REFERENCES

1. Homburg R. Clomiphene citrate—end of an era? A mini-review. Hum Reprod. 2005;20(8):2043-51.
2. Thessaloniki ESHRE/ASRM-Sponsored PCOS Consensus Workshop Group. Consensus on infertility treatment related to polycystic ovary syndrome. Hum Reprod. 2008;23(3):462-77.
3. Kamath MS, Bhattacharya S. Demographics of infertility and management of unexplained infertility. Best Pract Res Clin Obstet Gynaecol. 2012;26(6): 729-38
4. Gibreel A, Maheshwari A, Bhattacharya S. Clomiphene citrate in combination with gonadotropins for controlled ovarian stimulation in women undergoing in vitro fertilization. Cochrane Database Syst Rev. 2012;11: CD008528.
5. Badawy A, Abdel Aal I, Abulatta M. Clomiphene citrate or anastrozole for ovulation induction in women with polycystic ovary syndrome? A prospective controlled trial. Fertil Steril. 2009;92(3):860-3.
6. Palomba S, Falbo A, Zullo F, Orio F Jr. Evidence-based and potential benefits of metformin in the polycystic ovary syndrome: a comprehensive review. Endocr Rev. 2009;30(1):1-50.
7. Baillargeon JP, Jakubowicz DJ, Iuorno MJ, Jakubowicz S, Nestler JE. Effects of metformin and rosiglitazone, alone and in combination, in nonobese women with polycystic ovary syndrome and normal indices of insulin sensitivity. Fertil Steril. 2004;82:893-902.
8. Brown J, Farquhar C. Clomiphene and other antioestrogens for ovulation induction in polycystic ovarian syndrome. Cochrane Database Syst Rev. 2016;12:CD002249.
9. Rostami-Hodjegan A, Lennard MS, Tucker GT, Ledger WL. Monitoring plasma concentrations to individualize treatment with clomiphene citrate. Fertil Steril. 2004;81(5):1187-93.

10. George K, Kamath MS, Nair R, Tharyan P. Ovulation triggers in anovulatory women undergoing ovulation induction. Cochrane Database Syst Rev. 2014;(1):CD006900.
11. Hughes E, Brown J, Collins JJ, Vanderkerchove P. Clomiphene citrate for unexplained subfertility in women. Cochrane Database Syst Rev. 2010;(1): CD000057.
12. Abdelazim IA, Makhlouf HH. Sequential clomiphene citrate/hMG versus hMG for ovulation induction in clomiphene citrate-resistant women. Arch Gynecol Obstet. 2013;287(3):591-7.
13. Hurst BS, Hickman JM, Matthews ML, et al. Novel clomiphene "stair step" protocol reduces time to ovulation in women with polycystic ovarian syndrome. Am J Obstet Gynecol. 2009;200:510.e1-510.e4.
14. Mitwally M, Casper R. Aromatase inhibitors in ovulation induction. Semin Reprod Med. 2004;22:61-78.
15. Tulandi T, Martin J, Al- Fadhli R, et al. Congenital malformations among 911 newborns conceived after infertility treatment with Letrozole or Clomiphene citrate. Fertil Steril. 2006;85:1761-5.
16. Franik S, Kremer JA, Nelen WL, Farquhar C. Aromatase inhibitors for subfertile women with polycystic ovary syndrome. Cochrane Database Syst Rev. 2014;(2):CD010287.
17. Al-Omari WR, Sulaiman W, Al-Hadithi N. Comparison of two aromatase inhibitors in women with clomiphene- resistant polycystic ovary syndrome. Intern J Gynecol Obstet. 2004;85:289-91.
18. Badawy A, Mosbah A, Shady M. Anastrozole or letrozole for ovulation induction in clomiphene-resistant women with polycystic ovary syndrome? A prospective controlled trial. Fertil Steril. 2008; 89(5):1209-12.
19. Dhaliwal LK, Suri V, Gupta KR, Sahdev S. Tamoxifen: an alternative to clomiphene in women with polycystic ovary syndrome. J Hum Reprod Sci. 2011;4(2):76-9.
20. Elnashar A, Abdelmageed E, Fayed M, Sharaf M. Clomiphene citrate and dexamethazone in treatment of clomiphene citrate-resistant polycystic ovary syndrome: a prospective placebo-controlled study. Hum Reprod. 2006; 21(7):1805-8.
21. George SS, George K, Irwin C, et al. Sequential treatment of metformin and clomiphene citrate in clomiphene-resistant women with polycystic ovary syndrome: a randomized, controlled trial. Hum Reprod. 2003;18(2): 299-304.
22. Balen AH, Morley LC, Misso M, et al. The management of anovulatory infertility in women with polycystic ovary syndrome: an analysis of the evidence to support the development of global WHO guidance. Hum Reprod Update. 2016;22(6):687-708.
23. Vanky E, Stridsklev S, Heimstad R, et al. Metformin versus placebo from first trimester to delivery in polycystic ovary syndrome: a randomized, controlled multicenter study. J Clin Endocrinol Metab. 2010;95(12):E448-55.
24. Stabile G, Borrielli I, Artenisio AC, et al. Effects of the insulin sensitizer pioglitazone on menstrual irregularity, insulin resistance and hyperandrogenism in young women with polycystic ovary syndrome. J Pediatr Adolesc Gynecol. 2014;27(3):177-82.
25. Legro RS. Ovulation induction in polycystic ovary syndrome: current options. Best Pract Res Clin Obstet Gynaecol. 2016;37:152-9.

26. Brzechffa PR, Daneshmand S, Buyalos RP. Sequential clomiphene citrate and human menopausal gonadotrophin with intrauterine insemination: the effect of patient age on clinical outcome. Hum Reprod. 1998;13(8): 2110-4.
27. Song D, Shi Y, Zhong Y, et al. Efficiency of mild ovarian stimulation with clomiphene on poor ovarian responders during IVF\ICSI procedures: a meta-analysis. Eur J Obstet Gynecol Reprod Biol. 2016;204:36-43.
28. Aleyamma TK, Kamath MS, Muthukumar K, et al. Affordable ART: a different perspective. Hum Reprod. 2011;26(12):3312-8.
29. Baart EB, Martini E, Eijkemans MJ, et al. Milder ovarian stimulation for in-vitro fertilization reduces aneuploidy in the human preimplantation embryo: a randomized controlled trial. Hum Reprod. 2007;22(4):980-8.
30. Kato K, Takehara Y, Segawa T, et al. Minimal ovarian stimulation combined with elective single embryo transfer policy: age-specific results of a large, single-centre, Japanese cohort. Reprod Biol Endocrinol. 2012;10:35.

Chapter 2

Physiology and Pharmacology of Different Gonadotropins

Reena Gupta, Manish Banker

INTRODUCTION

Gonadotropins are hormones secreted by pituitary that have a stimulatory effect on gonads. This family includes follicle-stimulating hormone (FSH), luteinizing hormone (LH), and human chorionic gonadotropin (hCG). These hormones are central to the complex endocrine system that regulates normal growth, sexual development, and reproductive function. LH and FSH are secreted by the anterior pituitary gland, while hCG is secreted by the placenta in pregnant humans.

Gonadotropin therapy plays an integral role in ovarian stimulation for infertility treatments. It was introduced almost one century ago, and the last 25 years have yielded major advancements.

PHYSIOLOGY

The human ovarian follicular development depends on the synergistic and sequential effects of the two principal gonadotropins, FSH and LH. FSH stimulates the growth of a large preovulatory follicle that, because of its FSH-dependent maturation, is able to ovulate and to form a corpus luteum in response to the mid-cycle surge of LH.

At birth, ovaries contain 1–2 million follicles arrested at the primordial stage of development. But only about 400 follicles mature and ovulate during a woman's reproductive lifespan and rest of them undergo atresia.

Follicle development from the primordial to the pre-ovulatory stage takes several months.[1] The initial growth of the primordial follicles to preantral follicles is independent of pituitary gonadotropins. However, antrum formation requires tonic stimulation by FSH. These early antral follicles are FSH responsive and constitute a pool of available follicles that can be stimulated to grow. During the luteal-follicular transition phase, a selective rise in FSH occurs that must reach a critical threshold for recruitment of follicles. Although several follicles begin to grow during this phase because of mitogenic action of FSH on granulosa cells, only one is selected and the rest are destined to undergo atresia.

At the midfollicular phase, the dominant follicle reaches about 10 mm in diameter and is recognizable as the largest follicle in the ovary, which starts secreting estradiol at around 7th or 8th day of cycle. LH is capable of stimulating androgen-substrate production from theca cells, which is transformed to estrogen by FSH stimulated aromatase activity in granulosa cells (in accordance with two-cell-two-gonadotropin therapy). This rise in estradiol (and inhibin) leads to fall in FSH levels through negative feedback on the pituitary. The midfollicular fall in FSH concentration determines the atresia of less mature follicles that are unable to grow without adequate FSH concentrations. But the mature selected follicle continues to grow which is likely to be due to its increased sensitivity to FSH itself. It has been demonstrated that FSH induces LH receptor formation on pre-ovulatory follicle granulosa cells.[2] The action of LH on its receptors activates adenyl cyclase: the consequent production of cAMP represents an additive response to FSH.[3] Therefore, the maturing follicle reduces its dependency on FSH by acquiring LH receptors and LH responsiveness.[4-8] On the other hand, lower concentrations of FSH bring less mature follicles to atresia. When mid cycle LH surge occurs, the LH-follicle interaction disrupts granulosa cells in cumulus oophorus and induces final oocyte maturation, causes follicular rupture and finally luteinization of granulosa cells. hCG has been used as surrogate to LH for final oocyte maturation and ovulation in artificially stimulated cycles (Fig. 2.1).

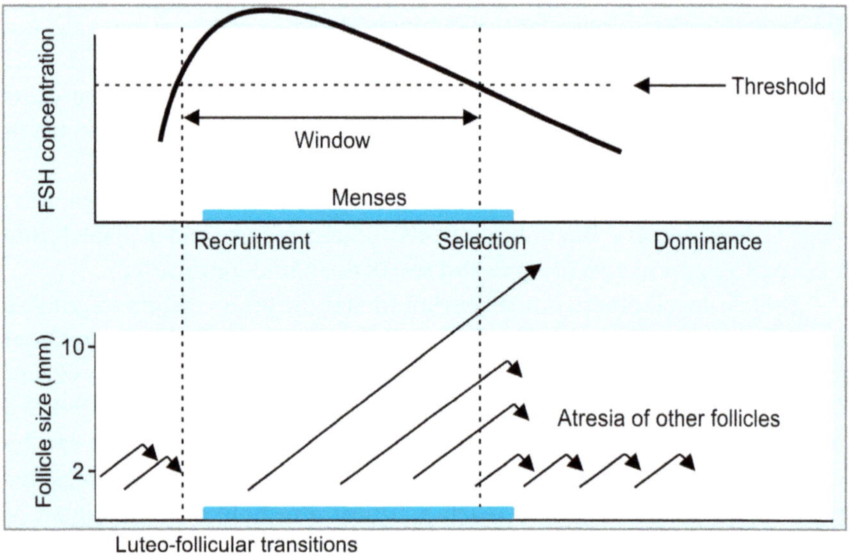

Fig. 2.1: Follicle-stimulating hormone (FSH) threshold and window concept in human follicle development.

To summarize, FSH acts on the early antral follicles to stimulate cell growth, steroidogenesis, and the expression of LH receptors. Subsequently, LH, in conjunction with FSH, acts on the FSH-stimulated follicle to maintain growth, and is eventually responsible for the process of ovulation and luteinization.

HISTORY OF GONADOTROPINS

Pharmaceutical preparations containing biologically active gonadotropins for ovulation induction have been available in the market for 75 years. It was Aschheim and Zondek, in 1927, who first discovered a substance in the urine of pregnant women which had the same action as the gonadotropic factor in the anterior pituitary.[9] They called this substance gonadotropin or "prolan". Furthermore, they believed that there were two distinct hormones, (1) prolan A and (2) prolan B now called as FSH and LH. They subsequently used their findings to develop a pregnancy test. In 1930, Zondek reported that gonadotropins were also present in the urine of postmenopausal women and in the same year, Cole and Hart found gonadotropins in the serum of pregnant mares.[10] However, it was only in 1937 that Cartland and Nelson were able to produce a purified extract of this hormone. In 1948, Stewart, Sano, and Montgomery discovered that gonadotropins in the urine of pregnant women were shown to originate from the chorionic villi of the placenta, rather than the pituitary, and subsequently designated it as "chorionic gonadotropin".[11] Within years, it became apparent that the use of gonadotropin extracts from non-primate sources was of limited clinical value owing to the development of antibodies that neutralized their therapeutic effect. Then, efforts were made to produce these gonadotropins from urine of postmenopausal women. The first urine extract of gonadotropin contained LH and FSH and was named Pergonal, inspired by the Italian words "per gonadi" (for the gonads). In 1961, with the use of Pergonal treatment, first pregnancy was reported in a patient with secondary amenorrhea. Urinary FSH and highly purified FSH became available after 1980s with the development of new technologies using specific monoclonal antibodies that bind to FSH and LH molecules in the human menopausal gonadotropin (hMG) material in such a way that unknown urinary proteins can be removed. In 2000, a major evolution occurred in the field of infertility with the development of recombinant FSH (rFSH) which had many advantages over urinary preparations. With this evolution of gonadotropins from pituitary to urinary to highly purified (HP) and most recently recombinant products the safety, purity and specific activity have increased progressively (Fig. 2.2).[12]

GONADOTROPIN STRUCTURE

The three gonadotropins, (1) FSH, (2) LH and (3) hCG, are glycoproteins composed of two noncovalently linked protein subunits, (1) the alpha and

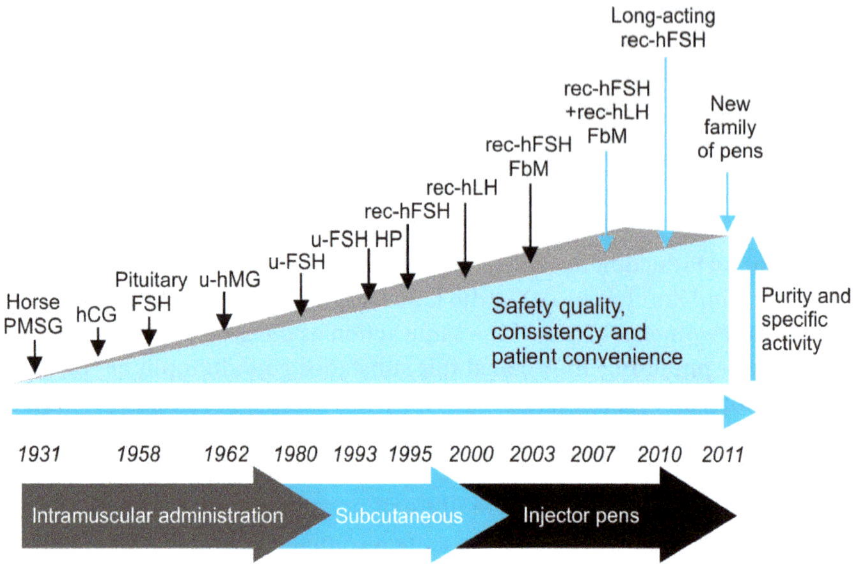

Fig. 2.2: Milestones in the development of gonadotropin preparations.
Source: Adapted from Leão R de BF, Esteves SC. Gonadotropin therapy in assisted reproduction: an evolutionary perspective from biologics to biotech. Clinics (Sao Paulo). 2014; 69(4):279-93.
(hFSH: Human follicle-stimulating hormone; hLH: Human luteinizing hormone; FbM: Filled-by-mass; hMG: Human menopausal gonadotropin; hCG: Human chorionic gonadotropin; PMSG: Pregnant mare's serum gonadotropin).

(2) beta subunits. The alpha subunit contains 92 amino acids (AA) and is identical in FSH, LH, and hCG. In contrast, the beta subunits are distinct and confer unique receptor specificity as well as differential biological properties. The subunits alone do not have any biological activity. It is the formation of heterodimers, by the attachment of carbohydrate moieties which is responsible for biological activity. The extent and pattern of glycosylation conveys the spectrum of different charges, bioactivities and half-lives for each glycoprotein. Glycoproteins have two basic types of glycosylation patterns: (1) O-linked glycosylation, which is characterized by a carbohydrate N-acetylgalactosamine (GalNAc) attached to the hydroxyl group of the amino acid serine or threonine, and (2) N-linked glycosylation, which is characterized by an N-acetylglucosamine (GlcNAc) attached to the amide group of asparagine (Asn). The oligosaccharides often terminate with sialic acid and/or sulfonated β1-4-linked GalNAc (SO_3-4GalNAc). Molecules with a large number of sulfonated GalNAcs disappear faster from the circulation than less-sulfonated isoforms due to their affinity for liver SO_3-4GalNAc receptors. On the other hand, the more the sialylation, the more is the half-life (Fig. 2.3).[13]

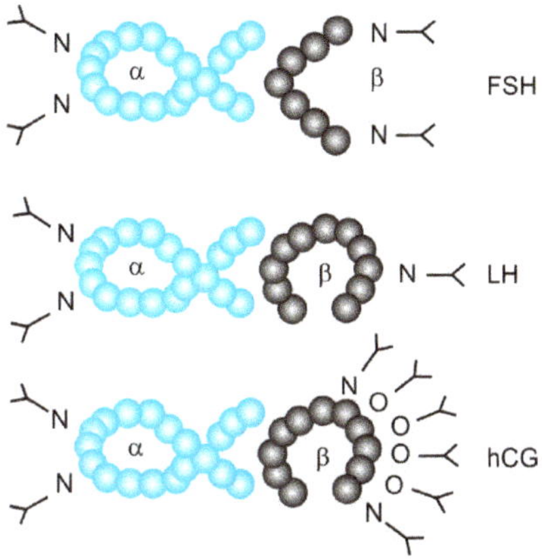

Fig. 2.3: Glycosylation patterns of FSH, LH and hCG. The alpha subunits of each hormone are identical in amino acid sequence and contain two sites of N-linked glycosylation. The beta subunit confers hormone specificity and contains variable amounts of N-linked glycosylation. LH beta subunit contains a single site of N-linked glycosylation, while FSH and hCG beta subunits contain two sites of N-linked glycosylation. In addition, hCG has an extended C-terminal that contains four sites of O-linked glycosylation.
(FSH: Follicle-stimulating hormone; LH: Luteinizing hormone; hCG: Human chorionic gonadotropin).
Source: Adapted from Esteves SC. Efficacy, efficiency and effectiveness of gonadotropin therapy for infertility treatment. Medical Express. 2015;2(3):1-11.

Follicle Stimulating Hormone

The beta subunit of FSH is composed of 111 amino acids. There are four asparagine-linked glycosylation sites (two on the alpha subunit and two on the beta subunit). Each subunit is attached to two carbohydrate moieties with variable compositions that, in turn, create different isoforms. These multiple forms of FSH differ in their plasma half-lives (range: 3–4 hours) due to variations in their binding potentials. When FSH isoforms have more sialic residues, they have decreased receptor affinity and therefore remain in circulation longer. The distribution of isoform types is under endocrine control, and the amount of sialic acid present is influenced mainly by estradiol (E_2) levels—the higher the estradiol levels, the less glycosylated the FSH, the shorter the half-life, but the greater the receptor affinity (Table 2.1). Therefore, the isoform profile is more acidic during the early follicular to mid-follicular phase of the menstrual cycle, but shifts to become more basic shortly before ovulation. These dynamic changes in sialylation are not mimicked by current controlled ovarian gonadotropin stimulation regimens. It is unknown whether such modifications in follicular stimulation protocols would affect oocyte quality.

Luteinizing Hormone

Although the alpha subunit of LH is identical to FSH and hCG, it is the beta subunit composed of 121 amino acids, which confers specific biologic

Table 2.1: Characteristics of follicle-stimulating hormone (FSH) isoforms.

Isoform	*E2 levels*	*Sialic acid content*	*In vivo half-life*	*Receptor affinity*	*Predominance*
Acid	Low	High	Long	Low	Early/mid-follicular and luteal phase
Basic	High	Low	Short	High	Late follicular/ preovulatory phase

Table 2.2: Structural characteristics of follicle-stimulating hormone (FSH), luteinizing hormone (LH) and human chorionic gonadotropin (hCG) molecules.

	Alpha subunit	*Beta subunit*	*N-linked glycosylation sites on alpha subunit*	*N-linked glycosylation site on beta subunit*	*O-linked glycosylation site on beta subunit*	*Carboxy-terminal segment*	*Terminal half-life*
FSH	92AA	111AA	2	2	0	Absent	3–4 hrs
LH	92AA	121AA	2	1	0	Absent	20–30 min
hCG	92AA	145AA	2	2	4	Present	24 hrs

activity and facilitates its interaction with the LH receptor. LH beta-subunits contain a single site with N-linked glycosylation (Asn 30) and fewer sialic acid residues (only 1 or 2) because of which LH has a short half-life of only 20–30 minutes (*see* Fig. 2.3).

Human Chorionic Gonadotropin

The beta subunit of LH and hCG has a similar amino acid sequence but, a notable difference is the presence of a long carboxyterminal segment with 24 amino acids containing four O-linked oligosaccharide sites in hCG (*see* Fig. 2.1). In addition, hCG beta subunits contain two sites of N-linked glycosylation compared with one in LH. Due to the higher number of both glycosylation sites and sialic acid residues (approximately 20) compared with LH, hCG has a markedly longer terminal half-life of 24 hours compared with approximately 30 minutes for LH. Due to the similarity in structure, hCG binds to the same receptor as LH.

The structural characteristics of three glycoproteins are illustrated in Table 2.2.

DIFFERENT GONADOTROPIN PREPARATIONS

Human Menopausal Gonadotropin (Menotropin)

Human menopausal gonadotropin, or menotropin, was first extracted from the urine of postmenopausal women in 1949.[14] Urine was originally obtained from an Italian nunnery, and at that time preparations contained varying amounts of FSH, LH, and hCG with only 5% of pure forms, i.e. only 5% of protein content was gonadotropins.[15] The specific activity of these products usually does not exceed 150 IU/mg protein. Human menopausal gonadotropin preparations have both FSH and LH activity, in equal amounts, but the latter is primarily derived from the hCG component present in postmenopausal urine and concentrated during purification. Generally, hCG is added to achieve the desired amount of LH-like biological activity.

The different proteins found in various hMG preparations include tumor necrosis factor binding protein 1, transferrin, urokinase, Tamm-Horsfall glycoprotein, epidermal growth factor and immunoglobulin related proteins. Urinary preparations are also found to have impurities such as prion proteins which are associated with transmissible spongiform encephalopathy (TSE) diseases, and if these Prion proteins are inactivated, it may also denature other proteins, including FSH. Local side effects, such as pain and allergic reactions are attributed to these non-gonadotropin proteins. Later, improvements in the purification techniques led to standardization of FSH and LH activities to 75 IU for each type of gonadotropin in 1963, as measured by standard in vivo bioassays (Steelman-Pohley assay). According to this assay an ampoule of hMG, which has 75 IU of FSH, may actually contain 60 and 90 IU.

In 1999, purified hMG gonadotropins were introduced, allowing its subcutaneous (SC) administration. Highly purified-hMG (HP-hMG) contains more hCG and less LH than does traditional hMG. Both conventional and HP-hMG are now commercially available in a FSH:LH ratio of 1:1.

Urinary Follicle-Stimulating Hormone (Urofollitropin)

In the 1980s, pure urinary FSH (uFSH) preparations were produced by removing LH with polyclonal antibodies but these preparations still contained high quantity of urinary proteins. Further technological advances made it possible to use highly specific monoclonal antibodies to extract FSH and produce highly purified-hFSH (HP-hFSH). The latter became commercially available in 1993. Such preparations contain less than 0.1 IU of LH and less than 5% of unidentified urinary proteins. FSH specific activity is approximately 10,000 IU/mg protein compared to 100–150 IU/mg protein in the earlier urinary hMG preparations. In addition, the enhanced purity of HP-hFSH enabled SC administration. Subcutaneous administration had better acceptance and tolerability among patients.

Recombinant Follicle-Stimulating Hormone

One of the major problems in the use of urinary-derived FSH preparation was limited supply of urinary products and because of their effective use in infertility the demand was constantly increasing. The other drawbacks were contamination due to presence of urinary proteins and the batch-to-batch variability in consistency which influences the real activity of the gonadotropins contained in the vials.

From 90s recombinant technology overcame these disadvantages of urinary gonadotropins and fulfilled the need for a more reliable source of FSH. To manufacture recombinant products, first the genes coding for the human FSH (hFSH) alpha subunit and beta-subunit were identified, which were then incorporated into the nuclear DNA of a host cell via a plasmid vector, using spliced DNA strings containing the FSH gene and segments of bacterial DNA. Initially *Escherichia coli* was tried as a host but structural complexity of human gonadotropins which required post-translational modification of the molecule by protein folding and glycosylation, made functional protein production impossible in *E. coli*. The Chinese hamster ovary cell line was then chosen as the host to produce gonadotropins because it is genetically stable, fully characterized and easily transfected with foreign DNA. Furthermore, it can be grown in cell cultures on a large scale and produce adequate levels of biologically active recombinant-hFSH (r-hFSH). In 1995, the first r-hFSH (follitropin alfa) was licensed for clinical use in the European Union. One year later, a similar r-hFSH (follitropin beta) was made available. In the manufacture of follitropin alfa, Serono (USA) used two separate vectors to construct an FSH-producing cell line, one vector for each subunit. Follitropin beta was manufactured by Organon Limited (Ireland), using a single vector containing the coding sequences of both subunit genes.

Initially a stable line of transformed cells was selected, which secreted high quantities of r-hFSH. These cell lines were used to establish a master cell bank (MCB), which then serves as a source of working cell banks (WCBs). The MCB consists of individual vials containing identical cells, which are cryopreserved until required. Thus a continuous supply of r-hFSH with guaranteed consistency from MCB to WCB is now available. MCBs and WCBs are routinely tested for sterility, mycoplasma and viral contamination.

Standardization of Gonadotropin Contents

Traditionally, quantification of gonadotropins was done by in vivo assays, most commonly used was Steelman-Pohley in vivo assay. FSH activity was quantified by rat ovarian weight gain and FSH vials or ampoules are subsequently filled according to the desired bioactivity, measured in IUs. However, this assay had many limitations: time consuming, cumbersome, uses large numbers of rats (ethical issues), and was limited in its precision—the European Pharmacopoeia defines an activity range (80–125% of the target value) within which an FSH batch is acceptable for clinical use.

Recent advances in the manufacturing process for r-hFSH follitropin alfa, enabled high batch to batch consistency in both isoform profile and glycan species distribution. The most significant advantage of this over other commercially available gonadotropins is that it permits FSH to be quantified by protein content (mass in µg) rather than by biologic activity. A physicochemical assay (SE-HPL) is used to assess the r-hFSH content in the active drug substance and the drug product. The final drug formulation is based on the r-hFSH protein content, thus ensuring a more precise content per vial [r-hFSH (FbM)].[16] The FbM r-hFSH preparation showed a 1.6% batch-to-batch variability using the physicochemical assay versus 10% variability obtained with the bioassay.[16]

Some clinical studies assessed the clinical implications of this improvement in drug manufacturing. FbM r-hFSH showed a better patient response consistency, improved control of follicular development, a reduced need for dose adjustment and fewer cancelled cycles, improved embryo quality and implantation rate with a trend to higher pregnancy rates, and fewer days of stimulation.[17,18] FbM r-hFSH is probably the most consistent r-hFSH in terms of protein content: this pharmaceutical FSH preparation is pure, low in degraded forms of FSH and has a consistent isoform profile.

Gonadotropin Preparations with LH Activity

At present, we have three groups of commercially available gonadotropin preparations containing LH activity:

1. Urinary hMG, in which LH activity is dependent on hCG rather than on pure LH glycoprotein
2. Pure LH glycoprotein produced by recombinant technology (lutropin alfa)
3. A combination of pure FSH and LH glycoproteins in a fixed ratio of 2:1 also manufactured by recombinant technology.

Recombinant hLH (r-hLH; lutropin alfa) came in the market in the year 2000 for use in women with gonadotropin insufficiency. The manufacturing process of r-hLH is similar to r-hFSH. It is administered subcutaneously in a dose of 75 IU. R-hLH is used not only to support follicular development during controlled ovarian stimulation (COS) in hypogonadotropic hypogonadic woman but also in other categories of female infertility, including poor responders, women over more than 35 years of age and hypo-responders.

Recombinant hLH has three major differences compared to urinary products containing LH activity:

1. It has higher purity and specific activity because it is manufactured using recombinant technology
2. It is associated with better dose precision due to filled-by-mass (FbM) technology that virtually eliminates batch-to-batch variation
3. Luteinizing hormone activity is derived directly from pure LH glycoprotein, unlike hMG, in which hCG is concentrated during purification or added to achieve the desired amount of LH-like biological activity.

In 2007, a new fixed combination of r-hFSH and r-hLH at 2:1 (150 IU + 75 IU) ratio was launched (follitropin alfa + lutropin alfa) as an alternative for those women who need LH supplementation. The 2:1 ratio of FSH and LH in a fixed dose combination was obtained by recombinant technology and vial filling using FbM. The bioequivalence of r-hFSH and r-hLH administrated alone or in combination has been found to be similar with the convenience of single injection.

Human Chorionic Gonadotropin

Human chorionic gonadotropin has been used traditionally to promote final follicular maturation in ovulation induction as a substitute for the mid-cycle LH surge. Due to structural and biological similarities, hCG and LH bind to and activate the same receptor. However, the luteotropic activity of hCG is markedly higher than that of LH due to its longer half-life and greater receptor affinity. Chorionic gonadotropins can be derived from urine of pregnant women or can be manufactured using recombinant technology. Currently, urinary hCG preparations are marketed in lyophilized vials with 5,000 or 10,000 IU for intramuscular use. Recombinant hCG (r-hCG) is available in prefilled syringes containing 250 μg of pure hCG, which is equivalent to approximately 6,500 IU of urinary hCG. Due to its higher purity, r-hCG is better tolerated and used subcutaneously, thus allowing patient self-administration. Nevertheless, the clinical efficacy of both urinary and recombinant preparations does not seem to differ. In a Cochrane meta-analysis comparing r-hCG versus urinary hCG for triggering final oocyte maturation no significant difference was detected in the live birth rate and incidence of ovarian hyperstimulation syndrome.[19]

Long-acting Follicle-Stimulating Hormone (Corifollitropin Alfa)

Corifollitropin alfa is a synthetic rFSH molecule containing a hybrid beta subunit, which provides a long plasma half-life of 65 hours while maintaining the pharmacodynamic properties of rFSH. It comprises an alpha subunit, which is identical to that of FSH and a beta subunit which is produced by the fusion of the C-terminal peptide from the beta-subunit of hCG (which provides a long half-life) to the beta subunit of FSH. The optimal dose is 100 mg for women less than 60 kg and 150 mg for women with a body weight of more than 60 kg. A single injection of corifollitropin alfa can replace first seven injections with standard daily gonadotropins and stimulation can then be continued with daily FSH injections, if required. This makes corifollitropin alfa potentially more patient friendly as it reduces the number of injections, leading to more acceptance amongst patients. The disadvantage of corifollitropin alfa is that it is not suitable in situations where monofollicular development is the goal. Moreover, the dose of corifollitropin alfa cannot be reduced during 1 week interval treatment in case of hyper-response.

Hence, it may not be suitable for patients with expected hyper-response such as polycystic ovary syndrome (PCOS) or prior history of ovarian hyperstimulation syndrome (OHSS). According to recent Cochrane review in 2015, which included six randomized controlled trials, a comparison of long-acting FSH versus daily FSH did not show evidence of difference in effect on overall live birth rate and OHSS.[20] There was no difference in the clinical pregnancy rate (any dose), ongoing pregnancy rate (any dose), multiple pregnancy rate (any dose), miscarriage rate (low or medium dose), ectopic pregnancy rate (any dose), congenital malformation rate, major or minor (low or medium dose). The authors concluded that the use of a medium dose (150–180 µg) of long-acting FSH is a safe treatment option and equally effective compared to daily FSH in women with unexplained subfertility. According to authors whether long-acting FSH is safe and effective for use in hyper- or poor responders still needs to be determined by further research.

Urinary versus Recombinant Preparations

Many meta-analysis and randomized trials have been done till date comparing the efficacy of urinary versus recombinant preparations, mostly concluding that both urinary and recombinant preparations have similar efficacy in terms of achieving a pregnancy or live birth per initiated cycle.[21-23] A recent Cochrane review in 2011, compared the effectiveness of recombinant gonadotropin (rFSH) with the three main types of urinary gonadotropins [i.e. (1) hMG, (2) FSH-P and (3) FSH-HP] for ovarian stimulation in women undergoing in vitro fertilization (IVF) or intracytoplasmic sperm injection (ICSI) treatment cycles.[24] It included 42 trials with a total of 9,606 couples. The review did not find any statistically significant difference in live birth rate on comparing rFSH to any of the other gonadotropins irrespective of the protocol used [28 trials, 7,339 couples, odds ratio (OR) 0.97, 95% confidence interval (CI) 0.87–1.08), suggesting that for a group with a 25% live birth rate using urinary gonadotropins the rate would be between 22.5% and 26.5% using rFSH. There was also no evidence of a difference in the OHSS rate (32 trials, 7,740 couples, OR 1.18, 95% CI 0.86–1.61).[24]

Although the live birth rate per initiated cycle is the most important end result in IVF studies, however in the present era of improved vitrification techniques and single embryo transfer, cumulative pregnancy rates could be better indicators of successful IVF, this in turn would depend upon the number of embryos formed and is directly proportional to the number of oocytes retrieved,[25] many studies recently have compared the efficacy of urinary gonadotropins with recombinant preparations in terms of oocyte yield. Revelli A et al. compared the efficacy of rFSH plus recombinant LH (rLH) with urinary hMG.[26] They found that the pregnancy rate in both groups progressively improved according to the number of oocytes retrieved. When comparing patients within the same subgroup of oocyte yield, both groups showed a comparable outcome up to the reported highest yield (>8) of oocytes.[26] However, when more than 8 oocytes were available, recombinant group had a significantly better pregnancy rate outcome.

Sykes et al. compared the cost-effectiveness of different gonadotropins, rFSH, highly purified uFSH-HP and hMG in IVF stimulation.[27] They calculated the cost-effectiveness ratios for "the average cost per ongoing pregnancy" and "incremental cost per additional pregnancy" for women entering into IVF treatment for a maximum of three cycles. The predicted cumulative pregnancy rate after three cycles was 57.1% for rFSH and 44.4% for both uFSH-HP and hMG. The cost of IVF treatment was more for rFSH, as compared to uFSH-HP and hMG for index cycle but when assessed in association with ongoing pregnancy rate and cumulative pregnancy rate the average cost per ongoing pregnancy was more favorable with rFSH than with either uFSH-HP or hMG. The other studies comparing urinary versus recombinant preparations have also concurred with these findings.[23,28-30]

ROLE OF LUTEINIZING HORMONE/HUMAN MENOPAUSAL GONADOTROPIN

In view of the concepts of LH threshold and LH ceiling, there has been a lot of debate on who are the candidates to be benefitted by adding LH or hMG.[31] Optimal follicular development is supposed to occur when LH is above a threshold of 1.1 IU/L and below a ceiling of 5.1 IU/L.[32,33] Most women undergoing COS for IVF have adequate endogenous LH levels and thus do not require LH supplementation as only 1% of LH receptors must be occupied to drive an adequate ovarian steroidogenesis. However, LH supplementation is must in hypogonadotropic hypogonadism patients as they do not have any endogenous LH. The other group of patients who have been shown to be benefitted by adding LH are those with poor ovarian reserve, advanced maternal age (>35 years), and ones who show suboptimal response on day 6 of stimulation with rFSH alone.[34-37] It has been hypothesized that these women would benefit from preparations containing LH, by an increase in androgen production for future aromatization into estrogens that could restore the follicular milieu and thus positively impact oocyte quality.

The MERIT group studied the effect of LH activity on IVF cycle outcomes and observed that, although the number of oocytes retrieved were more in rFSH group as compared to HP-hMG group (11.8 vs 10), there were more top-quality embryos with HP-hMG (11.3%) than with rFSH (9.0%; $p = 0.044$).[38,39] They found lower estradiol (E2) ($p = 0.031$) and higher progesterone ($p < 0.001$) levels with rFSH at the end of stimulation even after adjusting for follicular response. The ongoing pregnancy rate per cycle was 27% with HP-hMG and 22% with rFSH which was not statistically significant. The live birth, ongoing pregnancy and ongoing implantation rates for top-quality embryos were higher with HP-hMG than rFSH but did not reach statistical significance. The better implantation rates in the hMG group in this trial can be attributed to lower progesterone levels on the day of trigger, as the LH component in hMG converts the pregnenolone to androgens in theca cells which is later aromatized to estrogen. High serum progesterone on the day of trigger is found to be associated with reduced implantation rates due to detrimental effects on endometrium.[40,41] However, it has not been shown to have any adverse affect on embryo quality.[42]

Contrary to the above findings, Thuesen et al. confirmed that hCG/LH activity even increases the progesterone production during the follicular phase rather than reducing it.[43] Some authors have proposed that the cause of premature progesterone elevation might be due to enhanced FSH stimulation in ART cycles and is not related to type of gonadotropin used.[8,44]

CONCLUSION

Gonadotropins are the sine qua non for IVF. Since last few decades there have been continuous improvements in the manufacturing process of gonadotropins. Recombinant preparations are purer and safer than urinary-derived gonadotropins, and the introduction of FbM technology has virtually eliminated batch-to-batch variations, enabling accurate and consistent dosing.

As far as the outcome of treatment is concerned no clear evidence of difference has been demonstrated between urinary and recombinant products and not between hMG/addition of LH and pure FSH alone. The final decision for choosing gonadotropins should be made by the treating clinician taking into consideration the patient profile, personal experiences, affordability and availability of different preparations.

REFERENCES

1. Gougeon A. Regulation of ovarian follicular development in primates: facts and hypotheses. Endocr Rev. 1996;17(2):121-55.
2. Zeleznik AJ, Hillier SG. The role of gonadotropins in the selection of the preovulatory follicle. Clin Obstet Gynecol. 1984;27(4):927-40.
3. Goff AK, Armstrong DT. Stimulatory action of gonadotropins and prostaglandins on adenosine-3',5'-monophosphate production by isolated rat granulosa cells. Endocrinology. 1977;101(5):1461-7.
4. Fauser BC, Van Heusden AM. Manipulation of human ovarian function: physiological concepts and clinical consequences. Endocr Rev. 1997;18(1):71-106.
5. Willis DS, Watson H, Mason HD, et al. Premature response to luteinizing hormone of granulosa cells from anovulatory women with polycystic ovary syndrome: relevance to mechanism of anovulation. J Clin Endocrinol Metab. 1998;83(11):3984-91.
6. Campbell BK, Dobson H, Baird DT, et al. Examination of the relative role of FSH and LH in the mechanism of ovulatory follicle selection in sheep. J Reprod Fertil. 1999;117(2):355-67.

7. Sullivan MW, Stewart-Akers A, Krasnow JS, et al. Ovarian responses in women to recombinant follicle-stimulating hormone and luteinizing hormone (LH): a role for LH in the final stages of follicular maturation. J Clin Endocrinol Metab. 1999;84(1):228-32.
8. Filicori M, Cognigni GE, Pocognoli P, et al. Modulation of folliculogenesis and steroidogenesis in women by graded menotrophin administration. Hum Reprod. 2002;17(8):2009-15.
9. Rohde W. The contributions of Aschheim and Zondek to endocrinology. Pediatr Endocrinol Rev. 2010;7(4):323-7.
10. Walker D. Laboratory methods of equine pregnancy diagnosis. Vet Rec. 1977;100(19):396-9.
11. Stewart HL, Sano ME, Montgomery TL. Hormone secretion by human placenta grown in tissue culture. J Clin Endocrinol Metab. 1948;8(2):175-88.
12. Leão R de BF, Esteves SC. Gonadotropin therapy in assisted reproduction: an evolutionary perspective from biologics to biotech. Clinics (Sao Paulo). 2014;69(4):279-93.
13. Esteves SC. Efficacy, efficiency and effectiveness of gonadotropin therapy for infertility treatment. Medical Express. 2015;2(3):1-11.
14. Lunenfeld B. Historical perspectives in gonadotropin therapy. Hum Reprod Update. 2004;10(6):453-67.
15. Practice Committee of American Society for Reproductive Medicine, Birmingham, Alabama. Gonadotropin preparations: past, present, and future perspectives. Fertil Steril. 2008;90(5 Suppl):S13-20.
16. Bassett RM, Driebergen R. Continued improvements in the quality and consistency of follitropin alfa, recombinant human FSH. Reprod Biomed Online. 2005;10(2):169-77.
17. Hugues JN, Barlow DH, Rosenwaks Z, et al. Improvement in consistency of response to ovarian stimulation with recombinant human follicle stimulating hormone resulting from a new method for calibrating the therapeutic preparation. Reprod Biomed Online. 2003;6(2):185-90.
18. Balasch J, Fábregues F, Peñarrubia J, et al. Outcome from consecutive assisted reproduction cycles in patients treated with recombinant follitropin alfa filled-by-bioassay and those treated with recombinant follitropin alfa filled-by-mass. Reprod Biomed Online. 2004;8(4):408-13.
19. Youssef MA, Al-Inany HG, Aboulghar M, et al. Recombinant versus urinary human chorionic gonadotropin for final oocyte maturation triggering in IVF and ICSI cycles. Cochrane Database Syst Rev. 2011;(4):CD003719.
20. Pouwer AW, Farquhar C, Kremer JA. Long-acting FSH versus daily FSH for women undergoing assisted reproduction. Cochrane Database Syst Rev. 2015;(7):CD009577.
21. Jee BC, Suh CS, Kim YB, et al. Clinical efficacy of highly purified hMG versus recombinant FSH in IVF/ICSI cycles: a meta-analysis. Gynecol Obstet Invest. 2010;70(2):132-7.
22. Al-Inany HG, Abou-Setta AM, Aboulghar MA, et al. Highly purified hMG achieves better pregnancy rates in IVF cycles but not ICSI cycles compared with recombinant FSH: a meta-analysis. Gynecol Endocrinol. 2009;25(6): 372-8.
23. Devroey P, Pellicer A, Nyboe Andersen A, et al. A randomized assessor-blind trial comparing highly purified hMG and recombinant FSH in a GnRH antagonist cycle with compulsory single-blastocyst transfer. Fertil Steril. 2012;97(3): 561-71.

24. van Wely M, Kwan I, Burt AL, et al. Recombinant versus urinary gonadotrophin for ovarian stimulation in assisted reproductive technology cycles. Cochrane Database Syst Rev. 2011;(2):CD005354.
25. Vaughan DA, Leung A, Resetkova N, et al. How many oocytes are optimal to achieve multiple live births with one stimulation cycle? The one and done approach. Fertil Steril. 2017;107(2):397-404.e3.
26. Revelli A, Pettinau G, Basso G, et al. Controlled Ovarian Stimulation with recombinant-FSH plus recombinant-LH vs. human Menopausal Gonadotropin based on the number of retrieved oocytes: results from a routine clinical practice in a real-life population. Reprod Biol Endocrinol. 2015;13:77.
27. Sykes D, Out HJ, Palmer SJ, et al. The cost-effectiveness of IVF in the UK: a comparison of three gonadotrophin treatments. Hum Reprod. 2001;16(12):2557-62.
28. Lehert P, Schertz JC, Ezcurra D. Recombinant human follicle-stimulating hormone produces more oocytes with a lower total dose per cycle in assisted reproductive technologies compared with highly purified human menopausal gonadotrophin: a meta-analysis. Reprod Biol Endocrinol. 2010;8:112.
29. Wex J, Abou-Setta AM. Economic evaluation of highly purified human menopausal gonadotropin versus recombinant human follicle-stimulating hormone in fresh and frozen in vitro fertilization/intracytoplasmic sperm-injection cycles in Sweden. Clinicoecon Outcomes Res. 2013;5:381-97.
30. Levi Setti PE, Alviggi C, Colombo GL, et al. Human recombinant follicle stimulating hormone (rFSH) compared to urinary human menopausal gonadotropin (HMG) for ovarian stimulation in assisted reproduction: a literature review and cost evaluation. J Endocrinol Invest. 2015;38(5):497-503.
31. Shoham Z. The clinical therapeutic window for luteinizing hormone in controlled ovarian stimulation. Fertil Steril. 2002;77(6):1170-7.
32. Shoham Z, Smith H, Yeko T, et al. Recombinant LH (lutropin alfa) for the treatment of hypogonadotrophic women with profound LH deficiency: a randomized, double-blind, placebo-controlled, proof-of-efficacy study. Clin Endocrinol (Oxf). 2008;69(3):471-8.
33. Recombinant human luteinizing hormone (LH) to support recombinant human follicle-stimulating hormone (FSH)-induced follicular development in LH- and FSH-deficient anovulatory women: a dose-finding study. The European Recombinant Human LH Study Group. J Clin Endocrinol Metab. 1998;83(5):1507-14.
34. Laml T, Obruca A, Fischl F, et al. Recombinant luteinizing hormone in ovarian hyperstimulation after stimulation failure in normogonadotropic women. Gynecol Endocrinol. 1999;13(2):98-103.
35. De Placido G, Alviggi C, Perino A, et al. Recombinant human LH supplementation versus recombinant human FSH (rFSH) step-up protocol during controlled ovarian stimulation in normogonadotrophic women with initial inadequate ovarian response to rFSH. A multicentre, prospective, randomized controlled trial. Hum Reprod. 2005;20(2):390-6.
36. Lévy DP, Navarro JM, Schattman GL, et al. The role of LH in ovarian stimulation: exogenous LH: let's design the future. Hum Reprod. 2000;15(11):2258-65.
37. Hill MJ, Levens ED, Levy G, et al. The use of recombinant luteinizing hormone in patients undergoing assisted reproductive techniques with advanced reproductive age: a systematic review and meta-analysis. Fertil Steril. 2012;97(5):1108-14.e1.
38. Andersen AN, Devroey P, Arce J-C. Clinical outcome following stimulation with highly purified hMG or recombinant FSH in patients undergoing IVF: a randomized assessor-blind controlled trial. Hum Reprod. 2006;21(12):3217-27.

39. Ziebe S, Lundin K, Janssens R, et al. Influence of ovarian stimulation with HP-hMG or recombinant FSH on embryo quality parameters in patients undergoing IVF. Hum Reprod. 2007;22(9):2404-13.
40. Van Vaerenbergh I, Fatemi HM, Blockeel C, et al. Progesterone rise on HCG day in GnRH antagonist/rFSH stimulated cycles affects endometrial gene expression. Reprod Biomed Online. 2011;22(3):263-71.
41. Elgindy EA. Progesterone level and progesterone/estradiol ratio on the day of hCG administration: detrimental cutoff levels and new treatment strategy. Fertil Steril. 2011;95(5):1639-44.
42. Silverberg KM, Martin M, Olive DL, et al. Elevated serum progesterone levels on the day of human chorionic gonadotropin administration in in vitro fertilization cycles do not adversely affect embryo quality. Fertil Steril. 1994;61(3): 508-13.
43. Thuesen LL, Smitz J, Loft A, et al. Endocrine effects of hCG supplementation to recombinant FSH throughout controlled ovarian stimulation for IVF: a dose-response study. Clin Endocrinol (Oxf). 2013;79(5):708-15.
44. Kyrou D, Al-Azemi M, Papanikolaou EG, et al. The relationship of premature progesterone rise with serum estradiol levels and number of follicles in GnRH antagonist/recombinant FSH-stimulated cycles. Eur J Obstet Gynecol Reprod Biol. 2012;162(2):165-8.

Chapter 3

Stimulation Protocols for Intrauterine Insemination

Kalyani Shrimali, Ritu Hinduja

INTRODUCTION

Intrauterine insemination is one of the first lines of infertility treatments and assisted reproductive technologies (ART). It is the safest, least invasive, and cost-effective forms of assisted reproduction.

Ovarian stimulation aims at development of one or more of the ovarian follicles to reach the stage of maturity culminating in release of one or more mature oocytes ready for fertilization. Ovarian stimulation has been shown to significantly improve the outcome in IUI cycles. With the help of ovulation-inducing drugs, there is an increase in number of eggs for fertilization and also it helps patients with anovulatory cycles to overcome the subtle defect in the ovulatory function. When IUI is performed in unexplained subfertile couples, OI doubles the pregnancy rates, compared with IUI without OI.[1]

There are two mechanisms of ovarian stimulation: the first involves applying pharmacological agents that mimic endogenous gonadotropins (injectable gonadotropins) that directly stimulate ovarian follicular development through gonadotropin receptors; and the second involves pharmacological agents that manipulate and moderate endogenous gonadotropin production. These are the oral ovulation through moderating estrogen action, a major regulator of endogenous gonadotropin production.[2]

ORAL AGENTS FOR OVARIAN STIMULATION

Oral agents modulate estrogen action, hence endogenous gonadotropin production through direct effect on estrogen receptors, i.e. selective estrogen receptor modulators (SERMs), or through modulation of estrogen production (inhibition), i.e. aromatase inhibitors, or inhibition of the estrogen synthesis enzyme (the aromatase enzyme).

Clomiphene Citrate

Clomiphene citrate has been used as a first line ovulation inducing agent for over 40 years. CC is a nonsteroidal triphenylethylene derivative that exhibits both estrogen agonist and antagonist properties, i.e. SERM. CC mainly acts as antiestrogen.[3]

It is a SERM that stimulates endogeneous follicle-stimulating hormone (FSH) production and secretion by interrupting estrogen feedback to the hypothalamus and pituitary. Increased FSH release drives folliculogenesis at the level of ovary.[3]

Regimens of Clomiphene Citrate for Ovarian Stimulation

The regimen usually starts from the early follicular phase, that is second to the fifth day of the cycle for 5 days. There is no difference in pregnancy rate whether clomiphene is commenced on day 2, 3, 4, or 5 of the cycle, although there is perhaps a tendency to multiple follicular development the closer the agent is commenced to menses.

The dose required for achieving ovulation is dependent on the body weight. Although the effective dose of CC ranges from 50 mg/day to 250 mg/day. Most women respond to treatment with 50 mg (52%) or 100 mg (22%). Although higher doses are sometimes required, the success rates are usually very low (150 mg, 12%; 200 mg, 7%; 250 mg, 5%). Most women who fail to respond to 150 mg of CC will ultimately require alternative or combination treatments.[4,5] The usual recommended dose is 100 mg/day.

Pregnancy rates are highest in the early cycles of CC treatment (usually first three cycles) with a significant decline in the chance of achieving pregnancy beyond the third treatment cycle down to a very low chance beyond the sixth treatment cycle.[4]

Outcome[4]

- Pregnancy: 30%
- Failure (no pregnancy despite ovulation): 40%
- Resistance (no ovulation): 25%
- Antiestrogenic effect: 5%.

Generally speaking, failure to conceive after six ovulatory cycles of CC treatment should be regarded as a clear indication to expand the diagnostic evaluation to exclude other infertility factors or to change the treatment strategy when evaluation is already complete.[6]

Adverse Effects

Clomiphene citrate is in general a safe medication and usually well tolerated, with most of the side effects being relatively mild—multiple gestations, mild ovarian hyperstimulation being the most common. Other serious long-term adverse effects have been suggested, including increased risk of ovarian cancer.

- *Multiple gestation pregnancy*: The incidence reported for multiple pregnancy is approximately 8% with CC treatment. However, majority of multiple gestations are twins. Triplet and higher order pregnancies are rare.[7]

- Side effects such as vasomotor hot flashes are also noted. Unusual visual symptoms (visual blurring or persistent after-images) are also noted in 1% to 2% of patients taking CC, which are likely due to antiestrogenic effects of CC on the visual cortex.
- *Severe ovarian hyperstimulation syndrome*: The incidence of severe ovarian hyperstimulation syndrome (OHSS) is difficult to predict in CC-treated group; though mild OHSS is relatively common, but does not require active management most of the time.[6]
- *Ovarian cancer*: There is an uncertain association of ovarian cancer that has been suggested in the past. The recent subsequent studies have been reassuring but the question of whether the treatment with ovulation-inducing drugs increases risk of ovarian tumors or cancer still remains unsettled and cannot be summarily dismissed.[8-10] It is best to limit a patient's lifetime exposure to CC to 12 treatment cycles, as additional cycles may place the patient at increased risk of borderline ovarian tumors.[11]

Failure of Clomiphene Citrate Treatment

In anovulatory infertility, the failure is divided into two groups:

1. *Clomiphene resistance*: Patient who fails to ovulate with CC ovarian stimulation, i.e. failure to achieve ovulation. This could be due to one of the two main reasons; insulin resistance [(women with polycystic ovarian syndrome (PCOS)] and inappropriate indication for CC treatment, e.g. use in women with ovulatory dysfunction due to medical disorders or in women with WHO type I or III anovulation.
2. *Clomiphene pregnancy failure*: Patients who ovulate in response to CC treatment but do not achieve pregnancy. These may be related to a variety of other underlying infertility causes such as male factor, endometriosis or tubal factor or endometrial receptivity factors.

Clomiphene citrate exerts undesirable antiestrogenic effects in the periphery (endocervix, endometrium, ovary, ovum, and embryo) that can not be avoided due to long half-life of CC isomers. This could explain the discrepancy between ovulation and conception rates observed in CC-treated patients, i.e. explain the clomiphene treatment failure (ovulation but no pregnancy).

Aromatase Inhibitors

Aromatase inhibitors have been used for the last decade as adjunctive treatments in breast cancer. They block the conversion of testosterone and androstenedione to estradiol and estrone, respectively, and hence inhibit the estrogen-negative feedback on the hypothalamic-pituitary axis. This leads to increased gonadotropin secretion, which in turn leads to ovarian follicular growth and development.[12]

Letrozole is the commonly used aromatase inhibitors drug for ovulation induction. This is an off-label drug. According to the existing laws, the use of letrozole for OI alone is not allowed. Thus, it should be used only, if the local FDA approves it.

Ovulation and pregnancy rates with aromatase inhibitors such as letrozole and anastrozole appear to be promising, and these agents appear to have less antiestrogen effect on the endometrium, but the evidence on endometrial effects is conflicting, and most studies show equivalence with CC.[12-15]

The addition of letrozole to gonadotropin stimulation protocols decreases the gonadotropin requirement and increases the number of preovulatory follicles.[16,17]

Dosage

Letrozole is administered in doses of 2.5–5 mg/day for 5 days, starting from day 3 of the cycle.

Extended Letrozole Therapy

In a recent study conducted by Badawy et al., extended letrozole therapy (2.5 mg daily from day 1 of menses for 10 days) was used in CC-resistant PCOS women. They observed that the long letrozole protocol (10 days) can produce more mature follicles and subsequently, more pregnancies than the short letrozole therapy (5 days).[18]

Letrozole Step-up Protocol

Recently, a new protocol known as the letrozole step-up protocol has been reported by Mitwally et al. In this protocol, letrozole was administered in the step-up doses consisting of one, two, three, and four tablets of letrozole (2.5 mg) daily on menstrual cycle days 2, 3, 4, and 5, respectively. When compared with the standard CC protocol (CC 100 mg for 5 days, starting on day 3), the step-up letrozole protocol was associated with multifollicular development and a higher clinical pregnancy rates per treatment cycle (27.3% vs 11.8%, respectively).[19]

Adverse Effects

In 2005, Health Canada and the manufacturing company of letrozole issued a "Physician Warning Letter" on the off-label use of letrozole for fertility and the possibility of embryotoxicity, fetotoxicity, and teratogenicity found in rats.[20]

More recently, however, Tulandi et al.[21] retrospectively evaluated 911 newborns from letrozole and CC pregnancies. They found a 2.4% incidence of congenital malformations and chromosomal abnormalities in the letrozole group versus 4.8% in the CC group.[21]

Tamoxifen Citrate

It is used as an alternative to CC or with CC or in CC-resistant patients. It is structurally related to SERM which has weak estrogenic effect on cervical mucus and the endometrium. This drug also is used as an "off-label" drug.

Dosage: 20–40 mg/day to be started from day 2 to day 5.

Adverse Effects

Similar to CC but also noted slight increase in endometrial hyperplasia and endometrial carcinoma.[22]

Contraindication

Liver toxicity, pituitary failure, gonadal failure pregnancies, ovarian cyst, and abnormal uterine bleeding.

Gonadotropins

Use of gonadotropins has revolutionized the management of infertility.

Use of intramuscular gonadotropins began in the 1960s. Gonadotropins may be urinary derived (human menopausal gonadotropin or hMG) or manufactured using recombinant DNA technology (recombinant FSH or rFSH). Over the last decade, recombinant human FSH has been the main preparation, and it can be self-administered subcutaneously.[23] The rFSH is more expensive per unit dose but has been reported to have greater purity and, therefore greater efficacy of action.

Human menopausal gonadotropin also contains a degree of LH activity and some researcher claim that additional LH effect leads to better follicular/oocyte development and as a result, higher pregnancy rates compared to rFSH. However, there is no published evidence for this, particularly in IUI cycles where there is "background" pituitary production of FSH and LH. This is in contrast to ovarian stimulation for IVF where there is often concomitant pituitary down regulation using gonadotropin-releasing hormone (GnRH) analogs.

Gonadotropins are used to treat infertility caused by anovulation, usually after other less complicated and costly methods have failed. Two groups of anovulatory disorders may require gonadotropin therapy: (1) hypogonadotropic amenorrhea (HA, also known as hypogonadotropic hypogonadism, hypothalamic amenorrhea, or WHO type I amenorrhea); and (2) PCOS also known as hyperandrogenic amenorrhea or WHO type II amenorrhea.[24,25]

A recent Cochrane review (2007) on the available results of gonadotropins suggested that gonadotropins might be the most effective drugs when IUI is combined with ovarian hyperstimulation.[26]

Choice of Gonadotropins

The choice of gonadotropin to be used depends upon the day 2 plasma luteinizing hormone (LH)/FSH/estradiol (E2) levels. If serum LH is elevated, FSH containing gonadotropins are indicated, whereas if serum FSH is elevated (>10 mIU/mL), a combination of LH and FSH is used for ovarian stimulation. For ovarian stimulation in patients with hypogonadotrophic hypogonadism, a combination of LH and FSH is used.

Gonadotropin Regimens

Conventional regimen: In this protocol, a daily dose of 75–150 IU of gonadotropins is started from day 2 or day 3. Serial ultrasonography (USG) for follicular monitoring and serum E2 estimation is performed from day 8 onwards. This protocol has yielded acceptable pregnancy rates of up to 30%.

Low dose step-up: The use of a low dose step-up regimen of OI similar to that described by Franks and others (Messinis, 2005).[27] Following induction of menses with either progestogens or the oral contraceptive pill, FSH or hMG is commenced 2–3 days later at a dose no higher than 50–75 IU per day. The dose is not altered until there is no rise in the estradiol level or no increase in the follicle size on ultrasound assessment. If there is any evidence of an estrogen rise above baseline (even if no follicular development is seen), the existing dose is maintained and further assessment with ultrasounds and hormones are undertaken every 2–3 days. A rising estrogen level indicates follicular development. When there are 1–2 follicles, 17 mm in diameter or larger, and the estrogen level is about 1,200 pmol/L or 350 pg/mL; hCG 5,000–10,000 IU is administered (Fig. 3.1).

If no rise of estrogen above baseline is seen after 7 days of FSH/hMG, the dose can be cautiously increased by 25–50 IU per day above the previous

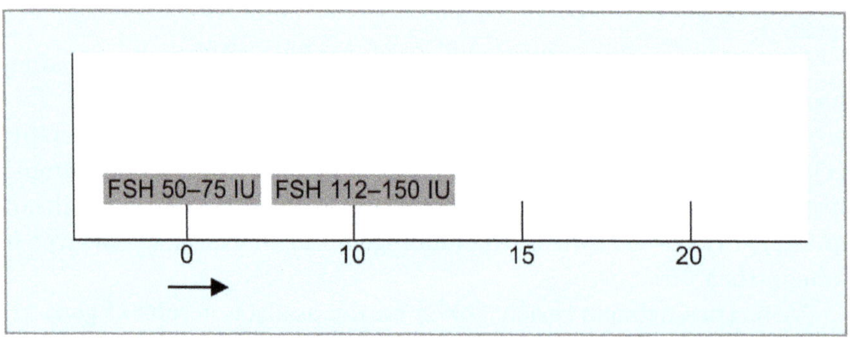

Fig. 3.1: Low dose step-up regimen.

dose. The process of further assessment 5–7 days later can be repeated, with further increases in FSH/hMG only being necessary in the absence of an estrogen/follicular response.

Step-down regimen: In a step-down protocol, hMG/FSH therapy at a daily dose of 150 IU is started on day 2 and continued till a dominant follicle of greater than 10 mm is observed on transvaginal sonography (TVS). After this, the dose is decreased to 112.5 units intramuscular (IM) per day for 3 days, followed by 75 units IM per day for the next 3 days. This dose is then continued till the day of human chorionic gonadotropin (hCG) injection. The rest of the regimen is the same as in the step-up regime.

In almost 15% to 20% of the cycles, which have been stimulated with gonadotropins or CC, the exaggerated estradiol level due to the multifollicular development often provokes higher LH levels during the follicular phase or an untimely LH hormone surge, which leads to cycle cancellation. Therefore, in order to avoid interference from endogenous gonadotropin secretion, a combination of gonadotropins and GnRH analogs have been used for ovulation induction. Although GnRH analogs are routinely used in IVF cycles, their routine use in IUI cycles is not recommended. A recent Cochrane review has concluded that GnRH analogs do not significantly improve pregnancy rates in IUI.

Gonadotropin-IUI is a successful treatment but the greatest risk lies with multiple pregnancy, as a result of multiple follicular development.

The aim of treatment is to develop one leading follicle but many times there are other smaller follicles. Additionally, most physicians would accept two codominant follicles as an appropriate result for triggering of ovulation. As a result, twin pregnancies are relatively common and represent about one-fifth of all ongoing pregnancies.

Unlike clomiphene, where pituitary FSH is initially stimulated and then gradually falls in serum level toward midcycle, gonadotropin injections maintain a constant level of serum FSH throughout the follicular phase. As a result the normal process of dominant follicle selection is overridden and even middle-sized follicles can contain an oocyte with the capacity to cause pregnancy. This leads to a higher risk of not only twins but also higher order multiple pregnancies.

OVULATION TRIGGER

The ovulation is triggered by the administration of hCG injection when the following conditions are met: (1) Leading follicle is 18–20 mm; (2) The number of follicles more than 16 mm is not more than 4 or follicles more than 12 mm are not more than 8 in number; (3) Serum E2 is not more than 1,500–2,000 pg/mL (serum E2 level is estimated only, if the total number of follicles exceed 12 and if there is a potential chance of OHSS).

CONCLUSION

Clomiphene citrate is an effective treatment for oligoovulation and anovulation. It helps to cause regular ovulation and increases pregnancy rates. It should be used only in properly selected patients and for the recommended amount of time. However, success rates with CC are low due to the antiestrogenic effects on the cervix (drying up the mucus) and endometrium.

Letrozole has been shown to be superior to clomiphene for patients with PCOS.

In women with infertility due to oligo or anovulation where treatment with CC or metformin is unsuccessful, fair evidence shows that gonadotropin treatment is effective.

Fair evidence shows that the pregnancy rate is higher with hypothalamic amenorrhea than it is with PCOS.

Protocols should attempt to minimize risk of multiple pregnancy and ovarian hyperstimulation syndrome.

REFERENCES

1. Guzick DS, Carson SA, Coutifaris C, et al. Efficacy of superovulation and intrauterine insemination in the treatment of infertility. National Cooperative Reproductive Medicine Network. N Engl J Med. 1999;340:177-83.
2. Mitwally MF, Casper RF. Chapter 1: Oral agents for ovarian stimulation. Section 1: Mild forms of ovarian stimulation. In: Aboulghar M, Rizk B (Eds). Ovarian Stimulation. New York, NY: Cambridge University Press; 2011. pp. 1-13.
3. Practice Committee of the American Society for Reproductive Medicine. Use of clomiphene citrate in women. Fertil Steril. 2004;82 Suppl 1:S90-6.
4. Garcia J, Jones GS, Wentz AC. The use of clomiphene citrate. Fertil Steril. 1977;28:707-17.
5. Athaullah N, Proctor M, Johnson NP. Oral versus injectable ovulation induction agents for unexplained subfertility. Cochrane Database Syst Rev. 2002;3: CD003052.
6. Usadi RS, Fritz MA. Chapter 68: Induction of ovulation with clomiphene citrate. In: Sciarra JJ (Ed). Gynaecology and Obstetrics. Philadelphia: Harper & Row; 1986.
7. Schenker JG, Yarkoni S, Granat M. Multiple pregnancies following induction of ovulation. Fertil Steril. 1981;35:105-23.
8. Venn A, Watson L, Lumley J, et al. Breast and ovarian cancer incidence after infertility and in vitro fertilization. Lancet. 1995;346:995-1000.
9. Modan B, Ron E, Lerner-Geva L, et al. Cancer incidence in a cohort of infertile women. Am J Epidemiol. 1998;147:1038-1042.
10. Silva I dos S, Wark PA, McCormack VA, et al. Ovarian stimulation drugs and cancer risks: a long term follow-up of British Cohort. Br J Cancer. 2009;100: 1824-31.
11. Rossing MA, Daling JR, Weiss NS, et al. Ovarian tumors in a cohort of infertile women. N Engl J Med. 1994;331:771-6.
12. Bayar U, Basaran M, Kiran S, et al. Use of an aromatase inhibitor in patients with polycystic ovary syndrome: a prospective randomized trial. Fertil Steril. 2006;86:1447-51.

13. Mitwally MFM, Casper RF. Use of aromatase inhibitor for induction of ovulation in patients with an inadequate response to clomiphene citrate. Fertil Steril. 2001;75:305-9.
14. Al-Fozen H, Al-Khadouri M, Tan SL, et al. A randomized trial of letrozole versus clomiphene citrate in women undergoing superovulation. Fertil Steril. 2004;82:1561-3.
15. Badawy A, Elnashar A, Totongy M. Clomiphene citrate or aromatase inhibitors for superovulation in women with unexplained infertility undergoing intrauterine insemination: a prospective randomized trial. Fertil Steril. 2009;92:1355-9.
16. Bancsi LF, Broekmans FJ, Eijkemans MJ, et al. Predictors of poor ovarian response in in vitro fertilization: a prospective study comparing basal markers of ovarian reserve. Fertil Steril. 2002;77:328-36.
17. Ng EH, Tang OS, Ho PC. The significance of the number of antral follicles prior to stimulation in predicting ovarian responses in an IVF programme. Hum Reprod. 2000;15:1937-42.
18. Badawy A, Mosbah A, Tharwat A, et al. Extended letrozole therapy for ovulation induction in clomiphene-resistant women with polycystic ovary syndrome: a novel protocol. Fertil Steril. 2009;92:236-9.
19. Mitwally MF, Said T, Galal A, et al. Letrozole step-up protocol: a successful superovulation protocol. Fertil Steril. 2008;89:S23-4.
20. Health Canada Endorsed Important Safety Information on Femara (letrozole). (2005). Health Canada website. Available from www.hc-sc.gc.ca/dhp-mps/medeff/advisories-avis/prof/_2005/femara_hpc-cps-eng.php [Accessed July 31, 2007].
21. Tulandi T, Martin J, Al-Fadhli R, et al. Congenital malformations among 911 newborns conceived after infertility treatment with letrozole or clomiphene citrate. Fertil Steril. 2006;85:1761-5.
22. Fritz MA, Speroff L. Clinical Gynecologic Endocrinology and Infertility. Baltimore: Lippincott Williams & Wilkins.
23. Guzick DS. Ovulation induction management of PCOS. Clin Obstet Gynecol. 2007;50:255-67.
24. Practice Committee of the American Society for Reproductive Medicine. Current evaluation of amenorrhea. Fertil Steril. 2006;86(Suppl 5):S148-55.
25. Reindollar RH, Novak M, Tho SP, et al. Adult-onset amenorrhea: a study of 262 patients. Am J Obstet Gynecol. 1986;155:531-43.
26. Cohlen BJ, Heineman MJ. Ovarian stimulation protocols (antiestrogens, gonadotropins with and without GnRH agonist/antagonist) for intrauterine insemination in women with subfertility. Cochrane Database Syst Rev. 2007;(2):CD005356.
27. Messinis I. Ovulation induction: a mini review. Hum Reprod. 2005;20:2688.

Chapter 4

Protocols for the Normoresponders

Sulbha Arora, Ashvini Deshmukh

INTRODUCTION

The first in vitro fertilization (IVF) baby was born from a natural or non-stimulated cycle.[1] However, it was soon realized that the success rates of natural cycle IVF were low, primarily due to the limited number of oocytes retrieved. To address this problem, stimulation of multiple follicular genesis by the ovaries was attempted by introducing urinary gonadotropin preparations. This resulted in a significant increase in both the number of oocytes retrieved as well as the success rates of IVF. Today, ovulation induction and controlled ovarian stimulation are integral parts of every assisted reproduction program.

As the popularity of ovarian stimulation grew, various problems started to surface. Premature luteinization and failure of synchronous follicular recruitment due to early dominant follicle selection were the two main problems limiting the success rates. Also, ovulation could occur at any time of the day, necessitating intensive monitoring and oocyte retrieval at inconvenient times of the day.[2] Gonadotropin-releasing hormone (GnRH) agonists were shown to result in pituitary downregulation and succeeded in overcoming these problems, becoming the next breakthrough in IVF treatment. Subsequently, GnRH antagonists, which have a similar function but require a shorter duration to achieve pituitary suppression (and prevent premature luteinizing hormone or LH surge) have been introduced and are now increasingly being used.

OBJECTIVES OF STIMULATION PROTOCOLS IN IN VITRO FERTILIZATION CYCLES

In stimulated cycles, our aim is to produce multiple follicles. In order to achieve this, we need to prevent dominant follicle selection. In natural cycles, estrogen secreted by the dominant follicle exerts a negative feedback on the pituitary that suppresses follicle-stimulating hormone (FSH) secretion below the threshold value, thereby causing atresia of the remaining follicles. In stimulated cycles, exogenous gonadotropins are used to achieve FSH levels above threshold during the phase of follicular recruitment to interfere with the selection of a single dominant follicle and encourage the growth of multiple follicles simultaneously.

Pituitary desensitization by using either GnRH agonists or GnRH antagonists, is an important part of IVF stimulation as it eliminates the possible interference by endogenous hormones, enabling synchronous follicular development. This prevents premature luteinization, and helps to reduce intensive and frequent monitoring allowing control over the timing of oocyte retrieval.

The LH surge is substituted by exogenous human chorionic gonadotropin (hCG), enabling clinics to time oocyte retrieval.

STIMULATION PROTOCOLS

- Long protocol: GnRH agonist + Gonadotropins FSH or human menopausal gonadotropin (hMG)
- Short (flare-up protocol): GnRH agonist + Gonadotropins
- Antagonist protocol: GnRH antagonist + Gonadotropins
  - Single dose
  - Multiple dose.

Various protocols have been used to achieve the goals of ovarian stimulation. The two agents used for downregulation include either the GnRH agonists or the GnRH antagonists. As the GnRH agonists cause an initial flare reaction, they need to be started earlier on, either in the mid-luteal phase of the previous cycle or at the start of the follicular phase. On the other hand, GnRH antagonists have an immediate suppressive effect, and therefore need to be started only toward the end of the follicular phase, that is just before the rise of the LH surge. They can be used either as a single dose or as multiple doses given daily.

Long Protocol

The long agonist protocol is the oldest stimulation protocol and has for many years also been the most common one to be used. It starts on day 21 of the previous cycle with a daily dose of GnRH agonist, which is then continued after the onset of menses and up to the day of trigger. Gonadotropin injections (hMG or FSH) are added with the onset of menses, that is, day 1 or 2 of the cycle. The gonadotropin doses are titrated by performing serial ultrasound measurements of the growing follicles. Follicular maturation is triggered by administering hCG, either urinary or recombinant, once at least three leading follicles have crossed 18 mm in diameter. Oocyte retrieval is scheduled 34.5 hours later (Fig. 4.1).

The advantage of this protocol is excellent cycle control, making it the desired protocol for first time patients as well as women with a previous normal response. However, the drawbacks include longer duration of injections, higher gonadotropin requirement and in turn added cost. Over

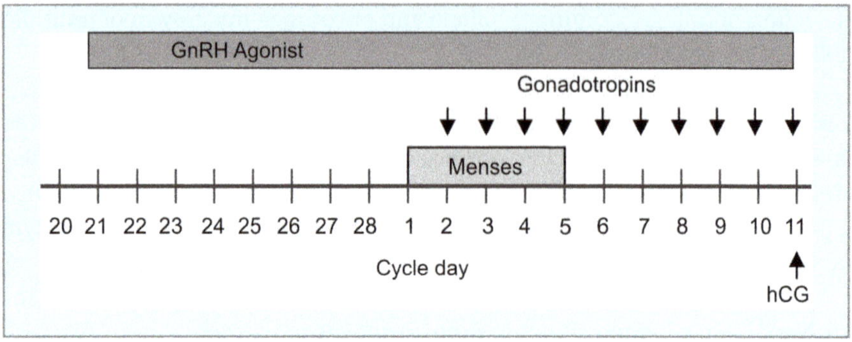

Fig. 4.1: Gonadotropin-releasing hormone (GnRH) agonist long protocol. (hCG: Human chorionic gonadotropin).

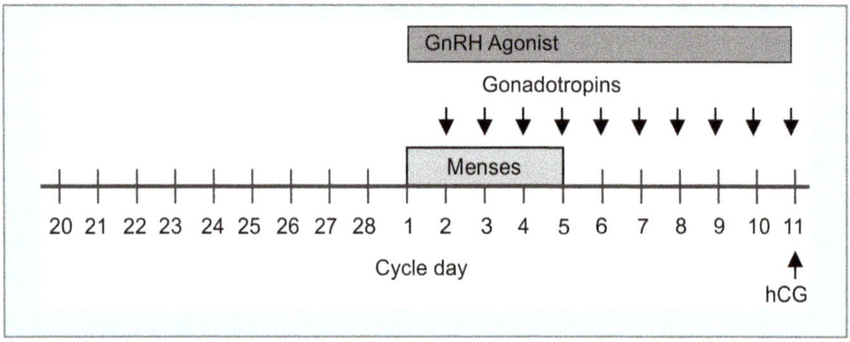

Fig. 4.2: Gonadotropin-releasing hormone (GnRH) agonist short protocol. (hCG: Human chorionic gonadotropin).

repeated cycles, patients start getting fed up of the sheer number of injections required and compliance levels start to fall. Due to these reasons, this protocol has largely given way to the newer, more patient-friendly antagonist protocols.

Short Protocol

In the short protocol, GnRH agonists are started in a daily dose along with the gonadotropin injections on day 1 or 2 of the cycle, that is, in the early follicular phase. The timing and administration of the trigger injection and the subsequent scheduling of the oocyte retrieval is as for the long protocol (Fig. 4.2).

The benefit of this protocol is the initial flare up reaction of the GnRH agonist, which causes the stimulation of FSH secretion by the pituitary gland in the first few days. As the pituitary gland has not yet been suppressed, this protocol results in better follicular recruitment than the long protocol. However, a significant drawback of this protocol is the high progesterone level at the start of the cycle, which may be due to the rescue of the corpus luteum from the previous cycle. Studies have shown a lower pregnancy rate with this protocol than the long protocol.[3] Therefore, although this was a favored protocol for poor responders in the past, its popularity has reduced with the advent of antagonist protocols.

GnRH Agonists used for Downregulation

Various different GnRH agonist preparations are available, and the choice of agent varies from one center to another based on the clinician's preference. They differ from each other mainly in potency and route of administration.

The most commonly used agents include buserelin, leuprorelin and triptorelin, which are administered in the form of a daily subcutaneous injection. Single dose subcutaneous depot preparations of the same are also available. Nafarelin and buserelin are available in the form of nasal sprays that needs to be administered in multiple daily doses. Although patient compliance with the intranasal route is better, the drawback is fluctuating absorption of the agent resulting in an unpredictable response. However, it does appear to be sufficient to prevent a spontaneous LH surge.

Meta-analyses of trials comparing the different preparations have shown no difference in either the efficacy of pituitary suppression or IVF outcomes, measured in terms of the number of oocytes retrieved and the pregnancy rates respectively. However, women treated with nafarelin required lower doses of gonadotropins and shorter duration of ovarian stimulation, compared to leuprorelin, triptorelin and buserelin.[4] On the other hand, the use of depot preparations of GnRH agonists was associated with increased requirements for gonadotropins and a longer time required for ovarian stimulation even though the IVF outcomes were not significantly different.

GnRH Antagonist Protocols

Although GnRH agonists have been the conventional agents used for down regulation over the years, they have certain drawbacks. They have an initial flare reaction, which implies that there is an initial agonist action before the receptors get blocked and the antagonist reaction begins. Thus they require a longer duration of 7–14 days to achieve adequate down regulation. This also merits a larger number of injections, unless a depot preparation is used. Also, due to profound suppression of the pituitary, menopausal side effects are not uncommon and higher doses of gonadotropins are required for stimulation. In contrast, the GnRH antagonists have an immediate pituitary suppressive action by blocking of the receptors, causing an immediate fall in circulating Serum FSH and LH levels within 8 hours of administration. This action makes them beneficial over the GnRH agonists.

In the antagonist protocol, gonadotropins are started from Day 2 of the cycle. The GnRH antagonist may be added in one of two ways: (1) In the fixed protocol, the antagonist is started from day 6 of the cycle regardless of follicular size, (2) In the flexible protocol, the antagonist is started once the leading follicle crosses 14 mm in diameter. The antagonist is then continued till the day of the hCG trigger.

The two different agents used are cetrorelix and ganirelix, administered in a dose of 0.25 mg subcutaeonus daily, and both are equally effective. The follicular monitoring, timing of trigger injection and oocyte retrieval are the same as the agonist protocols.

Fixed versus Flexible

A meta-analysis of randomized studies comparing the fixed and the flexible protocols[5] concluded that a trend toward higher pregnancy rates was observed with the fixed protocol, although the difference was not statistically significant. The flexible protocol was beneficial in terms of requiring lesser number of antagonist doses and lower gonadotropin requirement. At present there is not enough evidence supporting either one protocol over the other, and the choice of protocol is a matter of personal preference (Fig. 4.3).

Single versus Multiple Dose Protocols

The multiple-dose GnRH antagonist protocol involves the daily subcutaneous injections of 0.25 mg of antagonist from day 5 or 6 of stimulation (the fixed start) until administration of hCG. The single-dose protocol involves a single subcutaneous injection of 3 mg GnRH antagonist on day 7 or 8 of stimulation. This single dose provides 4 days of pituitary suppression. If the patient needs more days of stimulation, the daily 0.25 mg of antagonist injections are given until the hCG trigger. The monitoring, criteria for hCG administration and oocyte retrieval are similar to the agonist protocols.

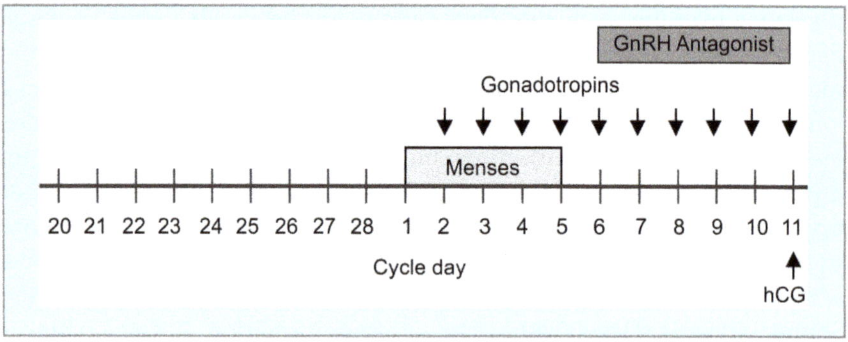

Fig. 4.3: Gonadotropin-releasing hormone (GnRH) antagonist fixed protocol. (hCG: Human chorionic gonadotropin).

GnRH Antagonists versus GnRH Agonists

Gonadotropin-releasing hormone antagonist protocols have several advantages over the agonist protocols. The shorter duration of treatment, lesser number of injections required and lower incidence of menopausal side effects render the antagonists more patient-friendly, thereby increasing compliance and reducing drop-out rates over repeated cycles. Cyst formation due to the initial flare-up reaction of the agonists is avoided when antagonists are used. Also, the gonadotropin requirement is higher when agonists are used as they can cause profound pituitary suppression. This allows the antagonist protocols to be less burdening financially as the gonadotropin requirement is correspondingly lower with their use. An important advantage, as shown in a 2007 Cochrane review,[6] is the significant reduction in the incidence of severe ovarian hyperstimulation syndrome (OHSS) in antagonist cycles as opposed to agonist cycles, as the former allow the use of a GnRH agonist trigger, eliminating the need of hCG which is known to aggravate the severity of OHSS.

On the other hand, the GnRH antagonist protocols are less programmable compared to the agonist protocols and this lack of flexibility may pose a problem at certain centers especially if planning batch IVF or if a couple has a tight traveling schedule. Although initially there was some skepticism about the possibility of lower success rates using antagonists, it is now well established that the success rates are not compromised by using the antagonist protocols. A large systematic review and meta-analysis that included results from 22 randomized controlled trials with 3,176 subjects found no significant difference in live birth rates between GnRH antagonists and agonists.[7]

OPTIMIZING OVARIAN STIMULATION

The response to stimulatory drugs during an IVF cycle depends on several factors: the number of recruitable follicles, their sensitivity to FSH as well as the bioavailability of FSH. While there are no strict criteria, "adequate response" to conventional ovarian stimulation usually means the retrieval of 8–10 oocytes. Failure to recruit an adequate number of follicles and retrieve 4–5 mature oocytes is termed "poor response," while recruitment of 20 or more follicles in high responders increases the risk of OHSS. Both are undesirable outcomes and hence an attempt is made to optimize ovarian stimulation to result in an adequate response.

The most important strategies to optimize ovarian stimulation include the following details.

Personalizing the Protocol

Different treatment protocols are suitable for different groups of women. The flare-up or antagonist protocols give better success rates in women with a poor ovarian reserve, e.g. patients with low antral follicle counts (AFCs) or low anti-Müllerian hormone (AMH) or women with a history of a poor response to the long protocol. The antagonist protocol has also been shown to reduce the risk of OHSS and may be the better choice in women at high risk of the same.

Optimal Starting Dose of Gonadotropin

In the first cycle, the important question is—what dose of gonadotropins will give an optimal response? Recent studies have demonstrated that predictive models can be useful in determining the optimal starting dose.[8]

A *standard patient* is one in whom we expect a normal response to ovarian stimulation and is usually defined as a patient aged less than 36 years, with a regular menstrual cycle, a normal basal FSH and a good AFC (>10 in both ovaries combined).

While the long protocol has so far been the oldest and the most popularly used protocol that gives good results in most "standard" patients, the GnRH antagonist protocol is more patient-friendly and is now increasingly being preferred by many centers for these "standard" patients.

Poor Responders

The long protocol gives poor results in patients with poor ovarian reserve, likely due to the profound pituitary suppression. While some studies have shown better results with the antagonist and microdose flare protocol in this group of patients, others have failed to demonstrate any benefit.

Many randomized trials have evaluated the use of various pituitary suppression regimens to improve outcome of poor responders undergoing IVF treatment. Sunkara et al.[9] conducted a systematic review of the trials of GnRH agonist long protocol, GnRH agonist short protocol and other pituitary suppression regimens in poor responders undergoing IVF/ICSI (intracytoplasmic sperm injection). A total of 680 women considered as poor responders were included in 9 randomized controlled trials. Meta-analyses of the results of these studies did not show a consistent benefit of any one pituitary suppression regimen over the others in improving outcome measures. In a 2008 study conducted by Lainas et al.,[10] 270 patients with a previous poor response were randomized to receive either the GnRH agonist flare protocol or the GnRH antagonist flexible protocol. They found that the flexible GnRH antagonist protocol was associated with significantly higher ongoing pregnancy rates compared to the GnRH agonist flare protocol in poor responders. In 2011, a meta-analysis of the published data was performed by Pu et al.[11] to compare the efficacy of GnRH antagonist versus GnRH agonist protocols for ovarian stimulation in IVF poor response patients. Fourteen eligible studies were included in this meta-analysis. They concluded that a clear advantage was gained in duration of stimulation with GnRH antagonists in poor ovarian responders undergoing IVF, although there was no statistical difference in the number of oocytes retrieved, the number of mature oocytes retrieved, the cycle cancellation rate and clinical pregnancy rate between GnRH antagonist and GnRH agonist protocols.

Over-Responders and Polycystic Ovarian Syndrome Patients

The GnRH antagonist protocol has the advantage of allowing GnRH agonist trigger to be used in place of hCG, thereby minimizing the incidence of OHSS in hyper-responders. Thus the antagonist protocol is preferred over the GnRH agonist long protocol in these patients. Women with polycystic ovarian syndrome (PCOS) are at risk of developing OHSS during ovarian stimulation. Current randomized controlled trials (RCTs) suggests that the flexible GnRH antagonist protocol is associated with a similar ongoing pregnancy rate, lower incidence of OHSS, lower gonadotropin requirement and shorter duration of stimulation, compared with GnRH agonist. The GnRH antagonist might be the treatment choice for patients with PCOS undergoing IVF.[12]

STARTING DOSE OF FSH/hMG

Safe and effective ovarian stimulation is a pivotal step in the success of assisted reproductive techniques (ART). It is important to categorize patients into normal, poor or high responders and accordingly select the starting dose so as to achieve an optimal yield of oocytes.[13] The appropriate starting dose usually depends on the clinician's experience rather than an objective calculated model.

The optimal yield of oocytes is also debatable. An appropriate response has been arbitrarily defined as retrieval of 8–10 oocytes as this should result in sufficient high quality embryos being available for transfer. In centers where cryopreservation is available the retrieval of 10–15 oocytes is considered a success as this allows multiple embryo transfer attempts per ovarian stimulation cycle and contributes to higher cumulative pregnancy rates.[14] While in centers where cryopreservation is not available or for patients who will not be able to afford it, choosing an appropriate dosage of gonadotropins that could yield a modest number of oocytes is considered crucial as it avoids oocyte and drug wastage.

At the same time, retrieval of less than 5 or more than 20 oocytes is regarded as an unfavorable response as the former would increase the incidence of cycle cancellation and the latter would increase the risk of OHSS.[15]

Many trials to develop a scoring system for calculating the appropriate gonadotropin dose have been attempted. Popovic-Todorovic in 2003 developed a model based on four predictors, the total number of antral follicles, total Doppler score, serum testosterone concentrations and smoking habit[8] but his scoring system was not widely adopted in clinical practice because of the inclusion of two predictive factors that are not measured routinely; Doppler score and testosterone concentrations. In addition smoking is not widespread in all communities to be included as a significant predictor of ovarian response.

In 2006, Howles and colleagues attempted another trial using a combination of 4 other variables that were identified as most important predictors of ovarian response. These included baseline serum FSH concentrations in the early follicular phase, body mass index (BMI), age and AFC.[16] These factors were modeled into a dosing algorithm to calculate the dose of recombinant FSH (rFSH) which was applied in a clinical trial in 2009.[17] Cancellation rate was high due to the application of a low starting dose of 75 IU for the stimulation of multiple follicular development in some cases which is an infrequent dose in routine clinical practice. In addition, the scoring system was very complicated. Olivennes and colleagues; the directors of the study advised modification of the algorithm and introduction of new variables that could yield a more practical model.

The main aspect of the "individualization" in IVF cycles is to offer every single patient the best therapy tailored on her own characteristics thus allowing a high chance of success and of course minimizing the risks deriving from ovarian stimulation. Choosing different doses of gonadotropins for different patients is the most important clinical decision in the personalization of therapy.[18] Usually clinicians choose the gonadotropin starting dose according to anamnesis and clinical criteria, the most important being the outcome of previous IVF cycles. If no previous cycles have been performed, the choice will be based on criteria as the women's age, BMI and markers of ovarian reserve.[19,20]

Currently used markers of ovarian reserve include FSH, AMH and AFC, with the last two markers having the best performance in predicting ovarian response to exogenous FSH.[21-23] AMH and AFC are nowadays considered two markers with similar diagnostic performance.[22-26] Indeed AMH and AFC actually measure the same thing: the pool of recruitable follicles. While AMH appears to have important advantages over AFC, as the lowest intra- and inter-menstrual cycle variability and the operator-independence, the great advantage of the AFC is the possibility of its measurement at the same moment in which clinicians examine the patient; hence, with great certainty we can assert that AFC will continue to be a widely used marker of ovarian reserve.

Rombauts performed a comprehensive search of the database in the Cochrane Library, MEDLINE, EMBASE, the NICE guidelines database and the reference lists of manuscripts.[27] A significant number of RCTs were identified that address the question of the FSH starting dose in expected normal responders. Using GnRH agonists for pituitary downregulation, five studies[28-32] compared a starting dose of 100 IU with 200 IU and three studies[33-35] compared a starting dose of 150 IU with 250 IU. Two studies were identified that used GnRH antagonists for pituitary suppression. One compared a starting dose of 150 IU with 200 IU,[36] whereas the other compared 150 IU with 225 IU.[37] All the studies were designed to detect differences in the number of oocytes collected and the total dose of FSH used and were of similar quality.

Taken together these RCTs suggest that higher starting doses do not lead to improved pregnancy rates, despite lower cancellation rates. One could argue that the higher oocyte numbers associated with higher starting doses will lead to more frozen embryos and therefore better cumulative pregnancy rates. However, 7 of the 10 RCTs found no significant difference. A higher number of frozen embryos was only found in 3 of the 5 studies comparing 100 versus 200 IU. Although it remains to be proven, it perhaps suggests that a starting dose of 100 IU may be associated with lower cumulative pregnancy rates per oocyte collection.

Even so, the improved egg yield was only apparent in younger patients, arguably those that need it the least. In a study by Out et al.[33] in the patient group of 30–33 years an average of four more eggs was collected (15 vs 11 eggs) if patients were given 250 IU instead of 150 IU. In the two other groups (34–36 years and 37–39 years) there was no difference. This observation was echoed by findings from the study from Yong et al.[34] They reported that approximately five more eggs were retrieved in women aged less than 33 years in the 225 IU compared with the 150 IU group, but in older women (≥33 years), the number of eggs retrieved in both groups was similar.

In view of the above, the higher rate of hormone-related side effects and extra cost associated with the higher dose protocol, it would be reasonable to conclude that most patients should start on a dose of 150 IU.

REGIMENS OF GONADOTROPIN USE

There are three regimens of gonadotropin use for ovarian stimulation:

1. In the *fixed dose regimen*, the gonadotropin dose is kept constant throughout the stimulation. If the optimal staring dose has been determined, this protocol is simple to follow and results in good outcomes.
2. In the "step-down" *regimen*, a high starting dose of gonadotropins (300–450 IU) is used for the first 2 days, followed by a dose reduction (150–225 IU/day). This enables supra-physiological levels of FSH required for maximal multifollicular recruitment during the critical period in the early follicular phase and seems to result in greater synchrony of follicles. The higher dose during the first few days theoretically increases the risk of over-response and OHSS, but the following dose reduction balances this risk.
3. In the "step-up" *regimen*, the starting dose of gonadotropin is low and is then gradually increased on cycle day 5 or later, depending on the response. This protocol can result in high FSH serum levels in the late follicular phase leading to an asynchronous development of multiple follicles, an undesirable outcome.[38]

TYPE OF GONADOTROPIN USED

At present, several different gonadotropin preparations are used for ovarian stimulation. Follicle-stimulating hormone (FSH)-containing gonadotropin preparations are as follows:

- Human menopausal gonadotropins
- Urinary FSH (uFSH)
- Highly purified urinary FSH (HP-uFSH)
- Highly purified hMG (HP-hMG)
- Recombinant FSH

Human menopausal gonadotropin, containing approximately equal amounts of FSH and LH, was the first commercially available gonadotropin preparation, purified from postmenopausal urine. In the early period, after the introduction of rFSH, studies indicated that rFSH was superior to uFSH. The common assumption that if rFSH was superior to uFSH, it should be superior to hMG and was evident in a meta-analysis. However, a subsequent meta-analysis comparing rFSH and hMG pointed in the opposite direction.[39,40] Then, uFSH became largely unavailable and HP-hMG was introduced into the market. Simultaneously, several studies demonstrated the importance of LH in ovarian stimulation and studies comparing rFSH and HP-hMG found either no evidence of benefit of one product over the other or HP-hMG to be more effective than rFSH. The argument against hMG is that the use of urine as a source raises concerns about potential contamination with pathogenic microorganisms. With respect to pharmaceutical quality, the increased purity and batch-to-batch consistency of the recombinant proteins can be considered a breakthrough.[41] In the current era of "prion scare", this may be an important argument in favor of rFSH. However, it is important to note that urinary-derived gonadotropins have been available since the beginning of the 1960s and, so far, prion or other infectivity has never been ascribed to them.

The clinical choice of the gonadotropin preparation to be used for ovarian stimulation should depend on availability, convenience, and costs.

MONITORING IVF CYCLES

Cycle monitoring is an essential part of any IVF protocol as it can indicate over- or under-response, enabling dose adjustments to optimize response. When performing ovarian stimulation in IVF cycles there are obvious reasons why the cycle has to be monitored: to evaluate if the dose of gonadotropins is optimal; to avoid OHSS and to find the optimal time for hCG administration. Of all the methods described for monitoring IVF cycles, ultrasound imaging of the utero-ovarian response to gonadotropins has become the clinically most useful. With the use of GnRH analogs, there seems to be less need for extensive hormonal monitoring of IVF cycles.[42] Ultrasound alone or in certain cases combined with one or two serum estradiol (E_2) measurements seems to be sufficient in the majority of women entering an IVF cycle.[43]

The aims of monitoring are:

- To assess the ovarian response
- To enable optimal ovarian response by tailoring the dose during the course of the stimulation
- To time the ovulation trigger and hence, the time of the ovum pick-up (OPU)
- To monitor other factors, which may have a negative impact on the success rates of IVF.

SHORT PROTOCOL/ANTAGONIST PROTOCOL/MINIMAL STIMULATION PROTOCOL

In these protocols, the stimulation begins from the early follicular phase. Hence, the first monitoring begins on the first or second day of the cycle to ensure optimal conditions as follows:

- Endometrium less than 4 mm
- Absence of ovarian cysts or follicles more than 9 mm
- Serum progesterone less than 1 ng/mL
- Absence of factors known to have a negative impact, such as endometrial polyps, hydrosalpinx (that may have been missed previously), etc.

The AFC is assessed and the type of protocol and the dose of gonadotropins are decided at this time based on the need for ovarian stimulation and the necessity to prevent ovarian hyperstimulation. In case, the first progesterone level is more than 1 ng/mL, a GnRH agonist can be administered to the patient and continued till the progesterone levels drop to less than 1 ng/mL. Ovarian stimulation can then be commenced with gonadotropins in conjunction with the GnRH analog as in the short protocol.

Monitoring is individualized based on the clinic protocol and the ovarian response. The pelvic scan is repeated at the discretion of the clinician. Usually no changes in the gonadotropin dose are made for the first 5 days of stimulation, and therefore the first follow-up scan is done on day 6. Subsequent scans are done every 2–3 days or more frequently depending on the patient's response. The follicles are mapped on a graph. The trigger is given once the leading three follicles reach 18 mm (measured in two dimensions and the average dimension is calculated). On the day of trigger, serum E_2 and serum progesterone are measured.

A 2008 Cochrane review[44] concluded on the basis of the existent material that there is no significant difference in pregnancy rates and live birth in cycles monitored using ultrasound and serum E_2 or those monitored by ultrasound alone.

Long Protocol

Gonadotropin-releasing hormone analogs, such as leuprolide, buserelin and triptorelin, are commenced in the luteal phase of the preceding cycle. It is imperative to confirm downregulation prior to ovarian stimulation. This is usually done on the first or second day of the period following the commencement of analog. Alternatively, this scan can be done after 10 days of analog administration.

The conditions to be met prior to the ovarian stimulation are:

- Endometrial thickness of less than or equal to 4 mm
- Absence of ovarian follicles more than 9 mm
- Serum estradiol level less than or equal to 50 pg/mL
- Absence of factors, known to have a negative impact, such as endometrial polyps, hydrosalpinx (that may have been missed previously).

In case downregulation is not achieved, the patient is advised to continue the analog and follow-up after a week. In case downregulation is confirmed, the ovarian stimulation can start; otherwise, the patient may need to continue the analog. The patient can also be offered to restart the treatment afresh in the next cycle.

The monitoring of ovarian response once downregulation is confirmed is the same as that in the other protocols. It is also important to confirm the availability of the husband on the day of scheduled OPU as also of the clinic and laboratory staff. In case a delay is desired, the analog is continued till such time that the stimulation can start.

DOSE ADJUSTMENT

Recommendations during Stimulation

Most experts believe that the best results are obtained in cycles where the dose of the gonadotropin is maintained rather than increased. Hence, estimating the correct starting dose is extremely important for optimal results. The effectiveness of dose increases, though widely practiced, does not seem to be based on the evidence. Several studies have shown that in patients receiving a step-up dosing of gonadotropin following a low response after 5 days of stimulation, the number of oocytes retrieved as well as the pregnancy rates remain significantly lower than in patients treated with a fixed dose.

Increase in Dose of Gonadotropins

This is done in case of inadequate or slow response, based on the number and size of follicles in each of the ovaries. The increase in the dose is generally in increments of 75 IU.

Reduction in Dose of Gonadotropins

This is done in case of an exaggerated response, in terms of the number of follicles being stimulated in the ovaries. The number of all the follicles should be counted diligently along with the dimensions. The dose reduction is similarly in decrements of 75 IU. A sharp reduction in the dose is generally not recommended.

Freezing All Embryos

Freezing of all the embryos or oocytes retrieved may be recommended in a few scenarios:

- Serum estradiol more than 3,500 pg/mL on the day of trigger
- Serum progesterone more than 1 ng/mL on any day during the ovarian stimulation
- Any unexpected uterine bleeding
- Hitherto undiagnosed hydrosalpinx seen on ultrasoundSignificant endometrial polyps (>1 cm).

Cancellation/Conversion to an Intrauterine Insemination Cycle

Conversion to an intrauterine insemination (IUI) cycle may be offered in case of a poor ovarian response (<3 follicles of size ≥ 12 mm). Cycle cancellation may be required in case of no response or a poor response where IUI is not a possibility such as bilateral tubal block. This has to be after appropriate counseling regarding the pros and cons of IVF versus IUI.

Cycle Monitoring—OHSS

Ovarian hyperstimulation syndrome is a rare but serious complication of ovarian stimulation. Therefore, one of the main aims of cycle monitoring is to prevent its occurrence. If ovarian over-response is recognized during cycle monitoring, the dose of gonadotropin is reduced or stopped (coasting). Frequent (even daily) monitoring is performed to continually assess the response. If the risk of OHSS seems to be very high, an agonist trigger is used instead of an hCG trigger, and all embryos are cryopreserved for subsequent transfer in a thaw cycle.

A randomized trial with a sufficiently large sample size to test the effects of different monitoring protocols on a rare outcome like OHSS is difficult. Nevertheless, the 2008 Cochrane review[44] mentioned earlier suggested that cycle monitoring using transvaginal ultrasound plus serum estradiol be retained as a precautionary good practice point.

CONCLUSION

Safe and effective ovarian stimulation is a pivotal step in the success of ART. It is important to categorize patients into normal, poor or high responders and accordingly select the starting dose so as to achieve an optimal yield of oocytes. Recombinant gonadotropins represent a very obvious technical progress in comparison with thc older urinary gonadotropins. This is evident in their relative ease of administration and lack of contamination. There is, however, no convincing evidence that rFSH improves the clinical outcome. The lower cost of urinary products represents a very significant factor in choosing a preferred gonadotropin. The clinical choice of the gonadotropin preparation to be used for ovarian stimulation should depend on availability, convenience and costs. A standard patient who is usually defined as a patient aged less than 36 years, with a regular menstrual cycle, a normal basal FSH and a good AFC (>10 in both ovaries combined) is usually treated with 150–225 IU/day as the starting dose. Patients with a poor response require a higher dose of 450 IU/day. Cycle monitoring is an essential part of any IVF protocol as it can indicate over- or under-response, enabling dose adjustments to optimize response. The best results are obtained in cycles where the dose of the gonadotropin is maintained rather than increased. Hence, estimating the correct starting dose is extremely important for optimal results.

REFERENCES

1. Steptoe PC, Edwards RG. Birth after the reimplantation of a human embryo. Lancet. 1978;2(8085):366.
2. Jones HW Jr, Jones GS, Andrews MC, et al. The program for in vitro fertilization at Norfolk. Fertil Steril. 1982;38(1):14-21.
3. Daya S. Gonadotropin releasing hormone agonist protocols for pituitary desensitization in in vitro fertilization and gamete intrafallopian transfer cycles. Cochrane Database Syst Rev. 2000;2:CD001299.
4. Wong JM, Forrest KA, Snabes SZ, et al. Efficacy of nafarelin in assisted reproductive technology: a meta-analysis. Hum Reprod Update. 2001;7(1):92-101.
5. Al-Inany H, Aboulghar MA, Mansour RT, et al. Optimizing GnRH antagonist administration: meta-analysis of fixed versus flexible protocol. Reprod Biomed Online. 2005;10(5):567-70.
6. Al-Inany HG, Abou-Setta AM, Aboulghar M. Gonadotrophin-releasing hormone antagonists for assisted conception: a Cochrane review. Reprod Biomed Online. 2007;14(5):640-9.
7. Kolibianakis EM, Collins J, Tarlatzis BC, et al. Among patients treated for IVF with gonadotrophins and GnRH analogues, is the probability of live birth dependent on the type of analogue used? A systematic review and meta-analysis. Hum Reprod Update. 2006;12(6):651-71.
8. Popovic-Todorovic B, Loft A, Bredkjaeer HE, et al. A prospective randomized clinical trial comparing an individual dose of recombinant FSH based on predictive factors versus a 'standard' dose of 150 IU/day in 'standard'patients undergoing IVF/ICSI treatment. Hum Reprod. 2003;18(11):2275-82.
9. Sunkara SK, Tuthill J, Khairy M, et al. Pituitary suppression regimens in poor responders undergoing IVF treatment: a systematic review and meta-analysis. RBM Online. 2007;15(5):539-46.
10. Lainas T, Sfontouris I, Papanikolaou E, et al. Flexible GnRH antagonist versus flare-up GnRH agonist protocol in poor responders treated by IVF: a randomized controlled trial. Hum Reprod. 2008;23(6):1355-8.
11. Pu D, Wu J, Liu J. Comparisons of GnRH antagonist versus GnRH agonist protocol in poor ovarian responders undergoing IVF. Hum Reprod. 2011;26(10):2742-9.
12. Lainas TG, Sfontouris IA, Zorzovilis IZ, et al. Flexible GnRH antagonist protocol versus GnRH agonist long protocol in patients with polycystic ovary syndrome treated for IVF: a prospective randomized controlled trial (RCT). Hum Reprod. 2010;25(3):683-9.
13. Al-Azemi M, Killick S, Duffy S, et al. Multi-marker assessment of ovarian reserve predicts oocyte yield after ovulation induction. Hum Reprod. 2011;26(2):414-22.

14. Tiitinen A. Prevention of multiple pregnancies in infertility treatment. Best Pract Res Clin Obstet Gynaecol. 2012;26(6):829-40.
15. Inge G, Brindsen P, Elder K. Oocyte number per live birth in IVF: were Steptoe and Edwards less wasteful? Hum Reprod. 2004;20(3):588-92.
16. Howles C, Saunders H, Alam V, et al. Predictive factors and a corresponding treatment algorithm for controlled ovarian stimulation in patients treated with recombinant human follicle stimulating hormone (follitropin alfa) during assisted reproduction technology (ART) procedures. An analysis of 1378 patients. Curr Med Res Opin. 2006;22(5):907-18.
17. Olivennes F, Howles C, Borini A, et al. Individualizing FSH dose for assisted reproduction using a novel algorithm: the CONSORT study. RBM Online. 2009;18(2):195-204.
18. La Marca A, Grisendi V, Giulini S, et al. Individualization of the FSH starting dose in IVF/ICSI cycles using the antral follicle count. J Ovarian Res. 2013;6(1):11.
19. Fauser BC, Diedrich K, Devroey P, et al. Predictors of ovarian response: progress towards individualized treatment in ovulation induction and ovarian stimulation. Hum Reprod Update. 2008;14(1):1-14.
20. Alviggi C, Humaidan P, Ezcurra D. Hormonal, functional and genetic biomarkers in controlled ovarian stimulation: tools for matching patients and protocols. Reprod Biol Endocrinol. 2012;10:9.
21. Broekmans FJ, Kwee J, Hendriks DJ, et al. A systematic review of tests predicting ovarian reserve and IVF outcome. Hum Reprod Update. 2006;12(6): 685-718.
22. La Marca A, Sighinolfi G, Radi D, et al. Anti-Müllerian hormone (AMH) as a predictive marker in assisted reproductive technology (ART). Hum Reprod Update. 2010;16(2):113-30.
23. Nelson SM, Yates RW, Fleming R. Serum anti-Müllerian hormone and FSH: prediction of live birth and extremes of response in stimulated cycles—implications for individualization of therapy. Hum Reprod. 2007;22(9):2414-21.
24. Broekmans FJ, de Ziegler D, Howles CM, et al. The antral follicle count: practical recommendations for better standardization. Fertil Steril. 2010;94(3): 1044-51.
25. La Marca A, Spada E, Sighinolfi G, et al. Age-specific nomogram for the decline in antral follicle count throughout the reproductive period. Fertil Steril. 2011;95(2):684-8.
26. Broer SL, Dolleman M, Opmeer BC, et al. AMH and AFC as predictors of excessive response in controlled ovarian hyperstimulation: a meta-analysis. Hum Reprod Update. 2011;17(1):46-54.
27. Rombauts L. Is there a recommended maximum starting dose of FSH in IVF? J Assist Reprod Genet. 2007;24(8):343-9.
28. Tan SL, Child TJ, Cheung AP, et al. A randomized, double-blind, multicenter study comparing a starting dose of 100 IU or 200 IU of recombinant follicle stimulating hormone (Puregon®) in women undergoing controlled ovarian hyperstimulation for IVF treatment. J Assist Reprod Genet. 2005;22(2):81-8.
29. Out HJ, Lindenberg S, Mikkelsen AL, et al. A prospective, randomized, double-blind clinical trial to study the efficacy and efficiency of a fixed dose of recombinant follicle stimulating hormone (Puregon®) in women undergoing ovarian stimulation. Hum Reprod. 1999;14(3):622-7.
30. Out HJ, David I, Ron-El R, et al. A randomized, double-blind clinical trial using fixed daily doses of 100 or 200 IU of recombinant FSH in ICSI cycles. Hum Reprod. 2001;16(6):1104-49.

31. Pruksananonda K, Suwajanakorn S, Sereepapong W, et al. Comparison of two different fixed doses of follitropin-beta in controlled ovarian hyperstimulation: a prospective randomized, double blind clinical trial. J Med Assoc Thai. 2004;87(10):1151-5.
32. Asian Purgeon Study Group, Hoomans EH, Mulder BB. A group-comparative, randomized, double-blind comparison of the efficacy and efficiency of two fixed daily dose regimens (100- and 200-IU) of recombinant follicle stimulating hormone (rFSH, Puregon®) in Asian women undergoing ovarian stimulation for IVF/ICSI. J Assist Reprod Genet. 2002;19(10):470-6.
33. Out HJ, Braat DD, Lintsen BM, et al. Increasing the daily dose of recombinant follicle stimulating hormone (Puregon) does not compensate for the age-related decline in retrievable oocytes after ovarian stimulation. Hum Reprod. 2000;15(1):29-35.
34. Yong PY, Brett S, Baird DT, et al. A prospective randomized clinical trial comparing 150 IU and 225 IU of recombinant follicle-stimulating hormone (Gonal-F*) in a fixed-dose regimen for controlled ovarian stimulation in in vitro fertilization treatment. Fertil Steril. 2003;79(2):308-15.
35. Latin-American Puregon IVF Study Group. A double-blind clinical trial comparing a fixed daily dose of 150 and 250 IU of recombinant follicle-stimulating hormone in women undergoing in vitro fertilization. Fertil Steril. 2001;76(5):950-6.
36. Out HJ, Rutherford A, Fleming R, et al. A randomized, double-blind, multicentre clinical trial comparing starting doses of 150 and 200 IU of recombinant FSH in women treated with the GnRH antagonist ganirelix for assisted reproduction. Hum Reprod. 2004;19(1):90-95.
37. Wikland M, Bergh C, Borg K, et al. A prospective, randomized comparison of two starting doses of recombinant FSH in combination with cetrorelix in women undergoing ovarian stimulation for IVF/ICSI. Hum Reprod. 2001;16(8):1676-81.
38. Andoh K, Mizunuma H, Liu X, et al. A comparative study of fixed-dose, step-down, and low-dose step-up regimens of human menopausal gonadotropin for patients with polycystic ovary syndrome. Fertil Steril. 1998;70(5):840-6.
39. Daya S, Gunby J, Hughes EG, et al. Follicle-stimulating hormone versus human menopausal gonadotropin for in vitro fertilization cycles: a meta-analysis. Fertil Steril. 1995;64(2):347-54.
40. Agrawal R, Holmes J, Jacobs HS. Follicle-stimulating hormone or human menopausal gonadotropin for ovarian stimulation in in vitro fertilization cycles: a meta-analysis. Fertil Steril. 2000;73(2):338-43.
41. Olijve W, de Boer W, Mulders JW, et al. Molecular biology and biochemistry of human recombinant follicle stimulating hormone (Puregon). Mol Hum Reprod. 1996;2(5):371-82.
42. Wikland M, Borg J, Hamberger L, et al. Simplification of IVF: minimal monitoring and the use of subcutaneous highly purified FSH administration for ovulation induction. Hum Reprod. 1994;9(8):1430-6.
43. Bergh C, Howles C, Borg K, et al. Recombinant human follicle stimulating hormone (r-hFSH; Gonal-F) versus highly purified urinary FSH (Metrodin HP): results of a randomized comparative study in women undergoing assisted reproductive techniques. Hum Reprod. 1997;12(10):2133-9.
44. Kwan I, Bhattacharya S, McNeil A, et al. Monitoring of stimulated cycles in assisted reproduction (IVF and ICSI). Cochrane Database Syst Rev. 2008;16(2):CD005289.

Chapter 5

Protocols for Poor Responders

Ritu Hinduja, Kalyani Shrimali

INTRODUCTION

In recent years, ground breaking research has been made in the field of assisted reproductive techniques in terms of clinical knowledge and technological development. Number of eggs retrieved is considered one of the fundamental steps to reach success in an in vitro fertilization (IVF) cycle. In patients defined "poor responders" the limited number of eggs obtained remains the main hurdle in optimizing the live birth rates. In fact, owing to the lower number of oocytes retrieved, there are fewer embryos to select and transfer, leading to lower pregnancy rates per transfer and lower cumulative pregnancy rates per cycle compared with normal responders.

The ESHRE working group on poor ovarian response has finally given a common definition of "poor responder", where at least two of the following three features must be present:

1. Advanced maternal age or any other risk factor for poor ovarian response
2. A previous poor ovarian response
3. An abnormal ovarian reserve test.[1]

Two episodes of poor ovarian response after maximal stimulation are sufficient to define a patient as poor responder in the absence of advanced maternal age or abnormal ovarian reserve testing. In such cases the refined definition should be "expected poor responder".

Many protocols have been proposed for management of poor ovarian response. Although high doses of gonadotropins have been used by vast majority of authors in the 1980s and early 1990s, results have been controversial and prospective randomized studies have shown little or no benefit.[2,3] In poor responders no superiority of recombinant follicle stimulating hormone has been proved compared to urinary gonadotropins.[4,5] Flare-up gonadotropin-releasing hormone (GnRH) agonist protocol has been proposed to producc better results than standard long luteal protocols.[6,7] GnRH antagonist did not hold true to its initial promise.[8] Adjuvant therapy with growth hormone (GH) or GH-releasing factors resulted in no significant improvement.[8-11] Corifollitropin alfa followed by highly purified human menopausal gonadotropin (HP-hMG) stimulation has shown promising results in two pilot studies[12,13] when used in young poor responders fulfilling the Bologna criteria. Finally, natural cycle IVF and mild or minimal stimulation IVF protocol have shown comparable result like those obtained in stimulated cycles in true poor responders.[14] However, well designed, large scale, randomized control trials are required to assess the efficacy of these different management strategies.

MAXIMAL GONADOTROPIN DOSAGE

The use of high doses of gonadotropins is the most extensively employed strategy to improve follicular response in "poor responders".[15-17]

The obvious clinical approach when the standard dose of gonadotropins (225–300 IU) fails to induce a proper multifollicular growth approach is to increase the dose. In the literature conflicting data are reported on the outcomes of this approach: some[18-20] but not all authors[21] did not report enhanced ovarian response and/or better pregnancy rates in prospective and retrospective studies when the starting dose of gonadotropins was increased up to 450 IU. It is today clear that these patients have a reduced ovarian reserve; the follicles that can be recruited are fewer and the gonadotropins, independently of the dosage administered, can only support the cohort of follicles receptive to stimulation without manufacturing follicles de novo.

It is not effective to increase the starting dose of gonadotropin after an unexpected poor response in the first IVF cycle.[16] It may increase the oocyte retrieval rates and embryo transfer (ET) rates, but will not add any significant improvement in the number of oocytes retrieved and the number of transferable embryos.

The only important benefit of increasing the dose is the low cancellation rate. Kovacs et al.[22] published a retrospective analysis of fresh ET cycles. Their analyses suggest detrimental influences of higher gonadotropin dose on the endometrium and confirmed the previously reported adverse association between higher dose and IVF outcome. Milder protocols may be of particular benefit in women ≤35 years of age. Low dose gonadotropin regimens have the benefit of reducing costs and risks of ovarian hyperstimulation without reducing the efficacy and in some cases, actually increasing the pregnancy rates.

GnRH ANALOGS

Combination of gonadotropins and GnRH agonists, started in the luteal phase of the previous cycle, has been considered the protocol of choice in normoresponders since the nineties. It lowers cancellation rate and raises the number of preovulatory follicles and the number of oocytes retrieved and good quality embryos for transfer, leading to better pregnancy rates.[23]

However, in poor responders this protocol could have a detrimental effect as it may induce an excessive ovarian suppression that could lead to a reduced or absent follicular response.[24,25]

In patients with poor ovarian reserve the following options could be resorted to:

- Decrease the length of suppression by decreasing the duration of GnRH agonist use (short and ultrashort, mini- and microdose flare-up regimens).[26-28]
- Lower or stop (after pituitary suppression) the dose of GnRH agonists initiated during the luteal phase.[29,30]
- Use the GnRH antagonists in combination with gonadotropins to prevent premature luteinizing hormone (LH) rise during the mid-late follicular phase.[31,32]

The efficacy of the microdose flare-up and multiple-dose antagonist protocols for poor-responder patients in intracytoplasmic sperm injection-embryo transfer (ICSI-ET) cycles was compared by Demirol and Gurgan. The microdose flare-up protocol seemed to have a better, with a significantly higher mean number of mature oocytes retrieved and higher implantation rate.[33]

Though short and ultrashort flare-up protocols are mostly used in poor responders for more than 20 years, prospective nonrandomized trials, or retrospective studies[34,35] were unable to demonstrate any significant benefit on the clinical outcome in this group of patients. The rationale to lower the dose of GnRH agonists or to stop it completely in the follicular phase is to obtain a reduction of the inhibitory direct effect of the GnRH agonist on the gonads.[36,37]

BIRTH CONTROL PILL PRIMING

Kovacs et al.[38] conducted a retrospective analysis which revealed no improvement in IVF cycle outcomes in poor responders who received oral contraceptive pills (OCP) to achieve hypothalamic-pituitary suppression instead of GnRH analogs. Duvan et al.[39] on the other hand compared OCP pretreatment plus microdose GnRH agonists in flare-up protocol and non-OCP microdose GnRH agonists in flare-up protocol among poor responder ICSI patients which reflected no benefit of OCP pretreatment.

GnRH ANTAGONIST

Several authors suggest the use of GnRH antagonists along with gonadotropins as a suitable protocol for poor responders because they are not administered during follicular stage so the suppression of endogenous gonadotropins is not present at that time in contrast to GnRH agonists which is a possible advantage during ovarian stimulation in poor responders.[40]

With GnRH antagonist the added benefit is that it is possible to assess the ovarian reserve by ultrasound on days 2/3 of the cycle in which ovarian stimulation is planned because there is absence of profound downregulation by GnRH agonist when resorting to a long protocol. This is beneficial in patients with a mean follicle count of less than five follicles as they are known to have significant cycle-to-cycle variability in antral follicle count from –2 to +5[41] to –3 to +7.[42]

CORIFOLLITROPIN ALFA

Corifollitropin alfa a new hybrid molecule with a prolonged half-life, supports the cohort of follicle receptive to stimulation for 7 days.[43] Corifollitropin can fully exploit the reduced ovarian reserve by rapidly increasing the serum follicle-stimulating hormone (FSH) concentration that consequently results in a significantly higher exposure of the small antral follicles to constant high levels of FSH during the early follicular phase.[44]

Polyzos et al.[44] conducted a retrospective study and compared laboratory and clinical results when corifollitropin alfa followed by recombinant FSH (rFSH) in combination with GnRH antagonist with conventional stimulation protocols in poor responder patients according to the "Bologna criteria" and reported similar results in both groups. Finally, promising pregnancy rates were reported in a retrospective pilot study in young (less than 40 years) poor responder patients following a combination of corifollitropin alfa with HP-hMG in a GnRH antagonist protocol.[45]

GnRH ANTAGONIST/LETROZOLE PROTOCOLS

Jovanovic et al.[46] evaluated the effect of adjunctive letrozole or clomiphene citrate (CC) in IVF stimulation protocols.

Supplementation with CC in poor responders showed significant improvements in E2, number of dominant follicles, oocytes retrieved, and number of embryos transferred. It significantly improved biochemical pregnancy rates while reducing cycle cancellations. Letrozole supplementation showed similar effects.[46] However, despite increasing oocyte yield and ET rates, the overall clinical and live birth rate in this population remained low and showed no measurable increase.[46]

ALTERNATIVE APPROACHES

Several alternative approaches have been proposed as adjuvants with the aim of strengthening the effect of exogenous gonadotropins in women with poor ovarian reserve.

ADDITION OF ESTRADIOL IN THE LUTEAL PHASE

A meta-analysis of eight selected studies reported a decreased risk of cycle cancellation and increased chances of clinical pregnancy in poor responder patients with, the addition of estradiol in the luteal phase with or without the simultaneous use of GnRH antagonist.[47]

The biological rationale might be that luteal estradiol priming could improve synchronization of the pool of follicles available to controlled ovarian stimulation.[48]

This meta-analysis has been strongly criticized because of important methodological pitfall randomized trials are needed before suggesting the addition of estradiol in the luteal phase.[49]

ADDITION OF RECOMBINANT LUTEINIZING HORMONE

Addition of recombinant LH during gonadotropin stimulation in poor responder patients has been suggested by some authors.[50]

However, two meta-analyses[51,52] showed that the addition of recombinant LH does not increase the number of oocyte retrieved, the total dose of FSH, the cancellation rates, and the ongoing pregnancy rates in poor responder patients.

A very recent meta-analysis of 40 randomized controlled studies,[53] on the other hand reported that significantly more oocytes were retrieved and significantly higher clinical pregnancy rates were observed with rFSH plus recombinant LH versus rFSH alone in poor responders.

ADDITION OF GROWTH HORMONE

It has been hypothesized that the use of GH might modulate the action of FSH on granulosa cells by upregulating the local synthesis of insulin-like growth factor-I (IGF-I).[54-56] The IGF-I amplifies the effect of FSH at the level of both granulosa and theca cells.[57,58] It has been suggested that addition of GH significantly increased the probability of live birth in poor responders by two recent meta-analyses of six randomized trials.[6,59] The frequency and dosage of GH varies from study to study. Up until now, there is not any robust data suggesting routine addition of GH in ovarian stimulation protocols for poor responders patients.[60,61] Because of the heterogeneity of the frequency and dosage of GH administered and the small number of patients enrolled in the studies, the recommendation of substituting ovarian stimulation with GH in poor responders is guarded.

ADDITION OF ANDROGENS

Theca cells produce androgens which play a critical role for an adequate follicular steroidogenesis and for a correct early follicular and granulosa cell development.[62] They are the substrate for the aromatase activity of the granulosa cells, which converts the androgens to estrogens. Androgens may increase FSH receptor expression in granulosa cells amplifying the effects of FSH and thus potentially enhance responsiveness of ovaries to FSH.[6,62,63] According to this hypothesis they may benefit poor responders when used as an adjuvant to gonadotropin for ovarian stimulation. A recent meta-analysis of four randomized controlled trials of adjuvant androgens [DHEA (dehydroepiandrosterone) and testosterone] in poor responder patients showed a significantly higher ongoing pregnancy rate in the androgen supplementation group.[64]

There is an urgent need of robust data from randomized controlled studies that could justify the widespread use of DHEA before ovarian stimulation in poor responders.[65]

ADDITION OF ASPIRIN

Increased intraovarian vascularity has been associated with improved delivery of gonadotropins and other growth factors required for folliculogenesis.[66,67] Poor ovarian response is associated with impaired ovarian blood flow.[68,69] Based on this rationale, by enhancing ovarian vascularization with vasoactive substances such as aspirin, the ovarian response could theoretically improve.[70]

However, the evidence supporting the effect of a low dose of aspirin in women undergoing IVF is poor and controversial.[71]

NATURAL CYCLES IN VITRO FERTILIZATION

Some authors suggest that natural cycles IVF was a valid option for poor responder patients because it has the same chance in terms of pregnancy and implantation rates.[72] Schimberni et al.[73] evaluated the IVF outcome in 500 patients and reported very encouraging results especially in young poor responders (less than 35 years). The pregnancy rate was 18% per started cycle, 29% per transfer, and 31% per patient in this group of women. In contrast, a recent paper studied the effect of natural cycles IVF in women defined as poor responders according to the "Bologna criteria": the data however showed that the cumulative live birth per patient does not exceed 8%.[74] The contradictory data can be very likely associated to the diversity of patients selected before the application of "Bologna criteria".

CONCLUSION

In the last two decades despite a large number of papers published suggesting the most efficient stimulation protocol for the management of patients with poor ovarian response, it still remains the most challenging task in the field of assisted reproduction.

The clear definition provided by expert committee ESHRE in Bologna in 2011 is highly appreciated. "Bologna criteria" can be considered an important step toward the identification of poor responder patients and consequently to find the most effective strategy in their management. Finally, we should consider the alternative strategies to be able to prevent the consequences of the poor ovarian response. Oocyte cryopreservation for fertility preservation before the ovarian reserve decline is an important option that must be offered. Available evidence indicates no harmful consequence of oocyte vitrification,[75,76] hence it is not just a possibility but a moral duty to fully exploit its potentials especially in the prevention of poor ovarian response.

REFERENCES

1. Ferraretti AP, La Marca A, Fauser BC, et al. ESHRE consensus on the definition of 'poor response' to ovarian stimulation for in vitro fertilization: the Bologna criteria. Hum Reprod. 2011;26(7):1616-24.
2. Keay SD, Liversedge NH, Mathur RS, et al. Assisted conception following poor ovarian response to gonadotrophin stimulation. Br J Obstet Gynaecol. 1997;104(5):521-7.
3. Ben-Rafael Z1, Bider D, Dan U, et al. Combined gonadotropin releasing hormone agonist/human menopausal gonadotropin therapy (GnRH-a/hMG) in normal, high, and poor responders to hMG. J In Vitro Fert Embryo Transf. 1991;8(1):33-6.
4. Jenkins JM, Davies DW, Devonport H, et al. Comparison of 'poor' responders with 'good' responders using a standard buserelin/human menopausal gonadotrophin regime for in-vitro fertilization. Hum Reprod. 1991;6(7):918-21.
5. Surrey ES, Schoolcraft WB. Evaluating strategies for improving ovarian response of the poor responder undergoing assisted reproductive techniques. Fertil Steril. 2000;73(4):667-76.
6. Kolibianakis EM, Venetis CA, Diedrich K, et al. Addition of growth hormone to gonadotrophins in ovarian stimulation of poor responders treated by in-vitro fertilization: a systematic review and meta-analysis. Hum Reprod Update. 2009;15(6):613-22.
7. Ferraretti AP, La Marca A, Fauser BC, et al. ESHRE consensus on the definition of "poor response" to ovarian stimulation for in vitro fertilization: the Bologna criteria. Hum Reprod. 2011;26(7):1616-24.
8. Benaglia L, Somigliana E, Vighi V, et al. Rate of severe ovarian damage following surgery for endometriomas. Hum Reprod. 2010;25(3):678-82.
9. Streuli I, de Ziegler D, Gayet V, et al. In women with endometriosis anti-Müllerian hormone levels are decreased only in those with previous endometrioma surgery. Hum Reprod. 2012;27(11):3294-303.
10. Raffi F, Metwally M, Amer S. The impact of excision of ovarian endometrioma on ovarian reserve: a systematic review and meta-analysis. J Clin Endocrinol Metab. 2012;97(9):3146-54.
11. De Vos M, Devroey P, Fauser BC. Primary ovarian insufficiency. Lancet. 2010;376(9744):911-21.
12. Fritz MA, Speroff L. Clinical Gynecologic Endocrinology and Infertility. Philadelphia, PA: Wolters Kluwer Health/Lippincott Williams & Wilkins; 2011.
13. Soto N, Iñiguez G, López P, et al. Anti-Müllerian hormone and inhibin B levels as markers of premature ovarian aging and transition to menopause in type 1 diabetes mellitus. Hum Reprod. 2009;24(11):2838-44.
14. Chang HH, Chen MJ, Lu MY, et al. Iron overload is associated with low anti-müllerian hormone in women with transfusion-dependent β-thalassaemia. BJOG. 2011;118(7):825-31.
15. Check JH. Advantages of using a lower vs. higher dosage of gonadotropins for follicular maturation including cycles of in vitro fertilization-embryo transfer. Clin Exp Obstet Gynecol. 2010;37(2):84-8.

16. Tutuncu L, Dundar O. Increasing the stimulation dose of rFHS in unexpected poor responders is not associated with better IVF outcome. Ginekol Pol. 2012;83(2):111-s5.
17. Kovacs P, Sajgo A, Kaali SG, Pal L. Detrimental effects of high-dose gonadotropin on outcome of IVF: making a case for gentle ovarian stimulation strategies. Reprod Sci. 2012;19(7):718-24.
18. Land JA, Yarmolinskaya MI, Dumoulin JC, et al. High-dose human menopausal gonadotropin stimulation in poor responders does not improve in vitro fertilization outcome. Fertil Steril. 1996;65(5):961-5.
19. Karande VC, Jones GS, Veeck LL, et al. High-dose follicle-stimulating hormone stimulation at the onset of the menstrual cycle does not improve the in vitro fertilization outcome in low-responder patients. Fertil Steril. 1990;53(3):486-9.
20. van Hooff MH, Alberda AT, Huisman GJ, et al. Doubling the human menopausal gonadotrophin dose in the course of an in-vitro fertilization treatment cycle in low responders: a randomized study. Hum Reprod. 1993;8(3):369-73
21. Hofmann GE, Toner JP, Muasher SJ, et al. High-dose follicle-stimulating hormone (FSH) ovarian stimulation in low-responder patients for in vitro fertilization. J In Vitro Fert Embryo Transf. 1989;6(5):285-9.
22. Kovacs P, Sajgo A, Kaali SG, et al. Detrimental effects of high-dose gonadotropin on outcome of IVF: making a case for gentle ovarian stimulation strategies. Reprod Sci. 2012;19(7):718-24.
23. Hughes EG, Fedorkow DM, Daya S, et al. The routine use of gonadotropin-releasing hormone agonists prior to in vitro fertilization and gamete intrafallopian transfer: a meta-analysis of randomized controlled trials. Fertil Steril. 1992;58(5):888-96.
24. Yoshimura Y, Nakamura Y, Ando M, et al. Direct effect of gonadotropin-releasing hormone agonists on the rabbit ovarian follicle. Fertil Steril. 1992;57(5):1091-7.
25. Kowalik A, Barmat L, Damario M, et al. Ovarian estradiol production in vivo. Inhibitory effect of leuprolide acetate. J Reprod Med. 1998;43(5):413-7.
26. Surrey ES, Bower J, Hill DM, et al. Clinical and endocrine effects of a microdose GnRH agonist flare regimen administered to poor responders who are undergoing in vitro fertilization. Fertil Steril. 1998;69(3):419-24.
27. Schoolcraft W, Schlenker T, Gee M, et al. Improved controlled ovarian hyperstimulation in poor responder in vitro fertilization patients with a microdose follicle-stimulating hormone flare, growth hormone protocol. Fertil Steril. 1997;67(1):93-7.
28. Padilla SL, Dugan K, Maruschak V, et al. Use of the flare-up protocol with high dose human follicle stimulating hormone and human menopausal gonadotropins for in vitro fertilization in poor responders. Fertil Steril. 1996;65(4):796-9.
29. Faber BM, Mayer J, Cox B, et al. Cessation of gonadotropin-releasing hormone agonist therapy combined with high-dose gonadotropin stimulation yields favorable pregnancy results in low responders. Fertil Steril. 1998;69(5):826-30.
30. Karande V, Gleicher N. A rational approach to the management of low responders in in-vitro fertilization. Hum Reprod. 1999;14(7):1744-8.
31. Craft I, Gorgy A, Hill J, et al. Will GnRH antagonists provide new hope for patients considered "difficult responders" to GnRH agonist protocols? Hum Reprod. 1999;14(12):2959-62.
32. Akman MA, Erden HF, Tosun SB, et al. Addition of GnRH antagonist in cycles of poor responders undergoing IVF. Hum Reprod. 2000;15(10):2145-7.
33. Demirol A, Gurgan T. Comparison of microdose flare-up and antagonist multiple-dose protocols for poor-responder patients: a randomized study. Fertil Steril. 2009;92(2):481-5.

34. Toth TL, Awwad JT, Veeck LL, et al. Suppression and flare regimens of gonadotropin-releasing hormone agonist: use in women with different basal gonadotropin values in an in vitro fertilization program. J Reprod Med. 1996;41(5):321-6.
35. Leondires MP, Escalpes M, Segars JH, et al. Microdose follicular phase gonadotropin-releasing hormone agonists (GnRH-a) compared with luteal phase GnRH-a for ovarian stimulation at in vitro fertilization. Fertil Steril. 1999;72(6):1018-23.
36. Yoshimura Y, Nakamura Y, Ando M, et al. Direct effect of gonadotropin-releasing hormone agonists on the rabbit ovarian follicle. Fertil Steril. 1992;57(5):1091-7.
37. Kowalik A, Barmat L, Damario M, et al. Ovarian estradiol production in vivo. Inhibitory effect of leuprolide acetate. J Reprod Med. 1998;43(5):413-7.
38. Kovacs P, Barg PE, Witt BR. Hypothalamic-pituitary suppression with oral contraceptive pills does not improve outcome in poor responder patients undergoing in vitro fertilization-embryo transfer cycles. J Assist Reprod Genet. 2001;18(7):391-4.
39. Duvan CI, Berker B, Turhan NO, et al. Oral contraceptive pretreatment doesnot improve outcome in microdose gonadotropin-releasing hormone agonist protocol among poor responder intracytoplasmic sperm injection patients. J Assist Reprod Genet. 2008;25(2-3):89-93.
40. Kenigsberg D, Littman BA, Hodgen GD. Medical hypophysectomy: I. Dose-response using a gonadotropin-releasing hormone antagonist. Fertil Steril. 1984;42(1):112-5.
41. Scheffer GJ, Broekmans FJ, Dorland M, et al. Antral follicle counts by transvaginal ultrasonography are related to age in women with proven natural fertility. Fertil Steril. 1999;72(5):845-51.
42. Bancsi LF, Broekmans FJ, Looman CW, et al. Predicting poor ovarian response in IVF: use of repeat basal FSH measurement. J Reprod Med. 2004;49(3):187-94.
43. van Schanke A, van de Wetering-Krebbers SF, Bos E, et al. Absorption, distribution, metabolism and excretion of corifollitropin alfa, a recombinant hormone with a sustained follicle-stimulating activity. Pharmacology. 2010;85(2):77-87.
44. Polyzos NP, Devos M, Humaidan P, et al. Corifollitropin alfa followed by rFSH in a GnRH antagonist protocol for poor ovarian responder patients: an observational pilot study. Fertil Steril. 2013;99(2):422-6.
45. Polyzos NP, De Vos M, Corona R, et al. Addition of highly purified HMG after corifollitropin alfa in antagonist-treated poor ovarian responders: a pilot study. Hum Reprod. 2013;28(5):1254-60.
46. Jovanovic VP, Kort DH, Guarnaccia MM, et al. Does the addition of clomiphene citrate or letrozole to gonadotropin treatment enhance the oocyte yield in poor responders undergoing IVF? J Assist Reprod Genet. 2011;28(11):1067-72.
47. Reynolds KA, Omurtag KR, Jimenez PT, et al. Cycle cancellation and pregnancy after luteal estradiol priming in women defined as poor responders: a systematic review and meta-analysis. Hum Reprod. 2013;28(11):2981-9.
48. Fanchin R, Salomon L, Castelo-Branco A, et al. Luteal estradiol pre-treatment coordinates follicular growth during controlled ovarian hyperstimulation with GnRH antagonists. Hum Reprod. 2003;18(12):2698-703.
49. Polyzos NP, Tournaye H. Poor ovarian responders: to meta-analyse or not, that is the question. Hum Reprod. 2014;29(3):634-5.
50. Hill MJ, Levens ED, Levy G, et al. The use of recombinant luteinizing hormone in patients undergoing assisted reproductive techniques with advanced reproductive age: a systematic review and meta-analysis. Fertil Steril. 2012;97(5):1108-14.e1.

51. Bosdou JK, Venetis CA, Kolibianakis EM, et al. The use of androgens or androgen-modulating agents in poor responders undergoing in vitro fertilization: a systematic review and meta-analysis. Hum Reprod Update. 2012;18(2):127-45.
52. Fan W, Li S, Chen Q, et al. Recombinant luteinizing hormone supplementation in poor responders undergoing IVF: a systematic review and meta-analysis. Gynecol Endocrinol. 2013;29(4):278-84.
53. Lehert P, Kolibianakis EM, Venetis CA, et al. Recombinant human follicle-stimulating hormone (r-hFSH) plus recombinant luteinizing hormone versus r-hFSH alone for ovarian stimulation during assisted reproductive technology: systematic review and meta-analysis. Reprod Biol Endocrinol. 2014;12:17.
54. Davoren JB, Kasson BG, Li CH, et al. Specific insulin-like growth factor (IGF) I- and II-binding sites on rat granulosa cells: relation to IGF action. Endocrinology. 1986;119(5):2155-62.
55. Hsu CJ, Hammond JM. Concomitant effects of growth hormone on secretion of insulin-like growth factor I and progesterone by cultured porcine granulosa cells. Endocrinology. 1987;121(4):1343-8.
56. Barreca A, Artini PG, Del Monte P, et al. In vivo and in vitro effect of growth hormone on estradiol secretion by human granulosa cells. J Clin Endocrinol Metab. 1993;77(1):61-7.
57. Adashi EY, Resnick CE, D'Ercole AJ, et al. Insulin-like growth factors as intraovarian regulators of granulosa cell growth and function. Endocr Rev. 1985;6(3):400-20.
58. Jia XC, Kalmijn J, Hsueh AJ. Growth hormone enhances follicle-stimulating hormone-induced differentiation of cultured rat granulosa cells. Endocrinology. 1986;118(4):1401-9.
59. Kyrou D, Kolibianakis EM, Venetis CA, et al. How to improve the probability of pregnancy in poor responders undergoing in vitro fertilization: a systematic review and meta-analysis. Fertil Steril. 2009;91(3):749-66.
60. Dor J, Seidman DS, Amudai E, et al. Adjuvant growth hormone therapy in poor responders to in-vitro fertilization: a prospective randomized placebo-controlled double-blind study. Hum Reprod. 1995;10(1):40–3.
61. Eftekhar M, Aflatoonian A, Mohammadian F, et al. Adjuvant growth hormone therapy in antagonist protocol in poor responders undergoing assisted reproductive technology. Arch Gynecol Obstet. 2013;287(5):1017-21.
62. Weil SJ, Vendola K, Zhou J, et al. Androgen receptor gene expression in the primate ovary: cellular localization, regulation, and functional correlations. J Clin Endocrinol Metab. 1998;83(7):2479-85.
63. Vendola KA, Zhou J, Adesanya OO, et al. Androgens stimulate early stages of follicular growth in the primate ovary. J Clin Invest. 1998;101(12):2622-9.
64. Sunkara SK, Coomarasamy A. Androgen pretreatment in poor responders undergoing controlled ovarian stimulation and in vitro fertilization treatment. Fertil Steril. 2011;95(8):e73-4.
65. Sunkara SK, Coomarasamy A, Arlt W, et al. Should androgen supplementation be used for poor ovarian response in IVF? Hum Reprod. 2012;27(3):637-40.
66. Weiner Z, Thaler I, Levron J, et al. Assessment of ovarian and uterine blood flow by transvaginal color Doppler in ovarian-stimulated women: correlation with the number of follicles and steroid hormone levels. Fertil Steril. 1993;59(4):743-9.
67. Bassil S, Wyns C, Toussaint-Demylle D, et al. The relationship between ovarian vascularity and the duration of stimulation in in-vitro fertilization. Hum Reprod. 1997;12(6):1240-5.

68. Pellicer A, Ballester MJ, Serrano MD, et al. Aetiological factors involved in the low response to gonadotrophins in infertile women with normal basal serum follicle stimulating hormone levels. Hum Reprod. 1994;9(5):806-11.
69. Battaglia C, Genazzani AD, Regnani G, et al. Perifollicular Doppler flow and follicular fluid vascular endothelial growth factor concentrations in poor responders. Fertil Steril. 2000;74(4):809-12.
70. Rubinstein M, Marazzi A, Polak de Fried E, et al. Low-dose aspirin treatment improves ovarian responsiveness, uterine and ovarian blood flow velocity, implantation, and pregnancy rates in patients undergoing in vitro fertilization: a prospective, randomized, double-blind placebo-controlled assay. Fertil Steril. 1999;71(5):825-9.
71. Nardo LG, Granne I, Stewart J, et al. Medical adjuncts in IVF: evidence for clinical practice. Hum Fertil (Camb). 2009;12(1):1-13.
72. Ubaldi FM, Rienzi L, Ferrero S, et al. Management of poor responders in IVF. Reprod Biomed Online. 2005;10(2):235-46.
73. Schimberni M, Morgia F, Colabianchi J, et al. Natural-cycle in vitro fertilization in poor responder patients: a survey of 500 consecutive cycles. Fertil Steril. 2009;92(4):1297-301.
74. Polyzos NP, Blockeel C, Verpoest W, et al. Live birth rates following natural cycle IVF in women with poor ovarian response according to the Bologna criteria. Hum Reprod. 2012;27(12):3481-6.
75. Noyes N, Porcu E, Borini A. Over 900 oocyte cryopreservation babies born with no apparent increase in congenital anomalies. Reprod Biomed Online. 2009;18(6):769-76.
76. Rienzi L, Cobo A, Paffoni A, et al. Consistent and predictable delivery rates after oocyte vitrification: an observational longitudinal cohort multicentric study. Hum Reprod. 2012;27(6):1606-12.

Chapter 6

The High Responder: Optimizing the Stimulation without Complications

Javier Martínez-Salazar Romero, Israel Ortega Sanchez, Juan Antonio García-Velasco

INTRODUCTION

Clinical practice has demonstrated that ovarian response to controlled-ovarian stimulation with gonadotropins may present a broad range of biological actions in women. In this sense, clinical and biologically consensus exists to distinguish women with normal, low and high or multifollicular response, although there is no generally accepted definition for these different types of response.

One might think that a high ovarian response is desirable for in vitro fertilization (IVF), since it would provide multiple oocytes and embryos for subsequent embryo development, leading to a better selection of good-quality embryos for transfer and thus, improving reproductive outcomes. However, it has been shown that an excessive ovarian response to gonadotropins might exert a deleterious effect on endometrial receptivity and thus, on reproductive outcomes.[1] On the other hand, the problem of an excessive high response is mainly related to the administration of high doses of gonadotropins. However, this is partly true, since it has been shown that patient´s individual characteristics might account for a high ovarian response, regardless of the gonadotropin dose. This is especially relevant in patients with multifollicular ovaries or diagnosed with a polycystic ovary syndrome (PCOS).

The narrow threshold of the ovarian response to ovarian stimulation in PCOS patients is known, and the boundary between the minimum effective dose of gonadotropins and the ones inducing excessive follicular development is so narrow that small dose modifications might induce high ovarian response and clinical complications, being ovarian hyperstimulation syndrome (OHSS) the most relevant one.

In order to improve the prediction and management of these complications, better diagnostic criteria have been established to better identify these patients and predict their ovarian response. Moreover, the incorporation of new therapeutic strategies, such as the use of GnRH antagonist protocols and the clinical application of oocyte/embryo vitrification in current routine practice have dramatically decrease the incidence of OHSS, without compromising the reproductive outcomes.

DEFINITION AND IDENTIFICATION OF HIGH RESPONDERS

Since the beginning of assisted reproduction it has been known the negative consequences and risks to which the high responder patients are exposed. Although, it has not been possible to reach a consensus on its definition. Over the past decade, several clinical criteria based on the number of follicles and serum estradiol levels obtained on the day of oocyte maturation have been proposed. Although a standard definition for high ovarian response is lacking, the clinical community has proposed that the following features must be present to define high ovarian response: more than 20 follicles in the final phase of stimulation, serum estradiol levels greater than 3,000 pg/mL and more than 15 oocytes obtained after oocyte retrieval.

Classically, the presence of risk factors such as age, body mass index, or the presence of polycystic ovaries have been used as good predictors of high ovarian response. According to the meta-analysis published by Broer et al.[2] these clinical markers together with the evaluation of the antral follicle count (AFC) by vaginal ultrasound, defined as the total number of follicles 2–10 mm in diameter at the beginning of the menstrual cycle, and determination of serum anti-Müllerian hormone (AMH) levels, are the best clinical markers to predict a high ovarian response in IVF with high sensitivity and specificity.

One of the most important advantages associated with the evaluation of AFC at the beginning of ovarian stimulation is that it presents limited intercycle variability, allowing a more accurate gonadotropin dose adjustment prior to the onset of ovarian stimulation. It has been proposed that an AFC more than 14 follicles per ovary might be a good predictor of high ovarian response, leading to a potential risk of developing OHSS.

Anti-Müllerian hormone is expressed in the granulosa cells of preantral and small antral follicles and is an excellent marker of ovarian reserve. Furthermore, it presents a low inter- and intracycle variability, allowing its evaluation at any time of the menstrual cycle. Evaluation of serum AMH levels prior to the onset of ovarian stimulation is a good predictor of ovarian response, allowing physicians to customize the stimulation protocol according to patient's individual characteristics. However, there is a lack of consensus on the cutt-off value of serum AMH level to define a high ovarian response. Based on our data, AMH levels less than 3 ng/mL (1 ng/mL = 7.14 pmol/L) might predict a high ovarian response, whereas levels greater than 7 ng/mL might predict a potential risk of developing OHSS.

Finally, the presence of more than 20 follicles greater than 14 mm at the end of the stimulation and/or serum estradiol levels greater than 3,000 pg/mL at the time of inducing oocyte maturation, are good predictors of high ovarian response, being useful to suspect a high risk of OHSS. However, the role of serum estradiol determination as a predictor of high ovarian response has recently been questioned.

CONSEQUENCES AND RISKS OF HIGH RESPONDERS

Ovarian Hyperstimulation Syndrome

The OHSS is the most important clinical complication in patients undergoing IVF, leading to potentially life-threatening situations, characterized by the presence of prolonged and persistent ovarian growth and accumulation of fluid in the serous cavities. It has been shown that the development of OHSS is directly related to the use of human chorionic gonadotropin (hCG) for triggering ovulation, which increases production of serum vascular endothelial growth factor and other mediators, such as ovarian renin-angiotensin system, interleukin-1 and interleukin-6, leading to increased vascular permeability.

Clinically, patients developing OHSS may present a broad range of clinical manifestations, including abdominal distension and pain, nausea and vomiting, oliguria and edema in the lower limbs. Regarding to laboratory abnormalities, the development of OHSS may be characterized by the presence of increased hematocrit (>45%), leukocytosis (>15,000/mm^3), electrolyte disturbances (hyponatremia and hyperkalemia), increased liver enzymes, hypoalbuminemia and decreased creatinine clearance.

Although the evolution of OHSS is closely related to the levels of hCG, the underlying mechanisms of hCG clearance are still poorly characterized. Nowadays, OHSS can be classified into two forms:

1. *Early OHSS*: It appears between 3–7 days after hCG administration and is related with the exogenous hCG administration. It usually disappears within 10–14 days in the absence of pregnancy.
2. *Late OHSS*: It appears 10 days post-hCG administration and is related to the presence of gestation and endogenous production of trophoblastic hCG, which prolongs or aggravates the symptoms of the syndrome.

Oocyte and Embryo Quality

Currently, there is a controversy regarding oocyte and embryo quality in high responder patients, since a large number of immature oocytes and lower pregnancy rates together with higher miscarriage rates have been observed in these patients compared to normoresponders. Furthermore, patients diagnosed with PCOS should be differentiated from those non-PCOS high responder patients, since the presence of metabolic disturbances such as hyperandrogenism, low-grade inflammation, insulin resistance and obesity that might impair oocyte quality, leading to poorer reproductive outcomes.

There is growing evidence showing that hyperinsulinemia secondary to insulin resistance, might have a detrimental effect on oocyte quality, accounting for the lower implantation and pregnancy rates observed in these patients. This hyperinsulinemia-induced deleterious effect on oocyte quality has also been observed in PCOS fertile women donating their oocytes in an egg donation program.[3] Thus, the poorer reproductive outcomes observed in patients with hyperinsulinemia seem to be related with an impairment of oocyte quality, and not with the endometrial receptivity.

The presence of high rates of immature oocytes observed in most of high responder patients may be due to an alteration in the maturation of intermediate follicles, emerging as a potential cause of higher miscarriage rates in this case. Previously, it has been shown that there is an inverse relationship between the quality and the number of oocytes retrieved.[4] However, despite the presence of low oocyte quality and maturity that leads to lower fertilization rates, pregnancy rates are not necessarily impaired as embryo quality may not be affected.

Previously, it has been suggested that in high responder donors the aneuploidy rate for day 3 embryos rises up to 56.6%, after obtaining an average number of 25.9 oocytes.[5] However, it is not yet clear whether this increase in aneuploidy rate is due to the patient's characteristics or might be secondary to ovarian stimulation protocols. The abovementioned aneuploidy rate in high responder patients is in sharp contrast with the one observed in normoresponder patients (37.3%) and those undergoing moderate ovarian stimulations.[6] Taking these results into account, we may conclude that these patients present a high incidence of embryo aneuploidy due to high response to gonadotropin stimulation. Interestingly, Munne et al.[7] have demonstrated that normal donors present more than 50% of aneuploid embryos when tested by techniques of comparative genomic hybridization (CGH), and it has been suggested that the aneuploidy rate could be even greater in young donors.[8]

Currently, there is growing evidence demonstrating that embryo aneuploidy is closely related to the gonadotropin dose used in controlled ovarian stimulation. Our group conducted a crossover study[9] to evaluate the aneuploidy rate from embryos originated from donors with a previous cycle of high ovarian response. All donors underwent two cycles of ovarian stimulation with a GnRH-antagonist protocol, separated by at least 3 months. In the first cycle, ovarian stimulation was started with initial doses of recombinant FSH(rFSH) of 225 IU/day, being subsequently adjusted according to serum estradiol levels on day 5 of ovarian stimulation. However in the second cycle, a fixed rFSH dose of 150 IU/day was administered regardless of high estradiol levels on day 5 of stimulation. Out of the 32 donors initially included in the study, 10 had to be cancelled ovarian stimulation in the second cycle due to insufficient response. These results confirm a significant increase in fertilization rates and the number of chromosomally normal blastocysts in high responder donors receiving low doses of gonadotropins in the second cycle, although the live birth rates were similar in both stimulation protocols, since the higher number of oocytes and embryos counterbalanced the decline in egg quality.[6]

Endometrial Receptivity

Over the past decade, our group has demonstrated that high responder patients with elevated serum estradiol levels present impaired endometrial receptivity,[1] being eligible for embryo freezing to perform frozen-thawed embryo transfer in a subsequent cycle. Before the introduction of oocyte/embryo vitrification in the routine clinical practice, the use of the slow freezing protocol in cases of high ovarian response avoided the incidence of OHSS. However, this cryopreservation technique was associated with low survival rates and poor reproductive outcomes.

Recently, several studies have shown that high responder patients exhibits increased serum progesterone levels during ovarian stimulation. Classically, this finding has been associated with the occurrence of premature luteinizing hormone (LH) surge during ovarian stimulation, but some studies indicate that this increase in progesterone levels is linked to excessive exposure to FSH during the follicular phase,[10] which induces paracrine changes leading to increased progesterone production in the late follicular phase. The presence of a high number of follicles and proliferation of granulosa cells leads to a higher progesterone concentrations in patients with high estrogen levels on the day of hCG,[11] suggesting that high response is frequently associated with elevated serum progesterone levels.

The consequences of such a progesterone increase during ovarian stimulation have been controversial. Several authors have suggested that elevated progesterone levels might exert a deleterious effect on IVF outcomes,[12] however such an association has not been confirmed by others.[13] The presence of high progesterone concentrations induces secretory changes in the endometrium and premature acceleration of endometrial maturation that might alter the window of implantation, impairing the clinical outcomes. In a recent study evaluating the cut-off of serum progesterone levels on the day of hCG in IVF patients, our group demonstrated that values greater than 1.5 ng/mL were associated with a significant decrease in pregnancy rates (31% vs 19%).[14] Recently, a retrospective study published by our group evaluated the effect of serum progesterone levels on the day of hCG on clinical outcomes in 2,500 high responder patients, showing no differences in either implantation or pregnancy rates. However, there was a trend to lower implantation rates when progesterone levels were greater than 1.8 ng/mL. These findings might be due to the fact that high responder patients present fast developing embryos, that might be synchronized with an advanced endometrium, presenting optimal implantation and pregnancy rates. It should be noted that this study was finished in 2011, when embryo vitrification and the use of GnRH antagonist protocols were fully established in routine clinical practice.[15] A recent meta-analysis supports this hypothesis; however, it should be viewed with caution due to the presence of selection bias in the included studies.[11] Regardless of whether clinical outcomes are affected or not, these patients should be recommended to vitrify their oocytes/embryos and postpone embryo transfer, due to the high risk of developing OHSS.

STIMULATION PROTOCOL IN HIGH RESPONDERS

For several years, the use of GnRH agonist, either long or short protocol, has been the gold standard in ART to inhibit pituitary gonadotropin secretion, inhibiting the appearance of a premature LH surge. However, it requires the use of hCG for oocyte maturation induction, increasing the risk of high responder patients to develop OHSS. To overcome this, several strategies have been developed over the past decade:

- Use of low doses of gonadotropins, which is associated with a potential risk of cycle cancellation due to absence of ovarian response
- Use of half the dose of hCG to induce final oocyte maturation
- Coasting, which involves delaying hCG administration, while maintaining administration of GnRH analoges until estrogen levels drop to "safe" values
- Embryo freezing, postponing frozen-thawed embryo transfer to a subsequent cycle. In the past, the slow freezing protocol yielded poorer reproductive outcomes compared to vitrification technique
- Cycle cancellation, avoiding hCG administration. This strategy is associated with psychological burden and financial implications for the patient.

The introduction of GnRH antagonists in stimulation protocols together with the incorporation of vitrification techniques in IVF laboratories represent one of the biggest breakthroughs in the management of these patients.

As previously discussed, both AMH levels and RFA allow us to predict high ovarian response in patients undergoing IVF using either GnRH agonists[2] or antagonist[16] protocols. It should be noted that GnRH antagonist protocol effectively suppresses endogenous LH secretion, while reducing the duration of ovarian stimulation and the dose of gonadotropins, leading to a reduction of complexity and cycle costs for the patient. Thus, the use of GnRH antagonist emerges as a safer approach to treat patients at risk of developing a high ovarian response compared to the GnRH agonist protocol, while maintaining similar ongoing and live birth rates.[17] Furthermore, the use of GnRH antagonist allows us to perform the induction of oocyte maturation with GnRH agonist, preventing the occurrence of early onset OHSS related to hCG administration. Taken together, the GnRH antagonist protocol represents nowadays the gold standard for those IVF patients at risk of developing a high ovarian response.

Taking into account the negative implications of high ovarian response, such as the high number of follicles, elevated serum estrogen and progesterone levels during ovarian stimulation, one might think that using half the dose of gonadotropins (150 IU of rFSH) with subsequent dose adjustment according to estradiol levels on day 3 of ovarian stimulation, might represent a valid strategy for these patients. Regarding the type of gonadotropin, several studies have demonstrated that there are not significant differences in clinical outcomes when comparing the use of both the urinary and recombinant gonadotropins.[18] However, the fact that most of these patients at risk of high ovarian response present PCOS with elevated basal LH levels, has led physicians to use rFSH, avoiding the effect of LH of urinary gonadotropins. However, further studies are necessary to establish the best gonadotropin protocol to be used in these patients.

In PCOS patients diagnosed with insulin resistance and hyperinsulinemia, the use of adjuvant therapies targeting glucose metabolism such as metformin, might improve oocyte hormonal environment and thus, improve oocyte quality.[19] Thus, according to current evidence, the use of metformin in association with gonadotropins is recommended in PCOS patients with impaired glucose tolerance.[20]

GnRH ANALOGS, OOCYTE MATURATION AND ITS CONSEQUENCES

It has been known for years that administration of a bolus of GnRH agonist at the end of ovarian stimulation induces trigger of oocyte maturation and reduces the incidence of OHSS.[21] However, this approach is not a valid strategy for those women undergoing a GnRH agonist long protocol. With the emergence of GnRH antagonists, the use of GnRH agonist as an agent to trigger ovulation has gained in importance,[22] being a dose of 0.2 mg of triptorelin acetate the optimal dose to yield a normal oocyte retrieval and produce good quality embryos. However, this approach was associated with some drawbacks, including high miscarriage rates and low ongoing pregnancy rates, secondary to a profound luteal phase insufficiency refractory to conventional luteal phase support protocols.

The underlying mechanism of such a profound luteal phase insufficiency after GnRH agonist administration is the inhibition of gonadotropin secretion, mainly LH, after initial flare-up. Humaidan et al.[22] confirmed that LH levels in the luteal phase when administering GnRH agonist to trigger ovulation were lower than in those patients who received hCG. However, hCG-induced luteotropic effect is enough to sustain the luteal phase, while low LH levels after GnRH agonist administration were not enough to maintain proper luteal phase.

Strategies in High Responders at Risk of OHSS

Given this background, there was an urgent need to establish new strategies in high responder patients at risk of OHSS after triggering oocyte maturation with GnRH agonist, aimed to avoid luteal phase insufficiency and unacceptable clinical outcomes.

To overcome this, over the past decade several alternatives have been suggested, including embryo freezing and subsequent embryo transfer at a later stage (also called "cycle segmentation"), or rescuing the insufficient luteal phase to allow fresh embryo transfer.

Freezing of all Oocytes/Embryos: Cycle Segmentation

This approach was already known at the time when hCG was administered to induce oocyte maturation in a GnRH antagonist protocol when the patients were at high risk of OHSS. By that time, the technique of oocyte freezing was not yet available and the slow freezing protocol offered limited results, but it was an alternative to avoid the risk of developing a severe OHSS.

Vitrification technique involves ultra-fast freezing, small volume and high concentration of cryoprotectants, and allows cryopreservation of both oocytes and embryos, yielding excellent survival rates of about 95%. Moreover, there are not significant differences in terms of clinical outcomes when comparing fresh embryo transfer with vitrified embryo transfer after thawing.[23] These optimal results together with its efficiency and safety have led the cryopreservation programs to become a crucial part in the routine practice in IVF laboratories.[24]

Embryo vitrification allows physicians to perform the frozen-thawed embryo transfer in a subsequent cycle with excellent clinical outcomes, either in a natural cycle or following hormonal replacement therapy.[25] Indeed, some studies have reported an improvement in obstetric and perinatal outcomes when using vitrified embryos compared to those obtained in the fresh cycle.[26]

The policy of cycle segmentation avoids the occurrence of severe late onset OHSS. In 2014, in IVI-Madrid there was only one case of early OHSS and 4 cases of late OHSS out of a total of 1,789 IVF cycles. Despite the use of vitrification, there is still a potential risk of developing an early OHSS, due to individual biological variability.[27]

It is still controversial whether high responder patients should freeze their oocytes or embryos. Oocyte vitrification has the advantage of limiting the number of surplus embryos, which might be beneficial not only for patients who have moral conflicts to generate supernumerary embryos, but also for embryologists, since the number of cryopreserved embryos decreases.

To clarify this issue, our group conducted a study[28] aimed to evaluate the pregnancy outcomes of 96 high responder patients after oocyte or embryo vitrification. All the patients followed a GnRH antagonist protocol with subsequent trigger with GnRH agonist, being randomized into two different groups: Group 1, oocyte vitrification was performed and ICSI was postponed in a subsequent cycle; Group 2, embryo vitrification was performed after ICSI, being thawed and transferred in a subsequent cycle. Baseline clinical characteristics were comparable between both groups.

Regarding the laboratory outcomes, there were no differences in either the number of retrieved oocytes or the maturation rate. Interestingly, a higher number of fertilized oocytes was observed in group 2 versus group 1 (14.8 vs 10.7), as well as a higher number of transferable embryos in group 2 (6.4 ± 4.2) compared to group 1 (4.3 ± 2.7). However, no differences in either fertilization rate (68.3% vs 73.3%) or in the transferable embryo rate (27.9% vs 31.3%) were reported.

After the first embryo transfer, no significant differences in implantation, biochemical or clinical pregnancy rates (44% in group 1 vs 50% in group 2) were observed. However, a significant increase in the miscarriage rate was observed in group 2 versus group 1 (30.4% vs 4.5%). Interestingly, there were no cases of OHSS in both groups.

Embryo survival rates were similar in both groups (group 1, 87.5% and 89.4% in group 2). However, the oocyte survival rate in group 1 was 78.8%, slightly lower than the one published by our group,[23] possibly due to bad oocyte quality in these patients. This might be the cause of the difference in the number of transferable embryos in group 1, secondary to a lower number of mature oocytes for ICSI.

After three embryo transfers, clinical outcomes remained similar between groups, with live birth rates of 72% in group 1 compared to 69.6% in group 2. However, it should be noted that miscarriage rate remained higher in group 2 compared to group 1, 21.9% versus 9.7%, respectively. This finding is difficult to justify and, ruling out the potential deleterious effect of vitrification on cryopreserved embryos, the only plausible justification is that oocyte vitrification in group 1 might act as a filter of quality, while in Group 2 the oocytes generate embryos with limited evolutionary potential, commonly associated with pregnancy loss.

In view of these considerations, oocyte freezing should be recommended to these patients since it offers similar clinical results compared to embryo freezing, avoiding legal and ethical concerns of generating surplus cryopreserved embryos. Moreover, oocyte vitrification also allows to better determine the number of oocytes to be fertilized, depending on patient's characteristics. Those couples interested in limiting the number of embryos, due to medical or ethical reasons, single women or presence of chronic diseases, would be eligible for oocyte vitrification, whereas those couples interested in having more children would be eligible for embryo freezing.

Luteal Phase Rescue

Given the luteal phase insufficiency after triggering oocyte maturation with GnRH agonist, some authors have suggested new strategies to perform fresh embryo transfer in the same cycle, avoiding the use of vitrification (Table 6.1). Among them, the most important approach to rescue the luteal phase in high responder patients is focused on administration of low doses

Table 6.1: Strategies in high ovarian response. Final oocyte maturation with GnRHa.

GnRH agonist	*Day of oocyte retrieval*	*Oocyte/ embryo vitrification*	*Luteal phase support*	*Reference*
Yes	–	Yes	No	García-Velasco et al.[25]
Yes	1,500 IU hCG	No	6 mg oral estradiol + 600 mg of vaginal progesterone starting after ovarian retrieval	Humaidan et al.[29]
Yes	1,500 IU hCG	No	1500 IU hCG every 4 days starting on the day of oocyte retrieval	Kol et al.[30]
Yes	500 IU hCG	No	500 IU hCG every 3 days starting on the day of oocyte retrieval	Castillo et al.[31]
+hCG (<33 IU/kg) Dual triggering	–	No	6 mg oral estradiol + 800 mg vaginal progesterone	Shapiro et al.[32]
Yes	–	No	50 mg IM progesterone daily + 0.3 mg transdermic estradiol/day starting on the day oocyte retrieval	Engmann et al.[33]

of hCG, using 1,500 IU of hCG on the day of oocyte retrieval together with a conventional luteal phase support with progesterone and estradiol.[29] According to the current evidence, this protocol offers good pregnancy rates and low miscarriage rates, decreasing the number of cases of OHSS.[34] However, it has been shown that those patients with a high number of oocyte retrieval might develop an early OHSS due to hCG administration. Moreover, this strategy might be associated with a high risk of late OHSS in case a pregnancy occurs. Thus, this strategy should be viewed with caution when used in high responder patients, due to the potential risk of both and early and late OHSS.[35]

It has been proposed progesterone-free luteal phase support, using two subcutaneous bolus of 1,500 IU hCG separated by 4 days starting on the day of oocyte retrieval. However, this clinical approach seems to be more appropriate in cases of mild high ovarian response, since administration of hCG, even at low doses, might considerably increase the risk of these patients to develop OHSS.[30]

The administration of low doses of customized hCG (<33 IU/kg) and GnRH agonist on the day of oocyte triggering (dual triggering), together with luteal phase support based on 6 mg orally administered estradiol and 800 mg vaginal progesterone, have been associated with optimal clinical results and low incidence of OHSS.[32] However, further studies are need to better evaluate the effectiveness of this approach before being integrated in the routine clinical practice.

It had been evaluated the potential beneficial effect of combined administration of high doses of progesterone in combination with transdermic estradiol as luteal phase support, achieving clinical pregnancy rates of up to 53% without the appearance of OHSS.[30,33,36,37]

CONCLUSION

Despite current knowledge about etiology and physiopathology of high ovarian response, the management of patients undergoing IVF at high risk of developing OHSS still represents a challenge for physicians. The use of GnRH antagonist protocol with low doses of rFSH (100–150 IU/day) represents the gold standard in the management of patients with high ovarian response. In cases of an excessive ovarian response (>15 mature follicles on the day of oocyte maturation), administration of GnRH agonist to trigger final oocyte maturation together with oocyte vitrification avoids the development of both the early and late OHSS. Luteal phase rescue with hCG at low doses with or without steroids may represent an alternative for those women who want to undergo a fresh embryo transfer in the same cycle. In these cases, single embryo transfer should be recommended and the patient should be informed about the risk of developing late OHSS. However, it still remains unknown the best approach to rescue the luteal phase in those women receiving fresh embryo transfer after GnRH agonist trigger, as well as the patient profile that might benefit from this strategy.

REFERENCES

1. Simon C, Cano F, Valbuena D, et al. Clinical evidence for a detrimental effect on uterine receptivity of high serum oestradiol concentrations in high and normal responder patients. Hum Reprod. 1995;10(9):2432-7.
2. Broer SL, Dolleman M, Opmeer BC, et al. AMH and AFC as predictors of excessive response in controlled ovarian hyperstimulation: a meta-analysis. Hum Reprod Update. 2011;17(1):46-54.
3. Cano F, Garcia-Velasco JA, Millet A, et al. Oocyte quality in polycystic ovaries revisited: identification of a particular subgroup of women. J Assist Reprod Genet. 1997;14(5):254-61.
4. Giles J, Requena A, Garcia-Velasco JA, et al. GnRH analogue for the prevention of ovarian hyperstimulation syndrome: a pilot study. Fertil Steril. 2009;91(4 Suppl):1366-9.
5. Reis Soares S, Rubio C, Rodrigo L, et al. High frequency of chromosomal abnormalities in embryos obtained from oocyte donation cycles. Fertil Steril. 2003;80(3):656-7.
6. Labarta E, Bosch E, Alama P, et al. Moderate ovarian stimulation does not increase the incidence of human embryo chromosomal abnormalities in in vitro fertilization cycles. J Clin Endocrinol Metab. 2012;97(10):E1987-94.
7. Munne S, Ary J, Zouves C, et al. Wide range of chromosome abnormalities in the embryos of young egg donors. Reprod Biomed Online. 2006;12(3):340-6.
8. Keskintepe L, Sher G, Keskintepe M. Reproductive oocyte/embryo genetic analysis: comparison between fluorescence in-situ hybridization and comparative genomic hybridization. Reprod Biomed Online. 2007;15(3):303-9.

9. Rubio C, Mercader A, Alama P, et al. Prospective cohort study in high responder oocyte donors using two hormonal stimulation protocols: impact on embryo aneuploidy and development. Hum Reprod. 2010;25(9):2290-7.
10. Hofmann GE, Bentzien F, Bergh PA, et al. Premature luteinization in controlled ovarian hyperstimulation has no adverse effect on oocyte and embryo quality. Fertil Steril. 1993;60(4):675-9.
11. Griesinger G, Mannaerts B, Andersen CY, et al. Progesterone elevation does not compromise pregnancy rates in high responders: a pooled analysis of in vitro fertilization patients treated with recombinant follicle-stimulating hormone/gonadotropin-releasing hormone antagonist in six trials. Fertil Steril. 2013;100(6):1622-8. e1-3.
12. Bosch E, Valencia I, Escudero E, et al. Premature luteinization during gonadotropin-releasing hormone antagonist cycles and its relationship with in vitro fertilization outcome. Fertil Sterility. 2003;80(6):1444-9.
13. Yding Andersen C, Bungum L, Nyboe Andersen A, et al. Preovulatory progesterone concentration associates significantly to follicle number and LH concentration but not to pregnancy rate. Reprod Biomed Online. 2011;23(2):187-95.
14. Bosch E, Labarta E, Crespo J, et al. Circulating progesterone levels and ongoing pregnancy rates in controlled ovarian stimulation cycles for in vitro fertilization: analysis of over 4000 cycles. Hum Reprod. 2010;25(8):2092-100.
15. Requena A, Cruz M, Bosch E, et al. High progesterone levels in women with high ovarian response do not affect clinical outcomes: a retrospective cohort study. Reprod Biol Endocrinol. 2014;12:69.
16. Hamdine O, Eijkemans MJ, Lentjes EW, et al. Ovarian response prediction in GnRH antagonist treatment for IVF using anti-Müllerian hormone. Hum Reprod. 2015;30(1):170-8.
17. Al-Inany HG, Youssef MA, Aboulghar M, et al. Gonadotrophin-releasing hormone antagonists for assisted reproductive technology. Cochrane Database Syst Rev. 2011(5):CD001750.
18. Aboulghar M, Saber W, Amin Y, et al. Prospective, randomized study comparing highly purified urinary follicle-stimulating hormone (FSH) and recombinant FSH for in vitro fertilization/intracytoplasmic sperm injection in patients with polycystic ovary syndrome. Fertil Sterility. 2010;94(6):2332-4.
19. Legro RS. Metformin as adjuvant therapy to IVF in women with PCOS: when is intention-to-treat unintentional? Hum Reprod. 2011;26(8):2043-4.
20. Thessaloniki ESHRE/ASRM-Sponsored PCOS Consensus Workshop Group. Consensus on infertility treatment related to polycystic ovary syndrome. Hum Reprod. 2008;23(3):462-77.
21. Itskovitz-Eldor J, Kol S, Mannaerts B, et al. First established pregnancy after controlled ovarian hyperstimulation with recombinant follicle stimulating hormone and the gonadotrophin-releasing hormone antagonist ganirelix (Org 37462). Hum Reprod. 1998;13(2):294-5.
22. Humaidan P, Bredkjaer HE, Bungum L, et al. GnRH agonist (buserelin) or hCG for ovulation induction in GnRH antagonist IVF/ICSI cycles: a prospective randomized study. Hum Reprod. 2005;20(5):1213-20.
23. Cobo A, de los Santos MJ, Castello D, et al. Outcomes of vitrified early cleavage-stage and blastocyst-stage embryos in a cryopreservation program: evaluation of 3,150 warming cycles. Fertil Steril. 2012;98(5):1138-46 e1.
24. Mukaida T, Oka C. Vitrification of oocytes, embryos and blastocysts. Best Pract Res Clin Obstet Gynaecol. 2012;26(6):789-803.

25. Garcia-Velasco JA. Agonist trigger: what is the best approach? Agonist trigger with vitrification of oocytes or embryos. Fertil Steril. 2012;97(3):527-8.
26. Maheshwari A, Pandey S, Shetty A, et al. Obstetric and perinatal outcomes in singleton pregnancies resulting from the transfer of frozen thawed versus fresh embryos generated through in vitro fertilization treatment: a systematic review and meta-analysis. Fertil Steril. 2012;98(2):368-77. e1-9.
27. Fatemi HM, Popovic-Todorovic B, Humaidan P, et al. Severe ovarian hyperstimulation syndrome after gonadotropin-releasing hormone (GnRH) agonist trigger and "freeze-all" approach in GnRH antagonist protocol. Fertil Steril. 2014;101(4):1008-11.
28. Herrero L, Pareja S, Aragones M, et al. Oocyte versus embryo vitrification for delayed embryo transfer: an observational study. Reprod Biomed Online. 2014;29(5):567-72.
29. Humaidan P, Polyzos NP, Alsbjerg B, et al. GnRHa trigger and individualized luteal phase hCG support according to ovarian response to stimulation: two prospective randomized controlled multi-centre studies in IVF patients. Hum Reprod. 2013;28(9):2511-21.
30. Kol S, Humaidan P, Itskovitz-Eldor J. GnRH agonist ovulation trigger and hCG-based, progesterone-free luteal support: a proof of concept study. Hum Reprod. 2011;26(10):2874-7.
31. Castillo JC, Dolz M, Bienvenido E, et al. Cycles triggered with GnRH agonist: exploring low-dose HCG for luteal support. Reprod Biomed Online. 2010;20(2):175-81.
32. Shapiro BS, Daneshmand ST, Garner FC, et al. Comparison of "triggers" using leuprolide acetate alone or in combination with low-dose human chorionic gonadotropin. Fertil Steril. 2011;95(8):2715-7.
33. Engmann L, DiLuigi A, Schmidt D, et al. The effect of luteal phase vaginal estradiol supplementation on the success of in vitro fertilization treatment: a prospective randomized study. Fertil Steril. 2008;89(3):554-61.
34. Radesic B, Tremellen K. Oocyte maturation employing a GnRH agonist in combination with low-dose hCG luteal rescue minimizes the severity of ovarian hyperstimulation syndrome while maintaining excellent pregnancy rates. Hum Reprod. 2011;26(12):3437-42.
35. Seyhan A, Ata B, Polat M, et al. Severe early ovarian hyperstimulation syndrome following GnRH agonist trigger with the addition of 1500 IU hCG. Hum Reprod. 2013;28(9):2522-8.
36. Griffin D, Benadiva C, Kummer N, et al. Dual trigger of oocyte maturation with gonadotropin-releasing hormone agonist and low-dose human chorionic gonadotropin to optimize live birth rates in high responders. Fertil Steril. 2012;97(6):1316-20.
37. Orvieto R. Intensive luteal-phase support with oestradiol and progesterone after GnRH-agonist triggering: does it help? Reprod Biomed Online. 2012;24(6):680-1.

Chapter 7

Ovulation Trigger

Carlos Dosouto Capel, Haahr T, Peter Humaidan

INTRODUCTION

Ovulation trigger (OT) in assisted reproductive technology (ART) is a key factor for success, and OT agents aim at mimicking the final oocyte maturation of the natural cycle which is induced by the mid-cycle surge of gonadotropins [luteinizing hormone (LH) and follicle-stimulating hormone (FSH)]. However, stimulated in vitro fertilization (IVF) cycles are significantly different from the natural cycle due to the multifollicular development, supraphysiological follicular and luteal phase steroid level, and altered hypothalamic response due to either use of gonadotropin-releasing hormone (GnRH) analogs or to the supraphysiological steroid levels. A profound knowledge about pharmacokinetics and pharmacodynamics of all these agents enable fertility specialists to individualize OT to secure the correct timing of the oocyte retrieval as well as the most optimal luteal phase support (LPS).

The initial major OT agent used in ART as a surrogate of the natural mid-cycle LH surge was human chorionic gonadotropin (hCG) due to its molecular similarity with LH and, thus, its affinity for the luteinizing hormone/choriogonadotropin receptor (LHCG-R). hCG is an excellent OT agent, seen from data on pregnancy outcomes in IVF cycles in which either fresh or frozen embryo transfer (ET) was performed. However, the major disadvantage of hCG relates to the pharmacological characteristics which in some patients—mainly high responder patients—induces a high risk of ovarian hyperstimulation syndrome (OHSS). OHSS remains a potential cause of death in women undergoing ART and the OHSS incidence ranges from 0.18% to 1.40%,[1] albeit it is well-established that OHSS is grossly under-reported.[2] The condition is characterized by massive enlargement of the ovaries and the presence of ascites due to increased vascular permeability as a result of an hCG mediated up-regulation of vascular mediators.[3] OHSS occurs almost exclusively in the presence of prolonged LH activity which is seen after hCG trigger.[3,4] Furthermore, the severity of OHSS is proportional to the dose of hCG administered and the amount of follicles and corpora lutea (CL) obtained after ovarian stimulation, respectively.

During recent years, the gold standard hCG trigger for final oocyte maturation in IVF/ICSI (intracytoplasmic sperm injection) cycles has been challenged as first-line treatment with the introduction of the gonadotropin-releasing hormone agonist (GnRHa) trigger, which has been proven to almost eliminate the risk of OHSS.[5]

The most optimal strategy to prevent OHSS is the identification of high-risk patients before or during ovarian stimulation in order to modify the stimulation regimen accordingly, and subsequently plan the trigger agent, either hCG or GnRHa. Both trigger agents allow either a fresh transfer or a freeze all policy (segmentation); however, only GnRHa trigger and segmentation will result in the virtually "OHSS free clinic".[6] Until now, the majority of fertility clinics plan segmentation for subgroups of patients, predominantly OHSS high-risk patients, and consequently the vast majority of IVF patients still undergo fresh ET after hCG trigger. However, patients with 15 or more preovulatory follicles less than or equal to 11 mm run a significantly higher risk of developing OHSS after hCG trigger than patient with fewer follicles;[7] thus, it is important to take the number of preovulatory follicles into account when the trigger agent (hCG or GnRHa) and the subsequent handling of the luteal phase is determined.

NATURAL OVULATORY CYCLE

At the end of every nonconception cycle an involution of the corpus luteum occurs, followed by a significant drop in the ovarian luteal steroid levels. The drop has a positive feedback effect at the level of the GnRH hypothalamic pulse generator which induces an early follicular raise in FSH levels. This phenomenon is the basis for the complex recruitment process of a new follicular cohort, which eventually ends up with monofollicular growth. The raise in estradiol (E) secreted by the leading follicle at a certain threshold induces a positive pituitary feedback, resulting in a mid-cycle surge of LH, and to a lesser degree FSH. This surge of gonadotropins triggers the resumption of meiosis, ovulation, and luteinization. Although the LH activity is crucial for final oocyte maturation, FSH also plays a role for oocyte maturation and, moreover, induces LH receptor formation in the luteinizing granulosa-theca cells which secures the function of the future corpus luteum.[3,8] Activation of the ovulatory cascade and luteinization of granulosa and theca cells do not occur as a result of the duration of the mid-cycle surge of gonadotropins, but rather the intensity of the signal (i.e. magnitude of increase in cAMP).[9] The secretion of both gonadotropins in a natural cycle is characterized by a three phased curve with a total duration of approximately 48 hours.[10] From the time of luteinization, the CL among other substances releases steroid hormones like progesterone (P) and E, and the function of the CL is entirely dependent on the pulsatile LH secretion from the pituitary.[8,11] However, LH also plays an important role during the luteal phase by upregulating cytokines and growth factors such as fibroblast growth factor 2 (FGF2), vascular endothelial growth factor A (VEGFA) and activating endometrial LH receptors—all factors which support implantation and early neovascularization.[3,8]

The functional life span of the CL in a non-conception cycle is usually 14 ± 2 days. During this time the CL produces 25-50 mg of P daily and its activity drops if no implantation has occurred.[12] However, in a conception cycle after implantation, which occurs approximately 7 days after ovulation, the trophoblast gradually begins to secrete hCG, which binds to and activates the same receptor as LH, the LHCG-R, securing an optimal CL function until approximately the 7th week of gestation at the so called luteo-placental shift.[12] The steroid production, of mainly P during the mid-luteal phase is mandatory to induce endometrial gland secretory transformation, prevent uterine contractions and enhance implantation. P deficiency at this point leads to early pregnancy loss (EPL).[5,8]

TRIGGERING AGENTS

Human Chorionic Gonadotropin

Human chorionic gonadotropin is a dimeric glycoprotein which shares the alpha subunit with FSH, LH and thyroid-stimulating hormone. The beta subunit is unique and confers specificity for the receptor. Moreover, the glycosylation degree of each hormone is variable and determines the receptor binding affinity and circulating half-life.[13] There is considerable structural homology between hCG and human LH and both hormones stimulate the same receptor—the LHCG-R.[13] For more than 30 years hCG extracted from the urine of pregnant women has proven to be useful for OT.[14] Urinary preparations, however, have some disadvantages, first and foremost uncontrolled source and low purity.[15] In recent years, recombinant human chorionic gonadotropin (rhCG), a genetically engineered hCG was developed with high purity and a more optimal consistency. Both urinary and rhCG are used in doses ranging from 5,000 to 10,000 IU for OT.[16]

Gonadotropin-Releasing Hormone Agonist

Gonadotropin-releasing hormone agonist is a synthetic peptide modeled after the hypothalamic GnRH that interacts with the GnRH receptor to elicit its biological response, i.e. the release of LH and FSH. However, following the initial "flare" of gonadotropins, continued stimulation with GnRHa causes GnRH receptor downregulation and, thus, pituitary desensitization. GnRHa for OT is only possible in GnRH antagonist co-treated IVF/ICSI cycles or in cycles in which no GnRH analog is used during stimulation. GnRHa has an affinity coefficient 2-50 times higher than that of the endogenous GnRH for the GnRH receptor;[16] thus in a GnRH antagonist co-treated cycle a bolus of GnRHa will displace the GnRH antagonist from the receptor, inducing a flare of gonadotropins (LH and FSH) and subsequently, oocyte maturation and ovulation.[17] GnRHa most commonly used for OT are: leuprorelin, buserelin, nafarelin, and triptorelin.[18]

Kisspeptin

Kisspeptin (Kp), although until now not used in daily clinical practice, is an interesting peptide hormone which influences the human neuroendocrine regulation.[19] It is released in the hypothalamic infundibular nucleus and acts through the Kp receptor (KISS 1R) directly on GnRH neurons as a key regulator of GnRH-secretion, impacted by circulating E and P levels.[19,20] In humans, exogenously administered subcutaneous kisspeptin (1.6–12.8 nmol/kg)[21] induces a dose-dependent release of endogenous LH and to a lesser extent FSH.[19,22,23] In the first experimental trials the use of a kisspeptin trigger was associated with good results in terms of the oocyte maturity rate.[24] However, the luteal phase after kisspeptin trigger is even more impaired as compared to GnRHa trigger, as the LH surge elicited is significantly shorter and with lower amplitude than that induced by GnRHa trigger. This is contrasted by the long duration (6–10 days) of LH activity induced by an hCG trigger[21]. Thus, the future role of kisspeptin as an OT agent needs to be further determined.

OVULATION TRIGGER IN OVULATION INDUCTION CYCLES FOR INTRAUTERINE INSEMINATION OR PROGRAMMED INTERCOURSE

A combination of intrauterine insemination (IUI) or programmed intercourse (PI) after controlled ovarian stimulation (COS) or in spontaneous cycles remains an important first-line treatment option for indications like cervical factor, mild endometriosis, mild-to-moderate male factor, ovulatory dysfunction, and unexplained infertility.[25] In spontaneous cycles as well as in stimulated cycles hCG has been administered successfully as a substitute for the endogenous LH surge to induce final oocyte maturation.[26] Although pregnancy rates per cycle vary according to the indication, they are usually reported in a range from 8% to 22%.[27] GnRHa, although not commonly used, has also been proven useful for OT in IUI and ovulation induction (OI) cycles.[28] However, OT with GnRHa is followed by an inadequate production of P, which is not overcome with a standard LPS. Thus, the addition of luteal hCG was reported to be useful to overcome this deficiency.[29] Until now hCG still remains the most widely used OT in IUI or PI cycles.

OVULATION TRIGGER IN IVF/ICSI CYCLES

Stimulated IVF/ICSI Cycle Triggered with hCG

In controlled ovarian stimulation IVF cycles triggered with hCG, the early luteal supra-physiological steroid concentration (P and E) induces a negative feedback on the endogenous LH secretion by the pituitary. This results in a marked reduction in circulating LH levels and a subsequent disruption of the luteal phase, necessitating the use of LPS if ongoing pregnancies are to be obtained.[30] Thus, significant differences exist in the comparison between the luteal steroid levels of the natural cycle and the hCG triggered stimulated cycle due to the significantly longer half-life of hCG compared to LH.[26,31] As the endogenous LH level of the hCG triggered cycle is significantly reduced due to a negative feedback on the pituitary, the CL function relies completely on the exogenous administration of LH activity in the form of hCG.[5] However, at peri-implantation hCG levels and consequently P levels are decreasing, which makes exogenous P supplementation mandatory to overcome the peri-implantation gap that develops between the decrease of exogenous hCG activity and the increase in endogenous hCG production from an implanting embryo.[5]

Stimulated IVF/ICSI Cycles Triggered with GnRHa

Unlike the natural mid-cycle surge of gonadotropins which has three phases that last for a total of for 48 hours, the GnRHa-induced surge consists of two phases, only, with a duration of 24–36 hours. This results in a reduced total amount of circulating LH (and FSH) released after GnRHa trigger compared to the natural cycle.[4,5] Thus, the mean mid-luteal LH level of the natural cycle is approximately 6 IU/L whereas it is approximately 1.5 IU/L after GnRHa trigger.[5,10] This level is insufficient to support the function of the CL, leading to either implantation failure or early pregnancy loss in fresh ET cycles if a standard LPS is used.[5] After the initial introduction of the GnRHa trigger for IVF patients, several modified LPS policies have been suggested. One strategy is to administer exogenously administered steroid support (P + E). Another strategy is to boost the endogenous steroid support by adding LH activity either in the form of a small bolus of hCG after the initial trigger or by adding daily recombinant LH injections during the luteal phase.[11,32]

Although GnRHa trigger induces a luteal phase deficiency, the concomitant release of FSH may add further physiological benefits as FSH upregulates the LH receptors of the CL. Indeed, previous studies reported a higher maturity rate of oocytes and a lower incidence of empty follicle syndrome (EFS) when GnRHa trigger was compared to hCG trigger.[5,33-35] As for hCG triggered cycles, early luteal phase supra-physiological levels of P and E produced by multiple CL induce a negative feedback on the endogenous LH secretion, which after the initial flare-up will result in a CL demise and a short luteal phase. Moreover, a possible direct luteolytic action of GnRHa has previously been proposed, and data from in vitro studies suggested that GnRHa is capable of activating the apoptosis cascade in granulosa cells.[36-38] Taken together, due to significant differences in circulating LH activity during the early luteal phase induced by a GnRHa trigger compared to a hCG trigger and the natural mid-cycle surge of gonadotropins, an extended or modified LPS is mandatory to obtain optimal pregnancy rates after GnRHa trigger.[5,39]

Dual Trigger (GnRHa and hCG Trigger)

The use of GnRHa combined with low-dose hCG trigger, so called "dual trigger", was initially reported in a retrospective study including a total of 45 patients.[40] hCG was administered concomitantly with a bolus of GnRHa in a dose ranging from 1,000 IU to 2,500 IU, depending on body weight of the patient and the individual risk of OHSS development. The authors reported an ongoing pregnancy rate of 53.3% and no OHSS cases. The dual trigger concept was subsequently investigated in a randomized controlled trial (RCT), in which a total of 200 patients who had failed at least one previous IVF-ET cycle using a long GnRHa downregulation protocol were included. The study group was triggered with both GnRHa (triptorelin 0.2 mg SC) and hCG (5,000 IU), whereas the control group was triggered with hCG (5,000 IU) only. The authors reported a significant increase in ongoing pregnancy rate per cycle in the dual trigger group.[41] Later a retrospective study was conducted in patients at risk of OHSS with peak serum estradiol (E2) levels less than 4,000 pg/mL. The use of dual trigger with GnRHa and a fixed dose of 1,000 IU hCG was compared to GnRHa trigger alone. In both groups an intensive LPS consisting of 50 mg intramuscular P daily and 0.3 mg transdermal E2 patches every other day starting from the day after the oocyte retrieval was used. Additional oral E and intramuscular P were given to maintain levels above 200 pg/mL and 20 ng/mL, respectively. The authors reported significantly higher live birth rates after dual trigger, and only one mild OHSS case occurred in the dual trigger group compared to none in the GnRHa trigger, only, group.[42] Similar results were reported in a retrospective study which included a total of 187 normal responder patients and compared dual trigger (GnRHa + hCG 6,500 IU) to hCG 6,500 IU alone.[43]

Interestingly the dual trigger concept has been proposed for the genuine EFS, and as previously mentioned the concept has also been shown to be an applicable OT strategy to improve the number of oocytes retrieved, especially in patients with a suboptimal follicle:oocyte ratio in a previous cycle (<50%) or a low proportion of mature oocytes (<66%).[44-46] Dual trigger combines the advantages of both agents (GnRHa and hCG): the direct intrafollicular LH activity mediated by hCG, the simultaneous induction of an endogenous FSH surge mediated by GnRHa and the support of the early luteal phase LH activity mediated by hCG.[47] Thus, dual trigger for a subgroup of patients might overcome existing impairments in granulosa cell function, oocyte maturation or cumulus expansion, resulting in the successful retrieval of mature oocytes.[48]

SAFETY AND EFFICACY OF TRIGGERING AGENTS (hCG AND GnRHA)

Ovulation Trigger, Optimal Oocyte Count and OHSS

The optimal OT should result in an optimal LH activity surge and a subsequent P rise.[49] A rule of thumb is that an optimal OT policy should result in more than 75% mature oocytes without increasing the risk of OHSS development.[19] GnRHa trigger effectively reduces OHSS rates due to the shorter half-life of the endogenous LH secretion compared to the long acting LH activity after an hCG trigger—approximately 33 hours versus 6-10 days respectively.[50,51] However, due to the short half-life, GnRHa trigger results in a defective CL formation and a decrease in the release of vasoactive peptides such as VEGF.[52] Although recent publications reported isolated cases of OHSS after GnRHa trigger in freeze all cycles (segmentation),[53-55] OHSS after GnRHa trigger and segmentation is very rare and most probably related to unexpected mutations or polymorphisms of the GnRH, FSH or LH receptor.

In comparison with GnRHa triggered IVF cycles, the hCG triggered cycles have been reported to have equal or slightly lower number of mature oocytes retrieved.[5,56,57] The physiological background for this finding could be the result of a reduction in the release of EGF-like peptides after hCG trigger, which have been shown to be potent mediators of oocyte maturation.

Ovulation Trigger and Embryo Quality

Embryo quality can be measured by international score assessment, blastulation rate, aneuploidy rate, and above all the live birth rate. Good quality oocytes and embryos have been shown to be obtained after GnRHa as well as after hCG trigger as seen in the reproductive outcomes of oocyte donation frozen thawed cycles.[58-60] However, some earlier studies reported a negative impact on early embryonic development when a bolus of hCG was used for trigger.[61] The authors hypothesized that an exaggerated intrafollicular shift in steroids from androgens and estradiol to progesterone mediated by high concentrations of hCG in the theca cell might negatively affect the oocyte.[62,63] In general, there is a lack of solid evidence to show significant differences in embryo quality related to the trigger agent.

Ovulation Trigger and Endometrial Receptivity/Luteal Phase

The OT agents affect endometrial receptivity either through direct mechanisms or by affecting the physiology of the CL and its subsequent steroid production. Regarding the use of hCG for OT, some studies reported a potential negative impact of hCG on endometrial receptivity.[64-66] The average serum level of hCG in hCG triggered cycles is approximately 120 IU/L during the early luteal phase, slowly decreasing to 4–6 IU/L on day 6.[67] This supra-physiological LH activity level during the early luteal phase might hamper successful implantation due to interference with specific actions mediated by hyperglycosylated hCG (H-hCG) produced by the implanting embryo.[68] Moreover, after an hCG trigger, P levels peak significantly earlier than during natural cycle, in which P reaches its peak concentration during the mid-luteal phase. Hypothetically, this early P rise may lead to an endometrial advancement that might negatively impact endometrial receptivity at the time of implantation.[69] In contrast, after GnRHa trigger, the early to mid-luteal phase steroid level is closer to the physiological range.[5,30] Moreover, GnRH receptors are expressed in extra-pituitary tissue including the endometrium, and the use of GnRH antagonists results in inhibitory intracellular events on transforming growth factor-beta (TGF-β) pathway, interleukin-1β (IL-1β) and VEGF production.[70,71] In this aspect, earlier studies reported that the use of a mid-luteal bolus of GnRHa resulted in a significant improvement in implantation rates.[8,9] Thus, it was hypothesized that a mid-luteal bolus of GnRHa might displace the GnRHa attached to the endometrial GnRH receptor, activating the downregulated receptors and resulting in the upregulation of pro-implantation factors.[41]

Ovulation Trigger and Luteal Phase Symptoms

Human chorionic gonadotropin trigger results in a significant increase in luteal fluid retention and ovarian volume, which causes significantly more abdominal pain, bloating and discomfort. In contrast, GnRHa trigger is associated with less fluid retention,[72] reduced ovarian volume and reduced discomfort[52] and, thus, a higher patient convenience.[73]

LUTEAL PHASE AFTER OVULATION TRIGGER

In all fresh ET IVF cycles LPS is mandatory as previously described. LPS can be stratified into standard and modified.

Luteal Phase after hCG Triggered IVF/ICSI Cycles

In IVF/ICSI cycles triggered with hCG, there is a need for progesterone supplementation (either vaginal, intramuscular or subcutaneous) to avoid the peri-implantation gap in progesterone as mentioned earlier, however, there is no need for E supplementation.[74] The LPS used after hCG trigger is known as a standard LPS.

Luteal Phase after GnRHa Triggered IVF/ICSI Cycles

In IVF/ICSI cycles triggered with GnRHa, a standard LPS is not sufficient to counterbalance the luteal phase insufficiency induced by the trigger. In contrast, an intensive or modified LPS is mandatory. Thus, the early GnRHa trigger studies using a standard LPS found significantly lower implantation rates and significantly higher early pregnancy loss rates compared to hCG triggered cycles.[4,5,75,76] However, after the introduction of modifications of the standard LPS, subsequent trials showed good pregnancy and live birth rates.[77,78]

The use of hCG as a surrogate for LH activity to promote the endogenous steroid production by the remnant CL was recently referred to as "The European Approach".[78] Over the years, the main effort has been to find the minimum hCG dose needed to rescue the CL until the hCG produced by the implanting embryo covers the luteal LH activity deficiency without increasing the risk of OHSS.[56,77,78]

As it is physiologically plausible that a refractory period may occur after the initial GnRHa trigger, during which human granulosa cells do not respond to subsequent LH-like exogenous stimulation, a pilot RCT in which low dose hCG (1,500 IU) was administered at either 12 hours or 35 hours after GnRHa trigger was performed. The comparator was hCG trigger (10,000 IU).[77] Higher mid-luteal P levels and better pregnancy rates were reported in the 35 hours group compared with the 12 hours group. Importantly, no differences in pregnancy outcomes were seen between the GnRHa trigger 35 hours hCG group and hCG group. Thus, the ideal timing of the 1,500 IU hCG rescue bolus following GnRHa trigger seemed to be the day of the oocyte retrieval.

The CL rescue concept after GnRHa trigger was further explored in a small group of 12 OHSS high-risk patients, having 25 or more follicles more than or equal to 11 mm. Patients were administered a bolus of 1,500 IU hCG following GnRHa trigger, i.e. shortly after the oocyte retrieval, resulting in promising results in live birth rate (50%) and OHSS reduction.[79] In a subsequent RCT, a total of 302 normogonadotropic patients were triggered with either hCG or GnRHa followed by 1,500 IU hCG at 35 hours. Again, a non-significant difference in live birth rates between GnRHa and hCG trigger was seen: 24% versus 31%, respectively.[33] The OHSS rate (severe and moderate) was 2% in hCG group, whereas no OHSS cases occurred in the GnRHa group, despite the fact that more than one-third of the patients in each group were considered at risk of OHSS, above ≥ 14 follicles ≥ 11 mm.[7] Although not significant, a 7% difference in live birth rate in favor of hCG trigger encouraged the authors to further scrutinize their data, revealing an increase in early pregnancy losses in the subgroup of normal responders (< 14 follicles ≥ 11 mm) who were triggered with GnRHa. This finding prompted the authors to suggest an innovative concept of an individualized luteal phase support (iLPS) after GnRHa trigger, in which the luteal administration of hCG was correlated to the number of preovulatory follicles larger than 11 mm.[80]

Another LPS policy after GnRHa trigger was recently described as "The American Approach".[78] This approach is based on the luteal phase regimen used for oocyte recipients who are treated with intensive LPS using intramuscular P and transdermal or oral E after the transfer of donated oocytes. Thus, this concept disregards CL function and relies solely on exogenous LPS after GnRHa trigger. Over the years, pregnancy rates similar to those of hCG trigger have been reported, however, close luteal phase monitoring to maintain P levels above 20 ng/mL and E levels above 200 pg/mL is mandatory to obtain good reproductive outcomes.[42,52,81] Until now this protocol has mainly been reported for patients considered at high risk of OHSS development, and this particular subset of patients are known to have significantly increased LH levels during the luteal phase and a decreased sensitivity of the GnRH pulse generator to the inhibition by ovarian steroids,[82] which leaves the patient with higher endogenous serum LH levels in the luteal phase.

In conclusion, two main modified LPS strategies have been suggested for GnRHa triggered cycles:

1. A bolus of hCG administered either during the early luteal phase or at the time of trigger followed by a standard LPS. This strategy aims to rescue the CL with subsequent endogenous steroid production.[78]
2. Intensive daily exogenous E and P administration which disregards the CL function. To use this luteal phase concept close luteal phase monitoring of P and E2 levels is mandatory if good reproductive outcomes are to be obtained.[42,52,83]

SEGMENTATION (FREEZE ALL POLICY)

Recently a "freeze all" policy was proposed for all GnRHa triggered IVF cycles;[6,49,84] however, prior to implementing this concept, there are concerns that need to be addressed. Although laboratories worldwide develop fast, not all IVF units have an optimal cryopreservation program, which is clearly crucial for the success of a freeze all policy. In addition, a higher early pregnancy loss rate related to frozen-thawed cycles has been reported,[85] as well as a higher risk of epigenetic changes.[86] Moreover, religious, ethical and financial reasons may preclude a freeze all policy. Finally, the early embryonic stage is a vulnerable period in terms of epigenetic activity and, hypothetically, additional manipulations (freeze-thaw) might induce irreversible changes which only appear in adulthood.[87] Thus, a "freeze all" policy should be adopted with caution, and results from large long-term follow-up trials in children conceived as a result of frozen-thaw ET are mandatory before a "freeze all" policy can be advised as a first-line treatment. However, in OHSS risk patients the immediate benefits from segmentation already outweigh the known and unknown risks involved with this strategy.[88] This policy is also applicable in aging good ovarian reserve patients who due to biological aging have a high aneuploidy rate and for whom the retrieval of additional oocytes increases the chance of transferring one euploid embryo.

CONCLUSION

Success rates in ART improve day-by-day, due to the refinement of gonadotropins, OT concepts, *LPS* and laboratory techniques. Importantly, the stimulation protocol remains crucial to achieve the maximum number of mature oocytes to obtain a live birth with the minimum risk for the patient. In this aspect OT plays a crucial role, and individualization in OT strategy is important to minimize the risk of an IVF treatment without negatively affecting the reproductive outcome. Until now hCG and GnRHa have clinically proven their efficacy when used for ovulation trigger whereas more trials are needed to reveal the possible future role of kisspeptin as a trigger agent in IVF.

REFERENCES

1. Kupka MS, Ferraretti AP, de Mouzon J, et al. Assisted reproductive technology in Europe, 2010: results generated from European registers by ESHRE†. Hum Reprod. 2014;29:2099-113.
2. Humaidan P, Nelson SM, Devroey P, et al. Ovarian hyperstimulation syndrome: review and new classification criteria for reporting in clinical trials. Hum Reprod. 2016;31:1997-2004.
3. Humaidan P, Westergaard LG, Mikkelsen AL, et al. Levels of the epidermal growth factor-like peptide amphiregulin in follicular fluid reflect the mode of triggering ovulation: a comparison between gonadotrophin-releasing hormone agonist and urinary human chorionic gonadotrophin. Fertil Steril. 2011;95:2034-8.
4. Fauser BC, De Jong D, Olivennes F, et al. Endocrine profiles after triggering of final oocyte maturation with GnRH agonist after cotreatment with the GnRH antagonist ganirelix during ovarian hyperstimulation for in vitro fertilization. J Clin Endocrinol Metab. 2002;87:709-15.
5. Humaidan P, Bredkjaer HE, Bungum L, et al. GnRH agonist (buserelin) or hCG for ovulation induction in GnRH antagonist IVF/ICSI cycles: a prospective randomized study. Hum Reprod. 2005;20:1213-20.
6. Devroey P, Polyzos NP, Blockeel C. An OHSS-free clinic by segmentation of IVF treatment. Hum Reprod. 2011;26:2593-7.
7. Papanikolaou EG, Pozzobon C, Kolibianakis EM, et al. Incidence and prediction of ovarian hyperstimulation syndrome in women undergoing gonadotropin-releasing hormone antagonist in vitro fertilization cycles. Fertil Steril. 2006;85:112-20.
8. Tesarik J, Hazout A, Mendoza-Tesarik R, et al. Beneficial effect of luteal-phase GnRH agonist administration on embryo implantation after ICSI in both GnRH agonist- and antagonist-treated ovarian stimulation cycles. Hum Reprod. 2006;21:2572-9.
9. Pirard C, Donnez J, Loumaye E. GnRH agonist as luteal phase support in assisted reproduction technique cycles: results of a pilot study. Hum Reprod. 2006;21:1894-900.
10. Tavaniotou A, Albano C, Van Steirteghem A, et al. The impact of LH serum concentration on the clinical outcome of IVF cycles in patients receiving two regimens of clomiphene citrate/gonadotrophin/0.25 mg cetrorelix. Reprod Biomed Online. 2003;6:421-6.

11. Engmann L, Benadiva C, Humaidan P. GnRH agonist trigger for the induction of oocyte maturation in GnRH antagonist IVF cycles: a SWOT analysis. Reprod Biomed Online. 2016;32:274-85.
12. Duncan WC, McNeilly AS, Fraser HM, et al. Luteinizing hormone receptor in the human corpus luteum: lack of down-regulation during maternal recognition of pregnancy. Hum Reprod. 1996;11:2291-7.
13. Pierce JG, Parsons TF. Glycoprotein hormones: structure and function. Annu Rev Biochem. 1981;50:465-95.
14. Gemzell C. Induction of ovulation with human gonadotropins. Recent Prog Horm Res. 1965;21:179-204.
15. Penarrubia J, Balasch J, Fabregues F, et al. Recurrent empty follicle syndrome successfully treated with recombinant human chorionic gonadotrophin. Hum Reprod. 1999;14:1703-6.
16. Driscoll GL, Tyler JP, Hangan JT, et al. A prospective, randomized, controlled, double-blind, double-dummy comparison of recombinant and urinary HCG for inducing oocyte maturation and follicular luteinization in ovarian stimulation. Hum Reprod. 2000;15:1305-10.
17. Gonen Y, Balakier H, Powell W, et al. Use of gonadotropin-releasing hormone agonist to trigger follicular maturation for in vitro fertilization. J Clin Endocrinol Metab. 1990;71:918-22.
18. van Loenen AC, Huirne JA, Schats R, et al. GnRH agonists, antagonists, and assisted conception. Semin Reprod Med. 2002;20:349-64.
19. Skorupskaite K, George JT, Anderson RA. The kisspeptin-GnRH pathway in human reproductive health and disease. Hum Reprod Update. 2014;20:485-500.
20. Millar RP, Newton CL. Current and future applications of GnRH, kisspeptin and neurokinin B analogues. Nat Rev Endocrinol. 2013;9:451-66.
21. Jayasena CN, Abbara A, Comninos AN, et al. Kisspeptin-54 triggers egg maturation in women undergoing in vitro fertilization. J Clin Invest. 2014;124:3667-77.
22. Jayasena CN, Comninos AN, Veldhuis JD, et al. A single injection of kisspeptin-54 temporarily increases luteinizing hormone pulsatility in healthy women. Clin Endocrinol (Oxf). 2013;79:558-63.
23. Jayasena CN, Abbara A, Veldhuis JD, et al. Increasing LH pulsatility in women with hypothalamic amenorrhoea using intravenous infusion of Kisspeptin-54. J Clin Endocrinol Metab. 2014;99:E953-61.
24. Jayasena CN, Comninos AN, Narayanaswamy S, et al. Acute and chronic effects of kisspeptin-54 administration on GH, prolactin and TSH secretion in healthy women. Clin Endocrinol (Oxf). 2014;81:891-8.
25. Duran HE, Morshedi M, Kruger T, et al. Intrauterine insemination: a systematic review on determinants of success. Hum Reprod Update. 2002;8:373-84.
26. Kessler MJ, Reddy MS, Shah RH, et al. Structures of N-glycosidic carbohydrate units of human chorionic gonadotropin. J Biol Chem. 1979;254:7901-8.
27. Guzick DS, Carson SA, Coutifaris C, et al. Efficacy of superovulation and intrauterine insemination in the treatment of infertility. National Cooperative Reproductive Medicine Network. N Engl J Med. 1999;340:177-83.
28. Balasch J, Fabregues F, Tur R, et al. Further characterization of the luteal phase inadequacy after gonadotropin-releasing hormone agonist-induced ovulation in gonadotrophin-stimulated cycles. Hum Reprod. 1995;10:1377-81.
29. Penarrubia J, Balasch J, Fabregues F, et al. Human chorionic gonadotrophin luteal support overcomes luteal phase inadequacy after gonadotrophin-releasing hormone agonist-induced ovulation in gonadotrophin-stimulated cycles. Hum Reprod. 1998;13:3315-8.

30. Humaidan P, Kol S, Papanikolaou EG. GnRH agonist for triggering of final oocyte maturation: time for a change of practice? Hum Reprod Update. 2011;17: 510-24.
31. Mannaerts BM, Geurts TB, Odink J. A randomized three-way cross-over study in healthy pituitary-suppressed women to compare the bioavailability of human chorionic gonadotrophin (Pregnyl) after intramuscular and subcutaneous administration. Hum Reprod. 1998;13:1461-4.
32. Itskovitz J, Boldes R, Levron J, et al. Induction of preovulatory luteinizing hormone surge and prevention of ovarian hyperstimulation syndrome by gonadotropin-releasing hormone agonist. Fertil Steril. 1991;56:213-20.
33. Humaidan P, Ejdrup Bredkjaer H, Westergaard LG, et al. 1,500 IU human chorionic gonadotropin administered at oocyte retrieval rescues the luteal phase when gonadotropin-releasing hormone agonist is used for ovulation induction: a prospective, randomized, controlled study. Fertil Steril. 2010;93:847-54.
34. Lok F, Pritchard J, Lashen H. Successful treatment of empty follicle syndrome by triggering endogenous LH surge using GnRH agonist in an antagonist down-regulated IVF cycle. Hum Reprod. 2003;18:2079-81.
35. Oktay K, Türkçüoğlu I, Rodriguez-Wallberg KA. GnRH agonist trigger for women with breast cancer undergoing fertility preservation by aromatase inhibitor/FSH stimulation. Reprod Biomed Online. 2010;20:783-8.
36. Latouche J, Crumeyrolle-Arias M, Jordan D, et al. GnRH receptors in human granulosa cells: anatomical localization and characterization by autoradiographic study. Endocrinology. 1989;125:1739-41.
37. Minaretzis D, Jakubowski M, Mortola JF, et al. Gonadotropin-releasing hormone receptor gene expression in human ovary and granulosa-lutein cells. J Clin Endocrinol Metab. 1995;80:430-4.
38. Takekida S, Deguchi J, Samoto T, et al. Comparative analysis of the effects of gonadotropin-releasing hormone agonist on the proliferative activity, apoptosis, and steroidogenesis in cultured porcine granulosa cells at varying stages of follicular growth. Endocrine. 2000;12:61-7.
39. Humaidan P, Papanikolaou EG, Kyrou D, et al. The luteal phase after GnRH-agonist triggering of ovulation: present and future perspectives. Reprod Biomed Online. 2012;24:134-41.
40. Shapiro BS, Daneshmand ST, Garner FC, et al. Gonadotropin-releasing hormone agonist combined with a reduced dose of human chorionic gonadotropin for final oocyte maturation in fresh autologous cycles of in vitro fertilization. Fertil Steril. 2008;90:231-3.
41. Schachter M, Friedler S, Ron-El R, et al. Can pregnancy rate be improved in gonadotropin-releasing hormone (GnRH) antagonist cycles by administering GnRH agonist before oocyte retrieval? A prospective, randomized study. Fertil Steril. 2008;90:1087-93.
42. Griffin D, Benadiva C, Kummer N, et al. Dual trigger of oocyte maturation with gonadotropin-releasing hormone agonist and low-dose human chorionic gonadotropin to optimize live birth rates in high responders. Fertil Steril. 2012;97:1316-20.
43. Lin MH, Shao-Ying Wu F, Kuo-Kuang Lee R, et al. Dual trigger with combination of gonadotropin-releasing hormone agonist and human chorionic gonadotropin significantly improves the live-birth rate for normal responders in GnRH-antagonist cycles. Fertil Steril. 2013;100:1296-302.
44. Kasum M, Kurdija K, Oreskovic S, et al. Combined ovulation triggering with GnRH agonist and hCG in IVF patients. Gynecol Endocrinol. 2016;32:861-65.

45. Haas J, Zilberberg E, Dar S, et al. Co-administration of GnRH-agonist and hCG for final oocyte maturation (double trigger) in patients with low number of oocytes retrieved per number of preovulatory follicles—a preliminary report. J Ovarian Res. 2014;7:77.
46. Zilberberg E, Haas J, Dar S, et al. Co-administration of GnRH-agonist and hCG, for final oocyte maturation (double trigger), in patients with low proportion of mature oocytes. Gynecol Endocrinol. 2015;31:145-7.
47. Beck-Fruchter R, Weiss A, Lavee M, et al. Empty follicle syndrome: successful treatment in a recurrent case and review of the literature. Hum Reprod. 2012;27:1357-67.
48. Haas J, Ophir L, Barzilay E, et al. Standard human chorionic gonadotropin versus double trigger for final oocyte maturation results in different granulosa cells gene expressions: a pilot study. Fertil Steril. 2016;106:653-9.e1.
49. Shapiro BS, Daneshmand ST, Garner FC, et al. Evidence of impaired endometrial receptivity after ovarian stimulation for in vitro fertilization: a prospective randomized trial comparing fresh and frozen-thawed embryo transfer in normal responders. Fertil Steril. 2011;96:344-8.
50. Damewood MD, Shen W, Zacur HA, et al. Disappearance of exogenously administered human chorionic gonadotropin. Fertil Steril. 1989;52:398-400.
51. Yen SS, Llerena O, Little B, et al. Disappearance rates of endogenous luteinizing hormone and chorionic gonadotropin in man. J Clin Endocrinol Metab. 1968;28:1763-7.
52. Engmann L, DiLuigi A, Schmidt D, et al. The use of gonadotropin-releasing hormone (GnRH) agonist to induce oocyte maturation after cotreatment with GnRH antagonist in high-risk patients undergoing in vitro fertilization prevents the risk of ovarian hyperstimulation syndrome: a prospective randomized controlled study. Fertil Steril. 2008;89:84-91.
53. Ling LP, Phoon JW, Lau MS, et al. GnRH agonist trigger and ovarian hyperstimulation syndrome: relook at "freeze-all strategy". Reprod Biomed Online. 2014;29:392-4.
54. Fatemi HM, Popovic-Todorovic B, Humaidan P, et al. Severe ovarian hyperstimulation syndrome after gonadotropin-releasing hormone (GnRH) agonist trigger and "freeze-all" approach in GnRH antagonist protocol. Fertil Steril. 2014;101:1008-11.
55. Gurbuz AS, Gode F, Ozcimen N, et al. Gonadotrophin-releasing hormone agonist trigger and freeze-all strategy does not prevent severe ovarian hyperstimulation syndrome: A report of three cases. Reprod Biomed Online. 2014;29:541-4.
56. Humaidan P, Polyzos NP, Alsbjerg B, et al. GnRHa trigger and individualized luteal phase hCG support according to ovarian response to stimulation: two prospective randomized controlled multi-centre studies in IVF patients. Hum Reprod. 2013;28:2511-21.
57. Imoedemhe DA, Sigue AB, Pacpaco EL, et al. Stimulation of endogenous surge of luteinizing hormone with gonadotropin-releasing hormone analog after ovarian stimulation for in vitro fertilization. Fertil Steril. 1991;55:328-32.
58. Acevedo B, Gomez-Palomares JL, Ricciarelli E, et al. Triggering ovulation with gonadotropin-releasing hormone agonists does not compromise embryo implantation rates. Fertil Steril. 2006;86:1682-7.
59. Griesinger G, Kolibianakis EM, Papanikolaou EG, et al. Triggering of final oocyte maturation with gonadotropin-releasing hormone agonist or human chorionic gonadotropin. Live birth after frozen-thawed embryo replacement cycles. Fertil Steril. 2007;88:616-21.

60. Bodri D, Guillén JJ, Galindo A, et al. Triggering with human chorionic gonadotropin or a gonadotropin-releasing hormone agonist in gonadotropin-releasing hormone antagonist-treated oocyte donor cycles: findings of a large retrospective cohort study. Fertil Steril. 2009;91:365-71.
61. Hausdorff WP, Caron MG, Lefkowitz RJ. Turning off the signal: desensitization of beta-adrenergic receptor function. FASEB J. 1990;4:2881-9.
62. Dumesic DA. Reduced intrafollicular androstenedione and estradiol levels in early-treated prenatally androgenized female rhesus monkeys receiving follicle-stimulating hormone therapy for in vitro fertilization. Biol Reprod. 2003;69:1213-9.
63. Dumesic DA, Schramm RD, Peterson E, et al. Impaired developmental competence of oocytes in adult prenatally androgenized female rhesus monkeys undergoing gonadotropin stimulation for in vitro fertilization. J Clin Endocrinol Metab. 2002;87:1111-9.
64. Forman R, Fries N, Testart J, et al. Evidence for an adverse effect of elevated serum estradiol concentrations on embryo implantation. Fertil Steril. 1988;49:118-22.
65. Fatemi HM, Kyrou D, Bourgain C, et al. Cryopreserved-thawed human embryo transfer: spontaneous natural cycle is superior to human chorionic gonadotropin-induced natural cycle. Fertil Steril. 2010;94:2054-8.
66. Fanchin R, Peltier E, Frydman R, et al. Human chorionic gonadotropin: does it affect human endometrial morphology in vivo? Semin Reprod Med. 2001;19:31-5.
67. Trinchard-Lugan I, Khan A, Porchet HC, et al. Pharmacokinetics and pharmacodynamics of recombinant human chorionic gonadotrophin in healthy male and female volunteers. Reprod Biomed Online. 2002;4:106-15.
68. Cole LA. Hyperglycosylated hCG and pregnancy failures. J Reprod Immunol. 2012;93:119-22.
69. Andersen CY, Elbaek HO, Alsbjerg B, et al. Daily low-dose hCG stimulation during the luteal phase combined with GnRHa triggered IVF cycles without exogenous progesterone: a proof of concept trial. Hum Reprod. 2015;30:2387-95.
70. Luo X, Xu J, Chegini N. Gonadotropin releasing hormone analogue (GnRHa) alters the expression and activation of Smad in human endometrial epithelial and stromal cells. Reprod Biol Endocrinol. 2003;1(1):125.
71. Meresman GF, Bilotas MA, Lombardi E, et al. Effect of GnRH analogues on apoptosis and release of interleukin-1β and vascular endothelial growth factor in endometrial cell cultures from patients with endometriosis. Hum Reprod. 2003;18:1767-71.
72. Garcia-Velasco JA, Motta L, Lopez A, et al. Low-dose human chorionic gonadotropin versus estradiol/progesterone luteal phase support in gonadotropin-releasing hormone agonist-triggered assisted reproductive technique cycles: understanding a new approach. Fertil Steril. 2010;94:2820-3.
73. Cerrillo M, Rodríguez S, Mayoral M, et al. Differential regulation of VEGF after final oocyte maturation with GnRH agonist versus hCG: a rationale for OHSS reduction. Fertil Steril. 2009;91:1526-8.
74. Fatemi HM. The luteal phase after 3 decades of IVF: what do we know? Reprod Biomed Online. 2009;19 Suppl 4:4331.
75. Beckers T, Bernd M, Kutscher B, et al. Structure-function studies of linear and cyclized peptide antagonists of the GnRH receptor. Biochem Biophys Res Commun. 2001;289:653-63.

76. Kolibianakis EM, Schultze-Mosgau A, Schroer A, et al. A lower ongoing pregnancy rate can be expected when GnRH agonist is used for triggering final oocyte maturation instead of HCG in patients undergoing IVF with GnRH antagonists. Hum Reprod. 2005;20:2887-92.
77. Humaidan P, Bungum L, Bungum M, et al. Rescue of corpus luteum function with peri-ovulatory HCG supplementation in IVF/ICSI GnRH antagonist cycles in which ovulation was triggered with a GnRH agonist: a pilot study. Reprod Biomed Online. 2006;13:173-8.
78. Humaidan P, Engmann L, Benadiva C. Luteal phase supplementation after gonadotropin-releasing hormone agonist trigger in fresh embryo transfer: the American versus European approaches. Fertil Steril. 2015;103:879-85.
79. Humaidan P. Luteal phase rescue in high-risk OHSS patients by GnRHa triggering in combination with low-dose HCG: a pilot study. Reprod Biomed Online. 2009;18:630-4.
80. Fatemi HM, Polyzos NP, van Vaerenbergh I, et al. Early luteal phase endocrine profile is affected by the mode of triggering final oocyte maturation and the luteal phase support used in recombinant follicle-stimulating hormone-gonadotropin-releasing hormone antagonist in vitro fertilization cycles. Fertil Steril. 2013;100:742-7.
81. Iliodromiti Z, Antonakopoulos N, Sifakis S, et al. Endocrine, paracrine, and autocrine placental mediators in labor. Hormones. 2012;11:397-409.
82. McCartney CR, Eagleson CA, Marshall JC. Regulation of gonadotropin secretion: implications for polycystic ovary syndrome. Semin Reprod Med. 2002;20:317-26.
83. Iliodromiti S, Lan VT, Tuong HM, et al. Impact of GnRH agonist triggering and intensive luteal steroid support on live-birth rates and ovarian hyperstimulation syndrome: a retrospective cohort study. J Ovarian Res. 2013;6:93.
84. Ozgur K, Humaidan P, Coetzee K. Segmented ART—The new era in ART? Reprod Biol. 2016;16:91-103.
85. Tomas C, Alsbjerg B, Martikainen H, et al. Pregnancy loss after frozen-embryo transfer—a comparison of three protocols. Fertil Steril. 2012;98:1165-9.
86. Henningsen AK, Romundstad LB, Gissler M, et al. Infant and maternal health monitoring using a combined Nordic database on ART and safety. Acta Obstet Gynecol Scand. 2011b;90:683-91.
87. Rimoldi SF, Sartori C, Rexhaj E, et al. Vascular dysfunction in children conceived by assisted reproductive technologies: underlying mechanisms and future implications. Swiss Med Wkly. 2014;144:w13973.
88. Krishna D, Dhoble S, Praneesh G, et al. Gonadotropin-releasing hormone agonist trigger is a better alternative than human chorionic gonadotropin in PCOS undergoing IVF cycles for an OHSS free clinic: a randomized control trial. J Hum Reprod Sci. 2016;9:164-72.

Chapter 8

Luteal Phase Support: ART and Non-ART Cycles

Barbara Lawrenz, Human M Fatemi

INTRODUCTION

The luteal phase of a menstrual cycle is the time between ovulation and, in case of conception, the establishment of a pregnancy or otherwise the onset of menses. In a natural cycle under the influence of luteinizing hormone (LH) formation of the corpus luteum will occur after ovulation. The corpus luteum is characterized by the production of up to 40 mg progesterone/day and also estradiol. Progesterone induces the secretory transformation of the endometrium in the luteal phase, promotes local vasodilatation and relaxation of the uterine muscle.[1]

After conception the developing embryo will secret human chorionic gonadotropin (hCG), which has structural similarities with LH and activates the same receptor. The role of hCG produced by the embryo is to maintain the corpus luteum and its secretions until the shift of progesterone production from the corpus luteum to the placenta around 9 weeks of pregnancy has taken place.[2]

For a pregnancy to occur, a receptive endometrium, a functional embryo at blastocyst developmental stage and synchrony between the embryo and the endometrium is required.[3] Failure to achieve receptivity and synchrony results in infertility and this is also a limiting factor for success in in vitro fertilization (IVF)—treatment.

Endometrial receptivity is driven by time of progesterone exposure after sufficient exposure to estrogen. The so called "window of implantation" (WOI), i.e. the time frame in which the endometrium is receptive and able to support trophoblast-endometrial interactions, is very limited in time. In a natural and idealized 28-day-cycle, it is thought to occur during a time around day 22 to day 24.[4] It is assumed, that the WOI is constant in time in all women. However, displacement of the WOI might not be a rare cause in infertility patients, especially in the patients with repeated implantation failure.[5]

STEROID PRODUCTION OF THE OVARY IN NATURAL AND STIMULATED CYCLES

Throughout the menstrual cycle, the ovary is producing the steroid hormones estradiol and progesterone. They are essential for human reproduction, which is demonstrated by the fact, that pregnancies with oocyte donation can be achieved after preparation of the endometrium with estradiol and progesterone,[6] even in women without ovaries.

In a natural cycle, estradiol synthesis increases progressively from the dominant follicle and initiates LH surge. Even before the LH-surge, a small increase in progesterone levels is seen, which reflects the increasing LH pulse amplitude and frequency leading up to the surge. A LH surge of 24–36 hours is sufficient to initiate the resumption of oocyte meiosis, luteinization of granulosa cells, ovulation, and the initial phase of corpora lutea development. Progesterone and 17α-hydroxyprogesterone (17α-OHP) plasma concentrations increase rapidly after the LH surge or administration of hCG,[7] indicating the beginning of granulosa and theca cell luteinization. As well as granulosa cells, the thecal cells produce significant amounts of progesterone. The corpus luteum is producing up to 40 mg of progesterone per day and additional a significant amount of androgens and estradiol. This is unique to the corpus luteum of many primates, including humans.[8]

Progesterone biosynthesis requires two enzymatic steps: firstly the conversion of cholesterol to pregnenolone (P5), catalyzed by the enzyme cytochrome P450scc and secondly its subsequent conversion to progesterone, which is catalyzed by 3β-hydroxysteroid dehydrogenase (3βHSD).[9] Progesterone is further metabolized to androgens by the action of *CYP17* in the thecal cells under the influence of LH. This step takes only place in the thecal cell compartment. However, during early follicular phase, the enzymatic activity necessary to convert 17-OH-progesterone to androstenedione, is absent or very low. Therefore, this process leads to increasing concentrations of progesterone and estradiol, as the follicular diameter increases.[10]

Whereas in natural cycle with development of a single dominant follicle, mid-follicular follicle-stimulating hormone (FSH)-levels are declining toward ovulation,[11] in ovarian stimulation for IVF, multifollicular development is achieved by administration of high daily gonadotropin concentrations. Stimulation dosage usually remains unchanged throughout the stimulation duration, unless the patient's individual response requires a change in the dosage. Therefore ovarian stimulation will result in a large number of growing follicles and each follicle will contribute to the progesterone in the systemic circulation. Progesterone concentration often reflects the number of preovulatory follicles and patients with high estradiol concentrations have significantly more oocytes and significantly higher progesterone concentrations.[12]

In a natural cycle without conception luteolysis occurs due to a lack of hCG support. The corpus luteum undergoes a process of regression with the loss of functional and structural integrity[13] leading to a decrease in progesterone production. In case of conception, the trophoblast produces hCG which prevents the regression of the corpus luteum and stimulates corpus luteum progesterone production which is necessary for maintenance of the pregnancy until placental progesterone production is adequate. Despite the fact, that serum hCG is detectable around the time of implantation approximately day 8 after ovulation, the hormonal characteristics of conception and nonconception cycles are different from the early luteal phase. Both LH and E2 levels are significantly higher in conception cycles on day 4 and 5 after the LH peak in urine compared to nonconception cycles.[14]

Influence of Progesterone on the Endometrium in Natural and Stimulated Cycles

The physiologic effects of P are primarily mediated by interaction with the progesterone receptor (PR). There are two classic PR isoforms, PR-A and PR-B and PR-A is required for normal ovarian and uterine function.[15] They are identical in structure except that the PR-B isoform contains a 164-amino acid N-terminal sequence, which is lacking in the PR-A isoform.[16] After binding to the nuclear receptors, steroid receptors activate their transcription genes.

The mitogenic effect of progesterone in the stroma is mediated by upregulating as well, PR-A as PR-B isoforms of the receptor.[17,18]

The different histological appearances of the endometrium, depending on the influence of estrogen or progesterone, have already been studied by Noyes et al. in 1950.[19] Whereas the proliferative phase under the influence of estradiol does not allow recognition of sub-phases other than early, middle or late proliferative phase, progressive changes occur in the endometrium of the secretory phase. In the period 36–48 hours directly after ovulation, no changes of the endometrium are visible. Further on under the influence of progesterone, the epithelial glands and vasculature continue to grow and become spiral, whereas the endometrial thickness is relatively unchanged, resulting in a denser endometrium. The morphological changes, observed on histology for each specific day after ovulation, established the classic endometrial dating paradigm that still serves as the gold standard for clinical evaluation of luteal function.[20] An endometrial biopsy that shows a difference of more than 2 days between the histologic dating and actual day after ovulation is considered to be "out of phase".[21]

Comparison of endometrial steroid receptors and proliferation index between natural cycles and gonadotropin-releasing hormone (GnRH)-agonist/human menopausal gonadotropin(hMG)-stimulated cycles for IVF have revealed distinct alterations in endometrial maturation. In stimulated cycles, a more advanced secretory endometrial maturation combined with reduced estrogen receptors (ERs) and PR and a low proliferation index in glands and stroma has been found on the day of oocyte retrieval, when compared to endometrial maturation in natural cycles on the day of ovulation.

Endometrial biopsies taken 2 days after oocyte pickup (OPU) in stimulated cycles showed a further reduction in steroid receptors and proliferation despite a similar histological maturation as compared to biopsies from natural cycles on day 2 after ovulation.[22] It can be assumed that supraphysiological hormonal levels during stimulation lead to a reduced number of ER and PR and a low proliferation index in glands and stroma. Those functional endometrial alterations might affect the proliferative potential of the endometrium.[22] However, solely from the serum progesterone concentrations and/or the absolute value of serum progesterone increase, the exact endometrial development on the day of OPU in stimulated cycles cannot be predicted.[23]

Besides the aforementioned advancement of endometrial maturation, in patients with a progesterone level above 1.5 ng/mL on the day of hCG-administration, differences in endometrial gene expression profile were found, when compared to the gene expression pattern below this threshold.[24] These changes might explain the impairment of endometrial receptivity in the presence of elevated progesterone, reflected in the lower pregnancy rates reported in the literature.[25]

The influence of elevated progesterone levels on the endometrial gene expression pattern was also analyzed by Labarta et al.[26] In a study, comparing the endometrial dating as well as the endometrium gene expression pattern during the WOI in 12 healthy oocyte donors. Six patients had progesterone levels above respectively below the progesterone threshold of 1.5 ng/mL. Out of 370 genes, 140 were dysregulated by more than two-fold in women with high serum progesterone levels. A large number of those genes represent biological processes like cell adhesion, immune system and organ development. Therefore dysregulation of those genes could affect the endometrium and the implantation process.

Interestingly, at day 7 after trigger, no more endometrial advancement was found in the group with elevated progesterone levels on the day of final oocyte maturation. It was shown previously that no pregnancies are achieved in case of an endometrial advancement of more than 3 days, when the embryo transfer is performed on day 3.[23,27] However, the detrimental effect of elevated progesterone level on the day of final oocyte maturation subsidies when the transfer is delayed until the blastocyst stage.[28] This suggests that the endometrium could recover during the WOI period.

Endocrine Profile in IVF-Cycles after Oocyte Retrieval, Depending on the Type of Trigger

Ovulation induction in ovarian stimulation for IVF with GnRH-agonist protocols has to be performed by the administration of hCG to mimic the LH-surge, whereas within GnRH-antagonist-protocols the use of GnRH-agonist for final oocyte maturation is possible with the advantage of reducing the risk for ovarian hyperstimulation syndrome (OHSS). Due to the different ways of action of hCG and GnRH-agonist, different endocrine profiles are seen after oocyte retrieval procedure. Patients, who were triggered with only hCG or GnRH-agonist plus 1,500 IU hCG had lower LH-levels compared to patients, triggered with GnRH-agonist only. Progesterone-levels on day 5 after oocyte retrieval procedure were highest in patients triggered with either hCG alone or a combination of GnRH-agonist plus 1,500 IU hCG and lowest in patients after GnRH-agonist only without any luteal phase support. This difference is caused by the fact, that after hCG-application progesterone production of the theca cells is sustained to approximately at least 5 days due to the LH-activity and the half-life-time of hCG of more than 24 hours.[29,30] After GnRH-agonist trigger severe luteal phase insufficiency occurred due to low levels of endogenous LH and therefore of progesterone.[31]

LUTEAL PHASE SUPPORT IN ASSISTED REPRODUCTIVE TECHNIQUES

As previously described, progesterone will be produced by the corpus luteum after LH-surge in normal, unstimulated cycle. Correction of a dysfunctional corpus luteum with the symptoms shortened luteal phase and pre-menstrual spotting by administration of progesterone was first described in 1949[32] and a defective luteal phase was defined, if the serum mid-luteal progesterone levels are less than 10 ng/mL.[33] Prevalence of luteal phase defect (LPD) in natural cycles in normo-ovulatory patients with primary or secondary infertility was demonstrated to be about 8.1%.[34] However in 2012, the ASRM stated that there is no reproducible, physiologically relevant, and clinically practical standard to diagnose LPD or distinguish fertile from infertile women.[35] The minimum threshold of progesterone level that is essential for the maintenance of a pregnancy is unknown and successful pregnancies have been reported even when the concentration of progesterone was never above 15 nmol/L for the first 14 days.[36] After ovarian stimulation for IVF/intracytoplasmic sperm injection (ICSI)-treatment it seems that patients having a progesterone levels at the day of implantation of more than 30 ng/mL and estradiol-levels of more than 100 pg/mL, are more likely to have a viable and ongoing pregnancy compared to patients with hormone levels below those thresholds.[37]

In stimulated cycles for IVF, a defective luteal phase occurs in almost all patients[23,27,38] and different theories have been discussed.[39] However, the reason for the luteal phase insufficiency seen after controlled ovarian stimulation seems to be the multifollicular development achieved during the follicular phase, resulting in supraphysiological luteal levels of P and E2 which inhibit LH secretion by the pituitary via negative feedback actions at the level of the hypothalamic-pituitary axis.[40-44] Besides the defective luteal phase due to the supraphysiological levels of estradiol and progesterone the WOI might be shorter in IVF-cycles compared to a natural cycle.[45]

To counterbalance the luteal phase insufficiency after ovarian stimulation, different ways of luteal phase support can be applied. Either direct substitution of progesterone via different routes of administration or indirect substitution of progesterone via the stimulation of the remaining corpora lutea to sustain progesterone production.

WAYS OF PROGESTERONE ADMINISTRATION

Oral Progesterone

Natural progesterone is rapidly metabolized after oral intake and has been shown to be ineffective in inducing a sufficient secretory transformation. Synthetic progesterone derivates are associated with side-effects, especially regarding the impact on the lipids[46] and on the psyche[47] which will limit their use. Micronization of progesterone reduces the particle size and improves absorption and bioavailability.[48] After oral digestion of 200 mg micronized progesterone maximal progesterone concentrations within the range of luteal phase are reached within 2–4 hours and will remain elevated then for approximately 6–7 hours.[48] Even higher doses of micronized progesterone have failed to induce sufficient secretory transformation. It seems that progesterone metabolites produced by the first liver passage lead to cross-reactions and are therefore responsible for those high progesterone levels.

Progesterone Intramuscular

Progesterone is rapidly absorbed after intramuscular (IM) injection. High progesterone plasma concentrations are reached after approximately 2 hours and peak concentrations will be achieved after around 8 hours. To achieve serum progesterone concentrations, which are equivalent to those during luteal phase in natural cycle, injection of 25 mg progesterone is required. It has been suggested, that the IM site of the injection might serve as a depot with progesterone accumulation in the fat tissue, leading to more sustained serum concentrations of progesterone.[49] The disadvantage of IM application of progesterone is that injection is painful and daily injections are required to sustain sufficient progesterone concentrations. Also swelling, redness and even sterile abscess formation are not uncommon side-effects.

Vaginal Progesterone

Progesterone plasma concentrations reach maximal levels approximately 3–8 hours after vaginal application and then fall continuously over the next 8 hours. Compared to IM. Progesterone it is faster cleared out of the circulation. To achieve luteal phase plasma levels, higher dosages of vaginal progesterone are needed and in most cases, 300–600 mg of progesterone is administered daily divided into 2 or 3 dosages,[50] depending on the formula, e.g. tablets, creams, suppositories. Vaginal mucosa absorbs proteins and lipids, however absorption is influenced by the kind of formula preparation and absorption is enhanced after previous estrogenization.[51]

After vaginal administration of progesterone, the serum levels are lower compared to IM application and sometimes even lower than measured in a natural cycle. However, despite the low serum levels, adequate secretory endometrial transformation was achieved. This suggests that vaginally administered progesterone exerts a direct local effect on the endometrium before entering the systemic circulation, the so called "first uterine pass" effect. The mechanism behind the "first uterine pass" effect is not fully understood and different ways of action are discussed: absorption of progesterone into the rich venous or lymphatic vaginal system and/or possibly countercurrent transfer between uterovaginal lymph vessels or veins and arteries, direct drug diffusion through the tissues or even due to intraluminal transfer from the uterus to the vagina similar to sperm transport. As the vaginal route is effective in providing sufficient luteal phase support and additional almost without any side-effects, it is a valuable and nowadays the preferred route of progesterone administration.[52]

Human Chorionic Gonadotropin for Luteal Phase Support

With the application of hCG, no luteolysis occurs as the corpora lutea will be stimulated and will sustain progesterone production. For a long time, the hCG-administration was the standard luteal phase support, however the disadvantage of this approach is the possible development of OHSS, especially in the good responder patients.[53]

Timing of Luteal Phase Support with Progesterone

Timing of luteal phase support in assisted reproductive technology (ART)-cycles is crucial, as it has to be initiated before endogenous progesterone levels are decreasing or low. On the other hand, preovulatory exposure of the endometrium to progesterone may have a negative impact on the endometrial receptivity as already described.

When luteal phase support was started before oocyte retrieval, a decreased likelihood of pregnancy was found, when compared to start on the day of oocyte retrieval. When P was initiated on the evening of oocyte retrieval versus start on day 1–3 after oocyte retrieval, no difference in clinical PR was found. However, when progesterone administration was started on day 6, a decreased likelihood of pregnancy was found. Therefore, initiation of progesterone supplementation between the evening of oocyte retrieval and day 3 after retrieval seems to be ideal.[54]

Duration of Luteal Phase Support

In early pregnancy, the embryo is producing a significant and rapidly increasing amount of hCG which will replace a possible lack of endogenous LH after ovarian stimulation. Later on in the pregnancy, between 7 and 9 weeks, progesterone production will shift from the corpora lutea toward the placenta. Studies evaluating the duration of progesterone administration after a positive pregnancy test did not find any influence on the miscarriage rate and the delivery rate when progesterone application was continued or discontinued for 3 weeks after positive pregnancy test.[55,56]

Luteal Support after GnRH-Trigger

Meanwhile the use of GnRH-agonist for final oocyte maturation is common in high responder patients as development of OHSS can almost completely be avoided. Following the introduction of GnRH-agonist for final oocyte maturation in GnRH-antagonist protocols, the first large randomized controlled trials reported a very poor reproductive out-come with this approach. It was assumed, that the severity of the induced luteolysis by application of GnRH-agonist cannot be counterbalanced using standard luteal phase support with "only" progesterone administration.[57] The administration of hCG or high doses of steroids[58] is considered to be essential to prevent luteolysis.

There is an ongoing debate on the adequate luteal phase support in this scenario. Luteolysis occurs when LH support from the primate corpus luteum is withdrawn for more than or equal to 3 days,[59] hence corpus luteum function can be rescued, if LH activity is reinitiated within 3 days, suggesting that corpus luteum viability can be preserved without LH support for at least 72 hours.[60] In order to sustain progesterone production from the corpora lutea and therefore rescue the luteal phase different treatment options have been described.

Following the concept that GnRH-agonist-induced luteolysis can be reverted with the administration of hCG, low-doses of hCG can be given during luteal phase. However it was found, that the rescue of the corpora lutea for up to 3 days of gonadotropin deprivation is hCG dose dependent, i.e. more than or equal to 1,500 IU.[61] The approach of administration of 1,500 IU of hCG 35 hours after GnRH-agonist trigger result in comparable pregnancy rates in respect to hCG-trigger, but unfortunately with this dosage, OHSS in the high-responder-group occurred.[62,63] Other authors[64] applied low-dose hCG in different dosages in the luteal phase after GnRH-agonist triggering and could demonstrate that those dosages were effective in normalizing the reproductive outcome. Despite the low dosages of hCG, OHSS could not be completely avoided.

A proof-of-concept study evaluated a luteal phase support by application of daily low hCG-dosages (125 IU rhCG) from the day of OPU without the use of exogenous progesterone. Significant differences during the luteal phase were observed with progesterone levels being significantly higher in the groups receiving daily low-dose hCG supplementation.[65] Hence even with this low hCG dosage, OHSS occurred in 3% of the patients, hence no hospitalization was needed.

Ovarian hyperstimulation syndrome can be almost completely avoided by the use of GnRH-agonist (200 mg of GnRH-agonist nasal spray twice daily; a total of 400 mg/day) for luteal phase support after GnRH-agonist trigger without exogenous progesterone and midluteal progesterone levels of around 190 nmol/L (approximately 59.7 ng/mL) can be achieved.[66]

Luteal Phase Support in Insemination Cycles

Intrauterine insemination (IUI) is a frequently applied techniques to increase the probability of conception in couples with subfertility or unexplained infertility, however the necessity of luteal support is addressed only in a few studies.

Intrauterine insemination can be performed in either natural cycles or stimulated cycles by using clomifen-citrat or gonadotropins for stimulation.

In natural IUI-cycles it can be assumed, that no luteal phase insufficiency should be present and therefore there is no biological or empirical evidence that treatment with hCG or progesterone in the luteal phase is necessary or improves the pregnancy rate.[67] Nevertheless the addition of progesterone, hCG and/or other substances became established clinical practice even in the absence of any robust evidence of effectiveness.[68]

In patients, who undergo mild ovarian stimulation for IUI, it can be assumed that due to supraphysiological hormonal levels, endogenous LH will be low, leading possibly to a luteal phase insufficiency. However, it is crucial to differentiate between the kind of stimulation done, as after clomiphene citrate administration, an increase in LH pulse frequency will result in a significant increase of serum E2 and progesterone levels, with a lengthening of the luteal phase. A study, evaluating a beneficial impact of progesterone application in normo-ovulatory patients stimulated with clomiphene citrate for IUI, did not find higher ongoing pregnancy rates in patients receiving progesterone after IUI compared to those, who had no luteal phase support.[69] However, as after gonadotropin-stimulation, comparable to ovarian stimulation for IVF, supraphysiological hormonal levels will lead to suppression of endogenous LH, development of luteal phase insufficiency can be expected. It was shown, that after IUI in a gonadotropin-stimulated cycle, the chance of pregnancy and live birth is higher, when progesterone application is done after IUI.[70]

Luteal Phase Support in Frozen Embryo Transfer Cycles

Due to the improvement of the cryoconservation-techniques in the IVF-laboratory with the introduction of vitrification, worldwide more and more frozen embryo transfer (FET) or warmth oocyte embryo transfer-cycles are performed.[71] The advantage of this technique is to improve the chance of a pregnancy in patients with surplus oocytes or embryos without performing a new ovarian stimulation cycle.

To optimize the pregnancy rates, synchronization of the embryo development and the endometrium is crucial. A simple way of endometrium preparation is the use of the natural cycle with endogenous production of estradiol of the growing follicle. However, in a natural cycle the LH-surge has to be detected in order to plan the correct timing for the embryo thawing and embryo transfer. A study, designed to compare the pregnancy rates between natural cycles and modified natural cycles with application of hCG to end the follicular phase showed significantly higher pregnancy rates in the natural cycle. However, for the natural cycle, patients were monitored closely by blood tests to detect ovulation and plan the thawing and transfer of the embryo(s) accordingly. To define ovulation, LH surge was deemed to have begun when the concentration rose by 180% above the latest serum value available in that patient and continued to rise thereafter. Day 1 after the LH rise, a drop of E2 and concomitant rise of P more than 1.5 nmol/L confirmed the ovulation.[72] Unfortunately, detection of LH-surge with tests performed in the urine is too unreliable to be used for accurate planning of frozen embryo transfer.

In modified natural cycle for FET, hCG is administered to induce ovulation and luteinization. However, it seems that hCG-administration to end the follicular phase results in significant lower pregnancy rates compared to natural cycles with the detection of LH-surge. It is assumed, that hCG may have a negative effect on endometrium receptivity.[72,73]

A more common approach is the use of a hormonal-replacement cycle with the administration of exogenous estradiol and progesterone, as the advantages of this approach are that disturbances due to cycle-variation can be avoided and also planning of the embryo-transfer is possible, which will smoothen the work flow for the IVF-laboratory. Hormonal replacement cycle can be performed with or without co-treatment with GnRH-agonists.

Until now, the best approach for FET is still under discussion and there is an urgent need for randomized controlled trials to compare the correctly conducted natural cycle with correct determination of LH-surge and the hormonal replacement cycle.

CONCLUSION

Estradiol and progesterone are essential for human production. Whereas in a natural cycle, progesterone is produced by the corpus luteum, luteal phase of ovarian stimulation cycles for IVF/ICSI are mostly characterized by severe luteal phase insufficiency. Multifollicular follicle growth leads to unphysiological high hormonal levels, which inhibit LH secretion from the pituitary via negative feedback actions at the level of the hypothalamic-pituitary axis.

To counterbalance the luteal phase insufficiency after ovarian stimulation luteal phase support has to be applied, either by direct substitution of progesterone or indirect via the stimulation of the remaining corpora lutea to sustain progesterone production. Progesterone can be applied orally, as

IM injection or vaginally. The latter one is nowadays the preferred route of progesterone administration. hCG-administration has the disadvantage of a possible development of ovarian hyperstimulation syndrome, especially in a good responder patient. Luteal phase support should be initiated within 1-3 days after oocyte retrieval procedure and is not required any more after the progesterone production shifted to the placenta between 7 and 9 weeks of gestation. In case of final oocyte maturation with GnRH-agonist in a GnRH-antagonist protocol, the optimal luteal phase support is still under discussion.

REFERENCES

1. Bulletti C, de Ziegler D. Uterine contractility and embryo implantation. Curr Opin Obstet Gynecol. 2005;17:265-76.
2. Csapo AI, Pulkkinen MO, Ruttner B, et al. The significance of the human corpus luteum in pregnancy maintenance. I. Preliminary studies. Am J Obstet Gynecol. 1972;112:1061-7.
3. Simon C, Martın JC, Pellicer A. Paracrine regulators of implantation. Baillieres Best Pract Res Clin Obstet Gynaecol. 2000;14:815-26.
4. Bergh PA, Navot D. The impact of embryonic development and endometrial maturity on the timing of implantation. Fertil Steril. 1992;58:537-42.
5. Ruiz-Alonso M, Galindo N, Pellicer A, et al. What a difference two days make: "personalized" embryo transfer (pET) paradigm: a case report and pilot study. Hum Reprod. 2014;29:1244-7.
6. Devroey P, Pados G. Preparation of endometrium for egg donation. Hum Reprod Update. 1998;4:856-61.
7. Christenson LK, Devoto L. Cholesterol transport and steroidogenesis by the corpus luteum. Reprod Biol Endocrinol. 2003;1:90.
8. Devoto L, Fuentes A, Kohen P, et al. The human corpus luteum: life cycle and function in natural cycles. Fertil Steril. 2009;92:1067-79.
9. Chaffin CL, Dissen GA, Stouffer RL. Hormonal regulation of steroidogenic enzyme expression in granulosa cells during the peri-ovulatory interval in monkeys. Mol Hum Reprod. 2000;6:11-8.
10. Yding Andersen C, Bungum L, Nyboe Andersen A, et al. Preovulatory progesterone concentration associates significantly to follicle number and LH concentration but not to pregnancy rate. Reprod Biomed Online. 2011;23:187-95.
11. Fleming R, Jenkins J. The source and implications of progesterone rise during the follicular phase of assisted reproduction cycles. Reprod Biomed Online. 2010;21:446-9.
12. Kyrou D, Al-Azemi M, Papanikolaou EG, et al. The relationship of premature progesterone rise with serum estradiol levels and number of follicles in GnRH antagonist/recombinant FSH-stimulated cycles. Eur J Obstet Gynecol Reprod Biol. 2012;162:165-8.
13. Stocco C, Tellerıa C, Gibori G. The molecular control of corpus luteum formation, function and regression. Endocr Rev. 2007;28:117-49.
14. Chen J, Oiu O, Lohstroh PN, et al. Hormonal characteristics in the early luteal phase of conceptive and nonconceptive menstrual cycles. J Soc Gynecol Investig. 2003;10:27-31.
15. Kastner P, Krust A, Turcotte B, et al. Two distinct estrogen-regulated promoters generate transcripts encoding the two functionally different human progesterone receptor forms A and B. EMBO J. 1990;9:1603-14.
16. Wei LL, Gonzalez-Aller C, Wood WM, et al. 5'-Heterogeneity in human progesterone receptor transcripts predicts a new amino-terminal truncated. "C"-receptor and unique A-receptor messages. Molecular Endocrinol. 1990;4:1833-40.

17. Salmi A, Pakarinen P, Peltola AM, et al. The effect of intrauterine levonorgestrel use on the expression of c-JUN, oestrogen receptors, progesterone receptors and Ki-67 in human endometrium. Mol Hum Reprod. 1998;4:1110-5.
18. Tseng L, Zhu HH. Regulation of progesterone receptor messenger ribonucleic acid by progestin in human endometrial stromal cells. Biol Reprod. 1997;57:1360-6.
19. Noyes RW, Hertig AT, Rock J. Dating the endometrial biopsy. Fertil Steril. 1950;1:3-25.
20. Noyes RW, Hertig AT, Rock J. Dating the endometrial biopsy. Am J Obstet Gynecol. 1975;122:262-3.
21. Wentz AC. Endometrial biopsy in the evaluation of infertility. Fertil Steril. 1980;33:121-4.
22. Bourgain C, Ubaldi F, Tavaniotou A, et al. Endometrial hormone receptors and proliferation index in the periovulatory phase of stimulated embryo transfer cycles in comparison with natural cycles and relation to clinical pregnancy outcome. Fertil Steril. 2002;78:237-44.
23. Ubaldi F, Bourgain C, Tournaye H, et al. Endometrial evaluation by aspiration biopsy on the day of oocyte retrieval in the embryo transfer cycles in patients with serum progesterone rise during the follicular phase. Fertil Steril. 1997;67:521-6.
24. Van Vaerenbergh I, Fatemi HM, Blockeel C, et al. Progesterone rise on HCG day in GnRH antagonist/rFSH stimulated cycles affects endometrial gene expression. Reprod Biomed Online. 2011;22:263-71.
25. Bosch E, Valencia I, Escudero E, et al. Premature luteinization during gonadotropin-releasing hormone antagonist cycles and its relationship with in vitro fertilization outcome. Fertil Steril. 2003;80:1444-9.
26. Labarta E, Martínez-Conejero JA, Alamá P, et al. Endometrial receptivity is affected in women with high circulating progesterone levels at the end of the follicular phase: a functional genomics analysis. Hum Reprod. 2011;26:1813-25.
27. Kolibianakis EM, Devroey P. The luteal phase after ovarian stimulation. Reprod Biomed Online. 2002a;5:26-35.
28. Papanikolaou EG, Kolibianakis EM, Pozzobon C, et al. Progesterone rise on the day of human chorionic gonadotropin administration impairs pregnancy outcome in day 3 single-embryo transfer, while has no effect on day 5 single blastocyst transfer. Fertil Steril. 2009;91:949-52.
29. Damewood MD, Shen W, Zacur HA, et al. Disappearance of exogenously administered human chorionic gonadotropin. Fertil Steril. 1989;52:398-400.
30. Yen SS, Llerena O, Little B, et al. Disappearance rates of endogenous luteinizing hormone and chorionic gonadotropin in man. J Clin Endocrinol Metab. 1968;28:1763-7.
31. Fatemi HM, Polyzos NP, van Vaerenbergh I, et al. Early luteal phase endocrine profile is affected by the mode of triggering final oocyte maturation and the luteal phase support used in recombinant follicle-stimulating hormone-gonadotropin-releasing hormone antagonist in vitro fertilization cycles. Fertil Steril. 2013;100:742-7.
32. Jones GES. Some new aspects of management of infertility. JAMA 1979;141:1123.
33. Jordan J, Craig K, Clifton DK, et al. Luteal phase defect: the sensitivity and specificity of diagnostic methods in common clinical use. Fertil Steril. 1994;62:54-62.
34. Rosenberg SM, Luciano AA, Riddick DH. The luteal phase defect: the relative frequency of, and encouraging response to, treatment with vaginal progesterone. Fertil Steril. 1980;34:17-20.
35. Practice Committee of the American Society for Reproductive Medicine. Current clinical irrelevance of luteal phase deficiency: a committee opinion. Fertil Steril. 2015;103:e27-32.

36. Csapo AI, Pulkkinen M. Indispensability of the human corpus luteum in the maintenance of early pregnancy. Luteectomy evidence. Obstet Gynecol Surv. 1978;33:69-81.
37. Liu HC, Pyrgiotis E, Davis O, et al. Active corpus luteum function at pre-, peri- and postimplantation is essential for a viable pregnancy. Early Pregnancy. 1995;1:281-7.
38. Macklon NS, Fauser BC. Impact of ovarian hyperstimulation on the luteal phase. J Reprod Fertil. 2000;55:101-8.
39. Fatemi HM, Popovic-Todorovic B, Papanikolaou E, et al. An update of luteal phase support in stimulated IVF cycles. Hum Reprod Update. 2007;13:581-90.
40. Beckers NG, Macklon NS, Eijkemans MJ, et al. Nonsupplemented luteal phase characteristics after the administration of recombinant human chorionic gonadotropin, recombinant luteinizing hormone, or gonadotropin-releasing hormone (GnRH) agonist to induce final oocyte maturation in in vitro fertilization patients after ovarian stimulation with recombinant follicle-stimulating hormone and GnRH antagonist cotreatment. J Clin Endocrinol Metab. 2003;88:4186-92.
41. Fatemi HM. The luteal phase after 3 decades of IVF: what do we know? Reprod Biomed Online. 2009;19:4331.
42. Fauser BC, Devroey P. Reproductive biology and IVF: ovarian stimulation and luteal phase consequences. Trends Endocrinol Metab. 2003;14:236-42.
43. Tavaniotou A, Devroey P. Effect of human chorionic gonadotropin on luteal luteinizing hormone concentrations in natural cycles. Fertil Steril. 2003;80:654-5.
44. Tavaniotou A, Albano C, Smitz J, et al. Comparison of LH concentrations in the early and mid-luteal phase in IVF cycles after treatment with HMG alone or in association with the GnRH antagonist Cetrorelix. Hum Reprod. 2001;16:663-7.
45. Bourgain C, Devroey P. The endometrium in stimulated cycles for IVF. Hum Reprod Update. 2003;9:515-22.
46. Hirvonen E, Mälkönen M, Manninen V. Effects of different progestogens on lipoproteins during postmenopausal replacement therapy. N Engl J Med. 1981;304:560-3.
47. Dennerstein L, Burrows GD, Hyman GJ, et al. Hormone therapy and affect. Maturitas. 1979;1:247-59.
48. Norman TR, Morse CA, Dennerstein L. Comparative bioavailability of orally and vaginally administered progesterone. Fertil Steril. 1991;56:1034-9.
49. Nillius SJ, Johansson ED. Plasma levels of progesterone after vaginal, rectal, or intramuscular administration of progesterone. Am J Obstet Gynecol. 1971;110:470-7.
50. Devroey P, Palermo G, Bourgain C, et al. Progesterone administration in patients with absent ovaries. Int J Fertil. 1989;34:188-93.
51. Villanueva B, Casper RF, Yen SS. Intravaginal administration of progesterone: enhanced absorption after estrogen treatment. Fertil Steril. 1981;35:433-7.
52. Tavaniotou A, Smitz J, Bourgain C, et al. Comparison between different routes of progesterone administration as luteal phase support in infertility treatments. Hum Reprod Update. 2000;6:139-48.
53. Ludwig M, Diedrich K. Evaluation of an optimal luteal phase support protocol in IVF. Acta Obstet Gynecol Scand. 2001;80:452-66.
54. Connell MT, Szatkowski JM, Terry N, et al. Timing luteal support in assisted reproductive technology: a systematic review. Fertil Steril. 2015;103:939-46.
55. Nyboe AA, Popovic-Todorovic B, Schmidt KT, et al. Progesterone supplementation during early gestations after IVF or ICSI has no effect on the delivery rates: a randomized controlled trial. Hum Reprod. 2002;17:357-61.
56. Schmidt KL, Ziebe S, Popovic B, et al. Progesterone supplementation during early gestation after in vitro fertilization has no effect on the delivery rate. Fertil Steril. 2001;75:337-41.

57. Humaidan P, Bredkjaer HE, Bungum L, et al. GnRH agonist (buserelin) or hCG for ovulation induction in GnRH antagonist IVF/ICSI cycles: a prospective randomized study. Hum Reprod. 2005;20:1213-20.
58. Engmann L, Benadiva C. Agonist trigger: what is the best approach? Agonist trigger with aggressive luteal support. Fertil Steril. 2012;97:531-3.
59. Hutchison JS, Zeleznik AJ. The rhesus monkey corpus luteum is dependent on pituitary gonadotropin secretion throughout the luteal phase of the menstrual cycle. Endocrinology. 1984;115;1780-6.
60. Hutchison JS, Zeleznik AJ. The corpus luteum of the primate menstrual cycle is capable of recovering from a transient withdrawal of pituitary gonadotropin support. Endocrinology. 1985;117:1043-9.
61. Dubourdieu S, Charbonnel B, Massai MR, et al. Suppression of corpus luteum function by the gonadotropin-releasing hormone antagonist Nal-Glu: effect of the dose and timing of human chorionic gonadotropin administration. Fertil Steril. 1991;56:440-512.
62. Humaidan P. Luteal phase rescue in high-risk OHSS patients by GnRHa triggering in combination with low-dose HCG: a pilot study. Reprod Biomed Online. 2009;18:630-4.
63. Seyhan A, Ata B, Polat M, et al. Severe early ovarian hyperstimulation syndrome following GnRH agonist trigger with the addition of 1500 IU hCG. Hum Reprod. 2013;28:2522-8.
64. Castillo JC, Dolz M, Bienvenido E, et al. Cycles triggered with GnRH agonist: exploring low-dose HCG for luteal support. Reprod Biomed Online. 2010;20: 175-81.
65. Andersen CY, Elbaek HO, Alsbjerg B, et al. Daily low-dose hCG stimulation during the luteal phase combined with GnRHa triggered IVF cycles without exogenous progesterone: a proof of concept trial. Hum Reprod. 2015;30:2387-95.
66. Bar-Hava I, Mizrachi Y, Karfunkel-Doron D, et al. Intranasal gonadotropin-releasing hormone agonist (GnRHa) for luteal-phase support following GnRHa triggering, a novel approach to avoid ovarian hyperstimulation syndrome in high responders. Fertil Steril. 2016;106:330-3.
67. Ragni G, Vegetti W, Baroni E, et al. Comparison of luteal phase profile in gonadotrophin stimulated cycles with or without a gonadotrophin-releasing hormone antagonist. Hum Reprod. 2001;16:2258-62.
68. ESHRE Capri Workshop Group. Intrauterine Insemination. Hum Reprod Update. 2009;15:265-77.
69. Kyrou D, Fatemi HM, Tournaye H, et al. Luteal phase support in normo-ovulatory women stimulated with clomiphene citrate for intrauterine insemination: need or habit? Hum Reprod. 2010;25:2501-6.
70. Oktem M, Altinkaya SO, Yilmaz SA, et al. Effect of luteal phase support after ovulation induction and intrauterine insemination. Gynecol Endocrinol. 2014; 30:909-12.
71. Le Lannou D, Griveau JF, Laurent MC, et al. Contribution of embryo cryopreservation to elective single embryo transfer in IVF-ICSI. Reprod Biomed Online. 2006;13:368-75.
72. Fatemi HM, Kyrou D, Bourgain C, et al. Cryopreserved-thawed human embryo transfer: spontaneous natural cycle is superior to human chorionic gonadotropin-induced natural cycle. Fertil Steril. 2010;94:2054-8.
73. Montagut M, Santos-Ribeiro S, De Vos M, et al. Frozen-thawed embryo transfers in natural cycles with spontaneous or induced ovulation: the search for the best protocol continues. Hum Reprod. 2016;31:2803-10.

Chapter 9

Role of Luteinizing Hormone in Controlled Ovarian Stimulation

Carlo Alviggi, Alessandro Conforti, Giuseppe De Placido, Sandro C Esteves

INTRODUCTION

Physiologically, a fine interplay between follicle-stimulating hormone (FSH) and luteinizing hormone (LH) promotes follicle growth and maturation. According to the "two cells, two gonadotropin theory" FSH and LH regulate two distinct compartments. While FSH modulates proliferation of granulosa cells, LH exerts its activity in theca cells stimulating the androgen synthesis pathway. Nonetheless, evidence indicates that granulosa cells express LH receptors in late follicular phase, thus suggesting that LH has a role in the final steps of follicle maturation.[1] Despite its pivotal role in follicular growth on natural cycles, the effect of LH in stimulated cycle is more equivocal. It has been demonstrated that LH supplementation is not necessary during controlled ovarian stimulation (COS) for all in vitro fertilization (IVF) women.[2,3] For example, the addition of LH to COS does not seem to offer any benefit to young normogonadotropic women with an adequate ovarian response, irrespective of the type of gonadotropin-releasing hormone (GnRH) analog used. On the other hand, emerging data indicates that selected patients might benefit from exogenous LH supplementation.[4]

The purposes of this chapter are: (1) to illustrate the molecular and biologic action of LH, (2) to describe the gonadotropin preparations containing LH activity, and (3) to present the clinical evidence with regards the use of LH supplementation to selected patients undergoing COS.

STRUCTURE AND FUNCTION OF LUTEINIZING HORMONE

Luteinizing hormone is a pituitary glycoprotein hormone which together with FSH regulates gonadal function. LH is synthesized and secreted by gonadotrophs cells localized in the lateral portion of pituitary gland under stimulation of GnRH.[5] Through a calcium-dependent mechanism, GnRH stimulates LH and FSH synthesis using inositol 1,4,5 triphosphate and 1,2 diacylglycerol as second messengers. The LH molecule comprises two non-covalently linked protein subunits, alpha and beta maintained by internal disulfide bonds with molecular weights of approximately 30,000 Da.[6] The alpha subunit contains

92 amino acids (AA) and is identical in all glycoprotein hormones [LH, FSH, human chorionic gonadotropin (hCG), and thyroid-stimulating hormone (TSH)]. The alpha subunit is encoded by a single gene located on chromosome 6 (6q12-q21).[7] The beta subunit confers a unique receptor specificity as well as differential biological and immunological properties (Figs. 9.1A and B).[8] The LH beta subunit gene is located on chromosome 19 (19q13.32). Glycosylation, which is achieved by the attachment of carbohydrate moieties forming heterodimers, is fundamental for the differential spectrum of charges, bioactivities and half-lives of LH.[8,9] Moreover, the biological activity of LH is influenced by the addition of a sialic acid (sialylation) or sulfonic group (sulfonation) to the carbohydrate moieties.[8,10] The LH beta subunit has a single site of glycosylation (Asn 30) and few sialic acid residues (only 1 or 2) (Fig. 9.2). Native LH has a short half-life of only 20–30 minutes.[9,11] Pulsatile secretion of LH during the menstrual cycle varies: frequency is higher whereas amplitude is lower during follicular phase than the luteal phase. Moreover, LH bioactivity markedly differs: alkaline LH products with higher in vitro biological/immunological ratios are predominant in young women whereas long-lived acidic isoforms are found during menopause.[12,13]

This phenomenon is due to physiologic fluctuations in isoform profile during the menstrual cycle. Indeed, the degree of sialylation and sulfation

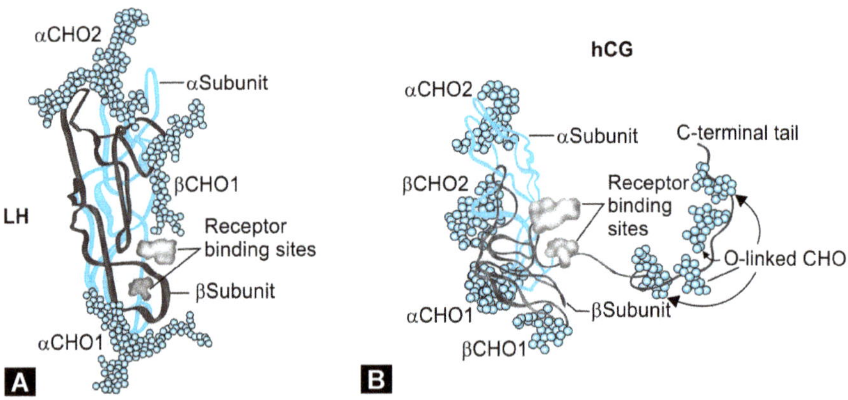

Figs. 9.1A and B: Luteinizing hormone and human chorionic gonadotropin molecules. (A) LH is a glycoprotein with two subunits, the alpha subunit (red), similar to that of FSH and hCG with two carbohydrate attachment sites, and the beta subunit (blue), with only one carbohydrate attachment site. The light purple balls represent the carbohydrate chains. (B) hCG is similar in its structural attributes to LH. A notable exception is the presence of a long carboxy-terminal segment that is O-glycosylated (O-linked CHO), conferring longer half-life to hCG. The alpha and beta subunits are represented in red and blue strands, respectively, whereas the light purple balls represent the carbohydrate chains.

(FSH: Follicle-stimulating hormone; hCG: Human chorionic gonadotropin; LH: Luteinizing hormone).

Source: Adapted with permission from Leao Rde B, Esteves SC. Gonadotropin therapy in assisted reproduction: an evolutionary perspective from biologics to biotech. Clinics (Sao Paulo). 2014;69:279-93.

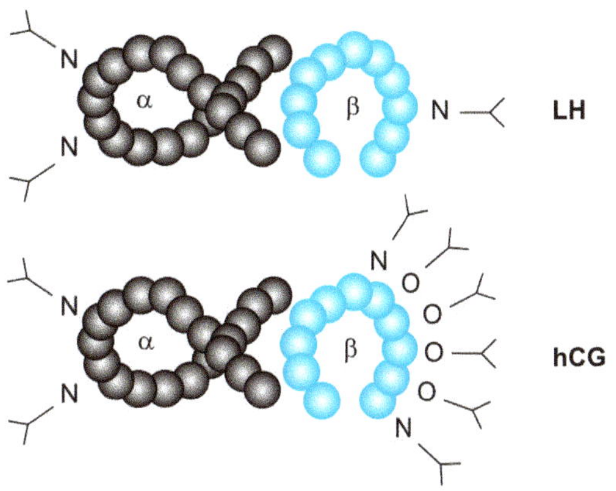

Fig. 9.2: Glycosylation patterns of LH and hCG. The alpha subunits of each hormone are identical in amino acid sequence and contain two sites of N-linked glycosylation. The beta subunit confers hormone specificity and contains variable amounts of N-linked glycosylation. LH beta subunit contains a single site of N-linked glycosylation, while hCG beta subunit contains two sites of N-linked glycosylation. Also, hCG has an extended C-terminal that includes four sites of O-linked glycosylation.
(LH: Luteinizing hormone; hCG: Human chorionic gonadotropin)
Source: Adapted with permission from Leao Rde B, Esteves SC. Gonadotropin therapy in assisted reproduction: an evolutionary perspective from biologics to biotech. Clinics (Sao Paulo). 2014;69:279-93.

affects LH half-life and determines in vivo and in vitro biopotency. More basic LH isoforms are observed at midcycle due to decreased sulfonation and increased sialylation. These changes increase LH half-life, thus explaining the increased levels of serum LH at this period. This shift in isoform profile seems to be physiologically important for ovulation triggering.[14]

Luteinizing hormone binds to specific G protein-coupled receptors (GPCRs) characterized by seven transmembrane domains and a large N-terminal extracellular region (Fig. 9.3).[15] As a distinctive feature of this glycoprotein hormone receptor, receptor activation requires that the hormone binds to the extracellular domain at the N-terminal region. Like FSH and TSH receptors, the LH receptor belongs to a large group of GPCRs. Whereas a single ligand activates FSH and TSH receptors, the LH receptor has both LH and hCG as its ligands.

The LH signaling pathway involves stimulation of adenylyl cyclase via G-protein receptor coupling, resulting in elevation of intracellular cAMP levels.[15] Furthermore, other second messengers are involved such as inositol triphosphate, calcium and mitogen-activated protein kinases.[16] LH receptors are expressed in both granulosa and theca cells. In the former, they reach their maximum concentration in preovulatory follicles. Antral follicles express these receptors at approximately 10% of the maximum.[17] Interestingly, recent data indicate that in granulosa cells, LH and FSH receptors can constitute functional heterodimer. This heterodimer could have specific functional characteristics, which differ from those of each homodimer.[15]

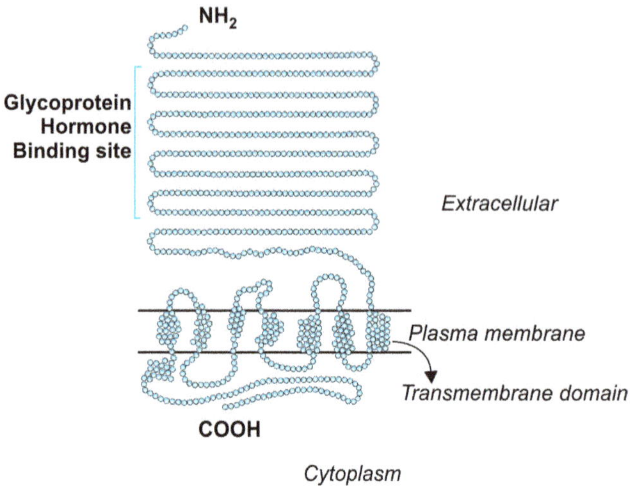

Fig. 9.3: LH/hCG receptor. LH receptors are included in the subgroup of G-protein coupled receptors. Such receptors are characterized by having seven-transmembrane domains and a large N-terminal extracellular region, which is the predominant site of hormone binding.

Metabolic and Physiological Function of Luteinizing Hormone

Luteinizing hormone is the central regulator of steroidogenesis in theca cells. The starting point of steroid biosynthesis is cholesterol, a carbon 27 (C27) steroid. Cholesterol is converted to pregnenolone (C21) by P450scc (CYP11A—cytochrome P450, family 11, subfamily A, polypeptide 1), whose regulation is mediated by steroidogenic acute regulatory protein (StAR).[10,18,19]

Pregnenolone metabolism is characterized by two routes. In the primary route (delta 5 pathway), pregnenolone is hydroxylated at the C17a and subsequently deacetalized to the androgen precursor dehydroepiandrosterone (DHEA). This action is mediated by CYP17 which has both hydroxylase and lyase activity. Lastly, DHEA is converted to androstenedione by 3 beta-hydroxysteroid dehydrogenase (3β-HSD).[19,20] In the secondary route of metabolism (delta 4 pathway), pregnenolone is converted to progesterone by the action of 3β-HSD. Progesterone is then converted to 17-hydroxyprogesterone by CYP17.[20] CYP17 is located exclusively in thecal and interstitial cells, whereas CYP19 (aromatase), which converts androgens to estrogens, is expressed only in granulosa cells. [20,21] Thus, aromatization of androgens to estrogens is carried out only granulosa cells induced by FSH receptor activation of the P450 aromatase (P450arom) gene. Androgens produced in the theca layer must diffuse into the granulosa layer to be converted to estrogens.

Theca and granulosa cells also secrete peptides that act as both autocrine and paracrine factors. Among these, insulin-like growth factor (IGF-I) and IGF-II, which are expressed in both granulosa and theca cells throughout folliculogenesis, are important in promoting follicular maturation.[22,23] IGFs enhance LH-mediated androgen production within the thecal compartment and FSH-mediated aromatization in granulosa cells.[24] Inhibin and activin are also two important modulators of steroidogenesis and follicle development. While inhibin stimulates androgen synthesis, activin has an opposite effect and sustains FSH action by increasing the expression of FSH receptors.[24]

Luteinizing hormone also acts in granulosa cells to stimulate progesterone production. Indeed, approximately 95% of progesterone is produced by the granulosa cells via the action of 3β-HSD that catalyzes the conversion of pregnenolone (delta-4 pathway); this pathway is under the influence of LH stimulation.[19,21,25] Peripheral concentrations of progesterone is limited by active liver metabolism. Progesterone can be further converted to 17-hydroxyprogesterone by CYP17 (delta-4 pathway). However, 17-hydroxyprogesterone is essentially the final product of delta-4 pathway in humans. The preovulatory rise in progesterone induces the positive feedback action of estrogen which in turn is the key factor to promote the midcycle LH peak in the natural cycle. Finally, progesterone also fosters a midcycle FSH surge, critical for supporting LH receptors expression in the granulosa layer.[26,27]

Role of Luteinizing Hormone during Folliculogenesis and Luteal Phase Support

During folliculogenesis LH plays two essential functions. The first, as explained in the previous session, consists in androgen production in the theca compartment. The second starts in the intermediate to late follicular phase[28,29] in which FSH induces LH receptor expression in the granulosa cells of developing follicles.[30] Progressively, the maturing follicle reduces its dependency on FSH by acquiring LH receptors and LH responsiveness.[31,32] FSH and LH cooperate in inducing the local production of various molecules necessary for follicular growth, including IGF-I, important for promoting follicular maturation,[23] and fibroblast growth factors which maintain calcium homeostasis and granulosa cell viability.[33] Additional growth modulators include endothelial-like growth factors (EGFs) that are also involved in granulosa cells proliferation, differentiation, and corpus luteum survival.[34,35] Finally, LH contributes to deselection of nondominant follicles. In fact, the developing follicles have specific LH requirements beyond which the maturation process is ceased.[1] In other words, each follicle has an established LH ceiling to continue the maturation process. LH ceiling may be higher in larger follicles and lower in those destined to atresia. Consequently, the increasing LH concentrations during folliculogenesis sustain progression of the leading follicles and favor degeneration of secondary follicles.[4] Notwithstanding, some investigators advocate that LH receptor expression governs the selection of dominant follicles; in other words, because small follicles do not express LH receptors, LH may indirectly promote their degeneration.[29,36]

During the luteal phase, LH sustains steroidogenic activity and corpus luteum.[37] Luteinizing hormone induces the up-regulation of growth factors, like vascular EGF-A,[37,38] which are implicated in luteal angiogenesis, and epidermal growth factor-like ligands (amphiregulin and epiregulin), which modulate apoptosis in luteinized human granulosa cells and sustains corpus luteum survival.[35] Furthermore, LH stimulates expression of cytokines involved in implantation[39] and seems to affect endometrial receptivity independently of ovarian functions.[40]

In conclusion, LH has a pivotal role in follicular development and maturation and is critical for maintaining corpus luteum function during the luteal phase.

GONADOTROPIN PREPARATIONS CONTAINING LUTEINIZING HORMONE ACTIVITY

Currently, there are three commercially available gonadotropin preparations containing LH activity: (1) conventional and highly purified human menopausal gonadotropin (hMG), in which LH activity is dependent on hCG rather than LH, (2) pure recombinant LH glycoprotein (lutropin alfa), and (3) a combination of recombinant FSH and LH in a fixed ratio of 2:1 also manufactured by recombinant technology (Table 9.1).

Menotropin

Human menopausal gonadotropin is obtained from the urine of postmenopausal women.[41,42] In the beginning, the preparations contained varying amounts of FSH, LH, and hCG, and only 5% of pure forms.[41,42] Improvements in the purification techniques standardized FSH and LH activities to 75 IU for each type of gonadotropin.

Luteinizing hormone activity in this preparation is primarily derived from hCG.[41,43] Sometimes hCG is added to achieve the desired amount of LH-like biological activity.[41]

At present, both conventional hMG and highly purified hMG (HP-hMG) are commercially available in vials containing FSH and LH at 1:1 ratio.[10] The enhanced purity of HP-hMG enabled subcutaneous delivery.[10]

Lutropin Alfa

Recombinant LH glycoprotein (lutropin alfa) was introduced in 2000. The manufacturing process of lutropin alfa involves recombinant technology in which the genes coding for human LH alpha and beta subunits are incorporated into the nuclear DNA of hamster ovary cells via a plasmid vector.[10]

Lutropin alfa is highly pure and has high biological activity (Table 9.1). It is presented in vials of 82.5 IU lyophilized pure glycoprotein powder to be reconstituted with a diluent before administration using a conventional

Table 9.1: Differences in luteinizing hormone (LH) activity among gonadotropin preparations.

	Purity (LH content)	*FSH activity (IU/vial)*	*LH activity (IU/vial)*	*hCG content (IU/vial)*	*Specific activity (LH/mg protein)*
Lutropin alfa	>99%	0	75	–	22,000
Follitropin alfa + lutropin alfa 2:1 ratio	>99%	150	75	–	22,000
HP-hMG	Unknown*	75	75*	~8	–

(FSH: Follicle-stimulating hormone; hCG: Human chorionic gonadotropin; HP-hMG: Highly purified human menopausal gonadotropin).
1 μg of lutropin alfa = 22 IU
*Derives primarily from the hCG component, which preferentially is concentrated during the purification process and sometimes was added to achieve the desired amount of LH-like biological activity.

syringe and needle (75 IU of lutropin alfa is delivered per vial). Lutropin alfa is intended for daily subcutaneous self-injections with good tolerability regarding pain at injection site. Due to the relatively short half-life (about one day), daily doses of lutropin alfa are needed during the stimulation period.[10,44]

Follitropin Alfa in Combination with Lutropin Alfa

A preparation containing both recombinant human follicle-stimulating hormone (r-hFSH) (follitropin alfa) and recombinant human luteinizing hormone (r-hLH) (lutropin alfa) at 2:1 ratio was introduced about 10 years ago.[45] The 2:1 ratio of FSH and LH in a fixed dose combination was obtained by recombinant technology and vial filling using protein mass (FbM). It is intended for daily subcutaneous injections and is presented in vials of lyophilized pure glycoprotein powder to be reconstituted with a diluent before administration using a conventional syringe and needle (150 IU of follitropin alfa and 75 IU of lutropin alfa is delivered per vial). This fixed 2:1 combination was demonstrated to be bioequivalent to r-hFSH and r-hLH administered separately, thus allowing the administration of both recombinant gonadotropins in a single injection.[46]

LUTEINIZING HORMONE SUPPLEMENTATION IN CLINICAL PRACTICE

On the one hand, fair evidence indicates that most normogonadotropic women do not need LH supplementation.[3,47] Indeed, residual circulating levels of endogenous LH after pituitary suppression are usually adequate to support multiple follicular growth in stimulated cycles.[48,49] It has been estimated that a minimum amount of LH is necessary to guarantee optimal follicle development during COS as only 1% of LH receptors need to be occupied to drive adequate ovarian steroidogenesis. According to some authors, the "LH window" for optimal androgen production of follicle maturation resides between 1.1 and 5.1 IU/L.[50,51]

On the other hand, there are distinct subgroups of women in which endogenous levels of LH are suboptimal during COS. For instance, patients with hypogonadotropic hypogonadism are not able to sustain adequate steroidogenesis by stimulation with FSH alone but resume sufficient estradiol production when LH is added.[50]

Moreover, response to FSH only-containing gonadotropins has shown to be suboptimal in normogonadotropic women with the following characteristics: (i) advanced reproductive age (≥35 years old),[52] (ii) poor ovarian reserve,[2,53] and (iii) highly suppressed levels of endogenous LH during COS.[54,55] Furthermore, normogonadotropic patients who require a high amount of FSH or show a steady response during COS, so-called "hyporesponders", seemed to benefit from LH supplementation.[56,57]

The possible clinical role of LH supplementation in the subgroups mentioned above could be explained by several factors, including reduced paracrine ovarian activity,[58] genetically-determined reduced LH bioactivity,[59] reduced androgen secretory capacity,[60] and decreased number of functional LH receptors.[61]

Furthermore, LH has also a direct effect on follicle growth and maturation, as already discussed, via different signaling pathways that positively impact oocyte quality.[62] Finally, recent data seemed to support the addition of LH for the prevention of ovarian hyperstimulation syndrome (OHSS),[63] as will be discussed later.

Hypogonadotropic Hypogonadism

The European Recombinant Human LH Study Group investigated the efficacy of recombinant LH in hypogonadotropic hypogonadal (WHO group I anovulation—LH levels of <1.2 IU/L; WHO group I anovulation).[50] Thirty-eight patients were randomized to receive 0, 25, 75, or 225 IU/day of r-hLH in addition to a fixed dose of r-hFSH (150 IU/day). In this study, r-hLH was able to promote a dose-related increase in estradiol and androstenedione. Furthermore, an increased ovarian sensitivity to FSH was observed in women who receive r-hLH. In detail, the proportion of women who developed follicles substantially increased according to the varying doses of r-hLH (42.8% in 25 IU, 77.8% and 80% in 75 IU and 225 IU, respectively).

A daily dose of 75 IU r-hLH was effective in the majority of women in promoting follicular development and endometrial growth.

The use of recombinant LH instead of HP-hMG seems to be the preferable option. In a recent randomized control trial, the efficacy of r-hFSH plus r-hLH in a 2:1 ratio was compared with HP-hMG urinary extract, in women with hypogonadotropic hypogonadism. In this study, pregnancy rates were significantly higher in r-hFSH + r-hLH group (55.6%) than in HP-hMG group in (23.3%) ($p = 0.01$).[64]

In conclusion, exogenous LH activity, preferably in the form of recombinant formulations, is mandatory in stimulation protocols applied to women with hypogonadotropic hypogonadism.

Advanced Age Women (More than 35-Year-Old)

The impact of LH administration on the ovarian response of advanced age women was studied using both the agonist and antagonist protocols.[52,65-70]

The addition of r-hLH to advanced age women undergoing COS has shown to offer advantages. Specifically, exogenous LH can increase androgen production, which levels are decreased in such patients.[71] As previously demonstrated, r-hFSH monotherapy cannot restore androgen synthesis in advanced age women.[72] LH supplementation may also counteract the increased apoptosis rate observed in granulosa cells,[62] which increases with aging. In detail, LH up-regulates several growth factors located in theca and granulosa,[73] thus exerting anti-apoptotic effects.[35] Lastly, recent studies demonstrated that endometrial LH receptors might modulate the embryo-endometrium crosstalk during implantation.[74] This phenomenon could partially explain the higher implantation rate observed in women of an advanced age supplemented with exogenous LH.[65]

The larger randomized controlled trial published to date comparing the effect of r-hLH during COS in GnRH antagonist cycles was carried out Bosch and colleagues. Their study involved 720 women undergoing their first or second IVF cycle.[65] The authors compared cycle outcome according to the use of r-hFSH or r-hFSH + r-hLH in an age-adjusted analysis. In the young population (up to 35-year-old), implantation rates and ongoing pregnancy rate per started cycle were similar. On the other hand, in older women (between 36–39 years), the implantation rate was significantly higher in the r-hFSH + r-LH group than in r-hFSH alone [odds ratio (OR) 1.56; 95% confidence interval (CI): 1.04–2.33, $p < 0.05$], albeit ongoing pregnancy rates per started cycle were not statistically different (33.5% versus 25.3%, $p > 0.05$).

Contrary results were reported by Konig et al. in a randomized controlled trial (RCT) involving 253 couples undergoing IVF/ICSI (intracytoplasmic sperm injection), and Vuong et al. in a RCT involving 240 women.[75] In the former, women of 35 years of age or greater received ovarian stimulation in a GnRH antagonist protocol with either r-hFSH or r-hFSH + r-hLH 150 IU/day starting on stimulation day 6. The intention-to-treat analysis revealed that implantation rates (18.8% vs 20.7%; mean difference 1.9%, 95% CI: –8.0 to 11.7) and clinical pregnancy rates (28.0% vs 29.7%; mean difference 1.5%, 95% CI: –9.4 to 12.7) did not differ between groups.

In the latter, Vuong et al. (2015)[70] conducted a RCT involving 240 women older than 34 years old (BMI < 28 kg/m^2 and ≤ 3 IVF attempts) who received ovarian stimulation with r-hFSH starting from cycle day 2 or day 3 in a GnRH antagonist protocol. On day 6, patients were randomized to either continue r-hFSH stimulation alone or r-hLH supplementation in a 2:1 r-hFSH/r-hLH ratio (150/75 IU/day). Live birth rates were not different between the groups (16.7% vs 17.5%, respectively), nor were the differences in the number of oocytes retrieved, implantation rate, miscarriage rate, and clinical pregnancy rate.

The discrepancies in the results between the study of Bosch et al. and the other two studies may be related to the different r-hLH timing adopted (day 1 in Bosch study versus day 6 in Konig and Vuong studies). Moreover, the latter enrolled women with various age ranges whereas Bosch et al. only included women up to 39 years old.

Likewise, several trials have investigated the effect of r-hLH in advanced age women using the GnRH agonist long protocol.[66-69,76,77]

A positive effect regarding implantation rate, clinical pregnancy rate, and live birth rate was observed by Marrs et al., Humaidan et al., and Matorras et al. trials.[68,69,76] On the other hand, no significant differences between r-hFSH alone regimen and r-FSH + r-hLH were detected by Fabregues et al. and Nyboe Andersen et al.[66,67,77] Moreover, Fabregues et al. reported significantly fewer oocytes retrieved and fewer MII oocytes in r-LH supplemented group than in the non-supplemented group. Notably, a positive effect of r-hLH was observed in those studies including only women between 35-year and 40-year-old.

The most recent systematic review and meta-analysis of the studies examining the age-related effect of LH supplementation in COS was conducted by Hill and colleagues in 2012.[52] The authors demonstrated that LH supplementation in women aged more than 34-year-old undergoing COS was beneficial. This meta-analysis included 7 RCTs (902 women) and compared COS using r-hFSH alone or in combination with r-hLH in both GnRH-agonist (5 trials) downregulation and GnRH-agonist micro-flare (2 trials). The dose and day of starting r-hLH supplementation varied among trials. Implantation (OR = 1.36; 95% CI: 1.05–1.78, $p < 0.05$) and clinical pregnancy rates (OR = 1.37; 95% CI: 1.03–1.83, $p < 0.05$) were significantly higher for women who received r-hLH in addition to r-hFSH compared with those in whom r-hFSH was administered alone.

In conclusion, evidence suggests that r-hLH supplementation has a positive effect on cycle outcome of older women between 35 years and 39 years. In women above 40 years old, it seems that the impact of age on ovarian reserve and oocyte quality (aneuploidy rates) become too relevant to be compensated by the r-hLH administration.

In antagonist regimen is preferable to adopt LH supplementation from the start of COS instead of the late follicular phase. Nevertheless, given the heterogeneity of the published data additional large RCTs are needed to drawn conclusive recommendations.

Poor Responders

The definition of poor responder women has been debated for several years. Up to 2010, 41 different definitions have been used in published RCTs. No more than three trials used the same definition, whereas even trials from the same research groups used different definitions. Only in 2011, an attempt to identify a specific definition of poor response was carried out. Nonetheless, even the new Bologna criteria were criticized for including heterogeneous populations with different characteristics and clinical prognosis.[78-80] Very recently, in 2016, another classification has been proposed by a panel of experts. This new classification introduced by the Poseidon group (Patient-Oriented Strategies Encompassing IndividualizeD Oocyte Number) advocates patient subgrouping according to low prognosis categories rather than poor ovarian response (POR).[79] Nonetheless, the utility of these new criteria in clinical practice is still under investigation.

As for poor responders, several RCTs and meta-analysis investigated the effect of r-hLH.[2,53,81-84] A meta-analysis by Mochtar et al. showed higher ongoing pregnancy rates (OR = 1.85; 95% CI: 1.1–3.11) in patients treated with r-hFSH plus r-hLH than r-hFSH alone. These authors pooled three RCTs including 310 participants. Another meta-analysis by Bosdou et al. which included 7 RCTs and 603 patients classified as poor responders, failed to detect differences in clinical pregnancy between patients receiving LH supplementation or not.[84] However, the definition criteria for poor responders was not uniform in the studies mentioned above. Moreover, even patients with adequate ovarian reserve but slow/hypo-response to gonadotropin stimulation were included as "poor responders". Lastly, the protocols of stimulation, LH dosage, and starting day of r-hLH differed or were not described, thus limiting the validity of the findings.

Recently, a large meta-analysis assessed the outcomes of r-hFSH plus r-hLH versus r-hFSH alone in poor responders undergoing ovarian stimulation in association with GnRH analogs for ART.[53] Although the studies included in meta-analysis were published prior to Bologna consensus, in 10 of the 14 studies, the definition of POR was aligned with Bologna criteria definition. In this meta-analysis, significantly more oocytes were retrieved (12 studies, n = 1077; weighted mean difference +0.75 oocytes; 95% CI: 0.14–1.36) and higher clinical pregnancy rates [14 studies, n = 1179; relative risk (RR): 1.30; 95% CI: 1.01–1.67; intention to treat population] were obtained with r-hFSH plus r-hLH versus r-hFSH

Collectively, the literature is mixed regarding the clinical effect of r-hLH supplementation in poor responder women. Although it seems that the number of oocytes retrieved and clinical pregnancy rates are higher in the poor responder population undergoing r-hFSH plus r-hLH stimulation, caution should be given to interpreting results for the extensive heterogeneity in the criteria with which the poor responder population is classified.

In addition, preliminary results from Efficacy and Safety of Pergoveris in Assisted Reproductive Technology (ESPART) study failed to find any differences in terms of oocytes retrieved between poor ovarian responders receiving fixed-ratio combination r-hFSH plus r-hLH and those receiving r-hFSH alone in women classified as poor responders according to Bologna criteria.[85]

Hypo-responders

The concept of "hypo-response" to COS has been proposed to identify normogonadotropic young women with normal ovarian reserve and at first hand with good prognosis for COS who turn out to (i) require high amounts of r-hFSH (e.g. >2,500 IU total dose) to obtain an adequate number (i.e. >4) of oocytes retrieved or (ii) who show a steady response during COS in terms of number of follicles and/or estradiol levels.[56,57] These women differ from classical poor responders because they are usually young (<39 years) and ovarian biomarkers [anti-Müllerian hormone (AMH)/antral follicle count (AFC)] are within normal ranges. The pathogenesis of hypo-response to FSH monotherapy is not entirely understood, but it has been hypothesized that hypo-response could be a genetically determined condition.[86,87] Some evidence indicates that this condition is associated with the presence of specific genetic polymorphism involving beta chain of LH (v-betaLH), and FSH receptor (FSH-R).[88,89]

The role of LH supplementation in hypo-responders was evaluated by Ferraretti and colleagues, who conducted a RCT involving 184 patients (age <38 years).[90] The mean number of oocytes retrieved was significantly lower in hypo-responders treated with r-hFSH step-up versus the group in which recombinant LH was added during ovarian stimulation. Pregnancy rates were also substantially higher in the group treated with r-hLH plus r-hFSH dose compared with both the patients receiving r-hFSH alone and hMG. Finally, live birth rates in r-hLH (40.7%) group was twofold higher than the r-hFSH alone group (22%); however, this difference did not reach statistical significance.

These results were confirmed later by De Placido and colleagues, in a multicenter RCT involving a total of 117 IVF/ICSI cycles.[56] In detail, the number of oocytes retrieved was significantly higher in the patients who received r-hLH supplementation (9.0 ± 4.3) compared with those in whom an increased dose of r-hFSH was administered (6.1 ± 2.6; $p < 0.01$). Furthermore, implantation and ongoing pregnancy rates were similar in "hypo-responders" treated with r-hLH and "normal responders" women.

Ruvolo et al. performed an RCT to verify whether r-hLH could improve oocyte quality in women with a hypo-response profile.[62] In this study, only women with a history of previous stimulation with high r-hFSH doses (>3,000 IU) was included. The apoptosis rate in cumulus cells was significantly lower in women who received r-hLH than those in the r-hFSH-alone group. Also, pregnancy and implantation rates were significantly higher in the r-hLH-supplemented group than in the non supplemented group.

Recently, a single center prospective study confirmed the results mentioned above.[91] The authors explored the effect of r-hLH supplementation in hypo-responders, according to the classification of De Placido et al.[56,57] Implantation rates were significantly higher in the r-hLH supplementation (36.1%) group than in the increased-dose r-hFSH group (15%, $p < 0.02$). The pregnancy rates were also higher in the former group than in the latter group.

In conclusion, these studies reinforced the idea that hypo-responders may benefit from LH supplementation. In this scenario, r-hLH can be started at the mid-follicular phase in the attempt to rescue the ongoing cycle or at stimulation day one in a subsequent cycle. The role of recombinant LH supplementation in hypo-responder women undergoing COS in association with the GnRH antagonist protocol remains to be established.

Deeply Suppressed Luteinizing Hormone Levels

Profound suppression of LH levels after GnRH agonist downregulation is found in 7–48% of normogonadotrophic women undergoing COS.[92-95] This variation might be related to the type of molecules and dosage adopted. For instance, intranasal administration of buserelin resulted in significantly less depressed levels of mid-follicular LH than subcutaneous administration. Also, suppressed steroidogenesis and follicular development seem to be more evident with buserelin than leuprolide acetate.[92,95]

Preliminary studies suggested that ovarian response and IVF cycle outcome could be impaired when mid-follicular serum LH levels are between 0.5 UI/L and 0.7 UI/L after downregulation with GnRH agonist.[96,97]

Westergaard and colleagues[93] observed that 49% women stimulated with r-hFSH after pituitary suppression with buserelin acetate (0.5 mg SC daily) achieved very low concentrations of LH for 14 days in the mid-follicular phase (<0.5 IU/L). Compared with the normal LH group, these women had significantly lower serum estradiol concentrations on stimulation day 8 (1349 ± 101 vs 2908 ± 225 pmol/L; $p < 0.001$). Furthermore, a fivefold higher risk of early pregnancy loss was observed in the low LH group (45% vs 9%; $p < 0.005$).

On the other hand, Fleming and colleagues[94] found that 26% of women treated with highly purified or recombinant FSH and GnRH agonist (type and dose not reported) had LH levels less than 0.7 IU/L on stimulation day 7. Nonetheless, no effect on pregnancy outcome was observed irrespective of the level of LH suppression.

Humaidan and colleagues also evaluated the effect of LH levels on stimulation day 8 on ovarian response and pregnancy outcome.[61] In this study, only 12% of the patients showed LH concentration below 0.5 IU/L. Notably, the frequency of fertilized oocytes was significantly lower in the group with profound LH suppression than the group with normal LH levels ($p < 0.05$). Likewise in the study of Fleming and colleagues, pregnancy and implantation rates were not significantly affected by profound mid-follicular LH suppression. Altogether, these data indicate that deeply-suppressed LH levels in GnRH agonist treated women could play a role on the ovarian response of stimulated cycles.

Nonetheless, the utility of LH supplementation in those women during COS is still a matter of debate. The only study specifically investigating this issue suggested that women with LH levels below 0.5 IU/L might benefit from r-hLH supplementation as regards the clinical pregnancy rates.[55] However, the higher number of embryos transferred in r-hLH (2.72 ± 0.22 vs 1.97 ± 0.91, $p < 0.001$) could have influenced the results of the study mentioned above. Interestingly, even studies carried out by the same group have shown conflicting results. For instance, in their first study Lisi et al. observed an increased implantation rate in women with levels of LH below 1.0 mIU/mL;[54] this effect, however, was not confirmed in their subsequent study.[98]

In conclusion, the evidence is not sufficiently high to suggest r-hLH supplementation in women with suppressed endogenous LH after of GnRH agonist suppression.

Luteinizing Hormone in the Prevention of Ovarian Hyperstimulation Syndrome

Many strategies have been proposed to prevent or limit the occurrence of OHSS.[99] Recently, the clinical utility of adding r-hLH to good prognosis normogonadotropic women undergoing ART has been investigated in a large RCT.[63] A possible explanation for the beneficial effect observed may relate to the fact that these selected patients achieved a "ceiling effect" after the addition of r-hLH, which resulted in a reduction of the number of selected follicles.[4] In this study, the authors investigated 999 infertile women aged less than or equal to 40 years old with basal FSH levels less than or equal to 12 mIU/m. The study population was randomized to receive r-hFSH alone ($n = 501$) or r-hFSH + r-hLH ($n = 498$). r-hLH supplementation was given at a dose of 75 IU/day from stimulation day 7 onward. The proportion of canceled cycles due to OHSS risk (8.3% vs 2.4%, $p < 0.001$) and clinical OHSS was significantly higher in the r-hFSH alone group than in the r-hFSH + r-hLH group (1.6% vs 0.2%, $p < 0.05$).

While these preliminary results are encouraging, more trials are necessary before a firm conclusion can be drawn.

CONCLUSION

Although FSH is the key gonadotropin to promote follicular recruitment and growth during COS, the importance of LH has been revisited. At present, the consensus is that most women have sufficient levels of endogenous LH to support ovarian stimulation with FSH alone. However, 15–40% of the patients undergoing ART have less sensitive ovaries, and fair evidence suggests that LH supplementation to FSH regimen can be advantageous during COS. Currently, three gonadotropin formulations deliver LH activity:

(1) hMG (with LH activity originated from hCG), (2) r-hLH, and (3) a fixed combination of r-hFSH and r-hLH at 2:1 ratio. The patients most likely to benefit from LH supplementation include (i) older patients (between 35 years and 39 years), (ii) hypo-responders and (iii) poor responders. The utility of recombinant LH supplementation in the prevention of OHSS syndrome need to be confirmed by further trials; however, the preliminary evidence is encouraging. Nevertheless, the specific requirements regarding LH dosages for optimal follicular development during the follicular phase of stimulated cycles has not been defined yet. Future clinical research should consider these aspects to aid in the development of better therapeutic strategies.

REFERENCES

1. Hillier SG, Whitelaw PF, Smyth CD. Follicular oestrogen synthesis: the 'two-cell, two-gonadotrophin' model revisited. Mol Cell Endocrinol. 1994;100:51-4.
2. Mochtar MH, Van der Veen, Ziech M, et al. Recombinant Luteinizing Hormone (rLH) for controlled ovarian hyperstimulation in assisted reproductive cycles. Cochrane Database Syst Rev. 2007;2:CD005070.
3. Kolibianakis EM, Kalogeropoulou L, Griesinger G, et al. Among patients treated with FSH and GnRH analogues for in vitro fertilization, is the addition of recombinant LH associated with the probability of live birth: a systematic review and meta-analysis. Hum Reprod Update. 2007;13:445-52.
4. Alviggi C, Clarizia R, Mollo A, et al. Who needs LH in ovarian stimulation? Reprod Biomed Online. 2011;22:S33-41.
5. Speroff L, Fritz M. Neuroendocrinology. In: Wilkins LW. (Ed). Clinical gynecologic Endocrinology and Infertility. 2005. pp. 157-99.
6. Palermo R. Differential actions of FSH and LH during folliculogenesis. Reprod Biomed Online. 2007;15:326-37.
7. Fiddes JC, Goodman HM. Isolation, cloning and sequence analysis of the cDNA for the alpha-subunit of human chorionic gonadotropin. Nature. 1979;281: 351-6.
8. Ulloa-Aguirre A, Espinoza R, Damian-Matsumura P, et al. Immunological and biological potencies of the different molecular species of gonadotrophins. Hum Reprod (Oxford, England). 1988;3:491-501.
9. Wide L, Naessen T, Sundstrom-Poromaa I, et al. Sulfonation and sialylation of gonadotropins in women during the menstrual cycle, after menopause, and with polycystic ovarian syndrome and in men. J Clin Endocrinol Metabol. 2007;92:4410-7.
10. Leao Rde B, Esteves SC. Gonadotropin therapy in assisted reproduction: an evolutionary perspective from biologics to biotech. Clinics (Sao Paulo, Brazil). 2014;69:279-93.
11. Campbell RK. Molecular pharmacology of gonadotropins. Endocrine. 2005;26: 291-6.
12. Fauser BC, Pache TD, Hop WC, et al. The significance of a single serum LH measurement in women with cycle disturbances: discrepancies between immunoreactive and bioactive hormone estimates. Clin Endocrinol. 1992;37:445-52.
13. Imse V, Holzapfel G, Hinney B, et al. Comparison of luteinizing hormone pulsatility in the serum of women suffering from polycystic ovarian disease using a bioassay and five different immunoassays. J Clin Endocrinol Metabol. 1992;74:1053-61.

14. Combarnous Y. Molecular basis of the specificity of binding of glycoprotein hormones to their receptors. Endocr Rev. 1992;13:670-91.
15. Costagliola S, Urizar E, Mendive F, et al. Specificity and promiscuity of gonadotropin receptors. Reproduction. 2005;130:275-81.
16. Themmen APN, Huhtaniemi IT. Mutations of gonadotropins and gonadotropin receptors: elucidating the physiology and pathophysiology of pituitary-gonadal function. Endocr Rev. 2000;21:551-83.
17. Jeppesen JV, Kristensen SG, Nielsen ME, et al. LH-receptor gene expression in human granulosa and cumulus cells from antral and preovulatory follicles. J Clin Endocrinol Metabol. 2012;97:E1524-31.
18. Alviggi C, Mollo A, Clarizia R, et al. Exploiting LH in ovarian stimulation. Reprod Biomed Online. 2006;12:221-33.
19. Wickenheisser JK, Nelson-DeGrave VL, McAllister JM. Human ovarian theca cells in culture. Trends Endocrinol Metab. 2006;17:65-71.
20. Smyth CD, Miro F, Whitelaw PF, et al. Ovarian thecal/interstitial androgen synthesis is enhanced by a follicle-stimulating hormone-stimulated paracrine mechanism. Endocrinology. 1993;133:1532-8.
21. Whitelaw PF, Smyth CD, Howles CM, et al. Cell-specific expression of aromatase and LH receptor mRNAs in rat ovary. J Mol Endocrinol. 1992;9:309-12.
22. Zhou J, Bondy C. Anatomy of the human ovarian insulin-like growth factor system. Biol Reprod. 1993;48:467-82.
23. Huang ZH, Clayton PE, Brady G, et al. Insulin-like growth factor-I gene expression in human granulosa-lutein cells. J Mol Endocrinology. 1994;12:283-91.
24. Speroff L, Fritz MA. Hormone biosynthesis, metabolism, and mechanisms of action. Steroidogenesis. In: Wilkins LW (Ed). Clinical Gynecologic Endocrinology and Infertility. Philadelphia: Lippincott Williams & Wilkins; 2005. pp. 109-16.
25. Miller WL. Steroidogenic enzymes. Endocr Dev. 2008;13:1-18.
26. Filicori M, Cognigni GE, Taraborrelli S, et al. Luteinizing hormone activity supplementation enhances follicle-stimulating hormone efficacy and improves ovulation induction outcome. J Clin Endocrinol Metab. 1999;84:2659-63.
27. Couzinet B, Brailly S, Bouchard P, et al. Progesterone stimulates luteinizing hormone secretion by acting directly on the pituitary. J Clin Endocrinol Metab. 1992;74:374-8.
28. Willis DS, Watson H, Mason HD, et al. Premature response to luteinizing hormone of granulosa cells from anovulatory women with polycystic ovary syndrome: relevance to mechanism of anovulation. J Clin Endocrinol Metab. 1998;83:3984-91.
29. Filicori M, Cognigni GE, Pocognoli P, et al. Current concepts and novel applications of LH activity in ovarian stimulation. Trends Endocrinol Metab. 2003;14: 267-73.
30. Zeleznik AJ, Hillier SG. The role of gonadotropins in the selection of the preovulatory follicle. Clin Obstet Gynecol. 1984;27:927-40.
31. Sullivan MW, Stewart-Akers A, Krasnow JS, et al. Ovarian responses in women to recombinant follicle-stimulating hormone and luteinizing hormone (LH): a role for LH in the final stages of follicular maturation. J Clin Endocrinol Metabol. 1999;84:228-32.
32. Campbell BK, Dobson H, Baird DT, et al. Examination of the relative role of FSH and LH in the mechanism of ovulatory follicle selection in sheep. J Reprod Fertil. 1999;117:355-67.
33. Peluso JJ, Pappalardo A, Fernandez G. Basic fibroblast growth factor maintains calcium homeostasis and granulosa cell viability by stimulating calcium efflux via a PKC delta-dependent pathway. Endocrinol. 2001;142:4203-11.

34. Park JY, Su YQ, Ariga M, et al. EGF-like growth factors as mediators of LH action in the ovulatory follicle. Science. 2004;303:682-4.
35. Ben-Ami I, Armon L, Freimann S, et al. EGF-like growth factors as LH mediators in the human corpus luteum. Hum Reprod. 2009;24:176-84.
36. Filicori M, Cognigni GE, Ciampaglia W. What clinical evidence for an LH ceiling? Hum Reprod. 2003;18:1556-7.
37. Wang TH, Horng SG, Chang CL, et al. Human chorionic gonadotropin-induced ovarian hyperstimulation syndrome is associated with up-regulation of vascular endothelial growth factor. J Clin Endocrinol Metabol. 2002;87:3300-8.
38. Sugino N, Kashida S, Takiguchi S, et al. Expression of vascular endothelial growth factor and its receptors in the human corpus luteum during the menstrual cycle and in early pregnancy. J Clin Endocrinol Metabol. 2000;85:3919-24.
39. Licht P, Russu V, Wildt L. On the role of human chorionic gonadotropin (hCG) in the embryo-endometrial microenvironment: implications for differentiation and implantation. Semin Reprod Med. 2001;19:37-47.
40. Tesarik J, Hazout A, Mendoza C. Luteinizing hormone affects uterine receptivity independently of ovarian function. Reprod Biomed Online. 2003;7:59-64.
41. Lunenfeld B. Historical perspectives in gonadotrophin therapy. Hum Reprod Update. 2004;10:453-67.
42. Beall SA, DeCherney A. History and challenges surrounding ovarian stimulation in the treatment of infertility. Fertil Steril. 2012;97:795-801.
43. Cole LA, Khanlian SA, Muller CY. Normal production of human chorionic gonadotropin in perimenopausal and menopausal women and after oophorectomy. Int J Gynecol Cancer. 2009;19:1556-9.
44. Practice Committee of American Society for Reproductive Medicine. Gonadotropin preparations: past, present, and future perspectives. Fertil Steril. 2008;90:S13-20.
45. Bosch E. Recombinant human follicular stimulating hormone and recombinant human luteinizing hormone in a 2:1 ratio combination. Pharmacological characteristics and clinical applications. Expert Opin Biol Ther. 2010;10:1001-9.
46. Picard M, Rossier C, Papasouliotis O, et al. Bioequivalence of recombinant human FSH and recombinant human LH in a fixed 2:1 combination: two phase I, randomised, crossover studies. Curr Med Res Opin. 2008;24:1199-208.
47. Esteves SC, Schertz JC, Verza S Jr, et al. A comparison of menotropin, highly-purified menotropin and follitropin alfa in cycles of intracytoplasmic sperm injection. Reprod Biol Endocrinol. 2009;7:111.
48. Loumaye E, Engrand P, Howles CM, et al. Assessment of the role of serum luteinizing hormone and estradiol response to follicle-stimulating hormone on in vitro fertilization treatment outcome. Fertil Steril. 1997;67:889-99.
49. Sills ES, Levy DP, Moomjy M, et al. A prospective, randomized comparison of ovulation induction using highly purified follicle-stimulating hormone alone and with recombinant human luteinizing hormone in in-vitro fertilization. Hum Reprod. 1999;14:2230-5.
50. Recombinant human luteinizing hormone (LH) to support recombinant human follicle-stimulating hormone (FSH)-induced follicular development in LH- and FSH-deficient anovulatory women: a dose-finding study. The European Recombinant Human LH Study Group. J Clinical Endocrinol Metab. 1998;83:1507-14.
51. Shoham Z, Smith H, Yeko T, et al. Recombinant LH (lutropin alfa) for the treatment of hypogonadotrophic women with profound LH deficiency: a randomized, double-blind, placebo-controlled, proof-of-efficacy study. Clin Endocrinol (Oxf). 2008;69:471-8.
52. Hill MJ, Levens ED, Levy G, et al. The use of recombinant luteinizing hormone in patients undergoing assisted reproductive techniques with advanced reproductive age: a systematic review and meta-analysis. Fertil Steril. 2012;97:1108-14.e1.

53. Lehert P, Kolibianakis EM, Venetis CA, et al. Recombinant human follicle-stimulating hormone (r-hFSH) plus recombinant luteinizing hormone versus r-hFSH alone for ovarian stimulation during assisted reproductive technology: systematic review and meta-analysis. Reprod Biol Endocrinol. 2014;12:17.
54. Lisi F, Rinaldi L, Fishel S, et al. Use of recombinant LH in a group of unselected IVF patients. Reprod Biomed Online. 2002;5:104-8.
55. Pezzuto A, Ferrari B, Coppola F, et al. LH supplementation in down-regulated women undergoing assisted reproduction with baseline low serum LH levels. Gynecol Endocrinol. 2010;26:118-24.
56. De Placido G, Alviggi C, Perino A, et al. Recombinant human LH supplementation versus recombinant human FSH (rFSH) step-up protocol during controlled ovarian stimulation in normogonadotrophic women with initial inadequate ovarian response to rFSH. A multicentre, prospective, randomized controlled trial. Hum Reprod. 2005;20:390-6.
57. De Placido G, Alviggi C, Mollo A, et al. Effects of recombinant LH (rLH) supplementation during controlled ovarian hyperstimulation (COH) in normogonadotrophic women with an initial inadequate response to recombinant FSH (rFSH) after pituitary downregulation. Clin Endocrinol. 2004;60:637-43.
58. Hurwitz JM, Santoro N. Inhibins, activins, and follistatin in the aging female and male. Semin Reprod Med. 2004;22:209-17.
59. Alviggi C, Clarizia R, Pettersson K, et al. Suboptimal response to GnRHa long protocol is associated with a common LH polymorphism. Reprod Biomed Online. 2009;18:9-14.
60. Piltonen T, Koivunen R, Ruokonen A, et al. Ovarian age-related responsiveness to human chorionic gonadotropin. J Clinical Endocrinol Metabol. 2003;88:3327-32.
61. Vihko KK, Kujansuu E, Morsky P, et al. Gonadotropins and gonadotropin receptors during the perimenopause. Eur J Endocrinol. 1996;134:357-61.
62. Ruvolo G, Bosco L, Pane A, et al. Lower apoptosis rate in human cumulus cells after administration of recombinant luteinizing hormone to women undergoing ovarian stimulation for in vitro fertilization procedures. Fertil Steril. 2007;87:542-6.
63. Caserta D, Lisi F, Marci R, et al. Does supplementation with recombinant luteinizing hormone prevent ovarian hyperstimulation syndrome in down regulated patients undergoing recombinant follicle stimulating hormone multiple follicular stimulation for IVF/ET and reduces cancellation rate for high risk of hyperstimulation? Gynecol Endocrinol. 2011;27:862-6.
64. Carone D, Caropreso C, Vitti A, et al. Efficacy of different gonadotropin combinations to support ovulation induction in WHO type I anovulation infertility: clinical evidences of human recombinant FSH/human recombinant LH in a 2:1 ratio and highly purified human menopausal gonadotropin stimulation protocols. J Endocrinol Invest. 2012;35:996-1002.
65. Bosch E, Labarta E, Crespo J, et al. Impact of luteinizing hormone administration on gonadotropin-releasing hormone antagonist cycles: an age-adjusted analysis. Fertil Sterility. 2011;95:1031-6.
66. Fabregues F, Creus M, Penarrubia J, et al. Effects of recombinant human luteinizing hormone supplementation on ovarian stimulation and the implantation rate in down-regulated women of advanced reproductive age. Fertil Steril. 2006;85:925-31.
67. Fabregues F, Iraola A, Casals G, et al. Evaluation of two doses of recombinant human luteinizing hormone supplementation in down-regulated women of advanced reproductive age undergoing follicular stimulation for IVF: a randomized clinical study. Eur J Obstet Gynecol Reprod Biol. 2011;158:56-61.
68. Marrs R, Meldrum D, Muasher S, et al. Randomized trial to compare the effect of recombinant human FSH (follitropin alfa) with or without recombinant

human LH in women undergoing assisted reproduction treatment. Reprod Biomed Online. 2004;8:175-82.
69. Matorras R, Prieto B, Exposito A, et al. Mid-follicular LH supplementation in women aged 35-39 years undergoing ICSI cycles: a randomized controlled study. Reprod Biomed Online. 2009;19:879-87.
70. Vuong TN, Phung HT, Ho MT. Recombinant follicle-stimulating hormone and recombinant luteinizing hormone versus recombinant follicle-stimulating hormone alone during GnRH antagonist ovarian stimulation in patients aged >/= 35 years: a randomized controlled trial. Hum Reprod. 2015;30:1188-95.
71. Davison SL, Bell R, Donath S, et al. Androgen levels in adult females: changes with age, menopause, and oophorectomy. J Clin Endocrinol Metabol. 2005;90:3847-53.
72. Welt CK, Jimenez Y, Sluss PM, et al. Control of estradiol secretion in reproductive ageing. Hum Reprod. 2006;21:2189-93.
73. Rimon E, Sasson R, Dantes A, et al. Gonadotropin-induced gene regulation in human granulosa cells obtained from IVF patients: modulation of genes coding for growth factors and their receptors and genes involved in cancer and other diseases. Int J Oncol. 2004;24:1325-38.
74. Gridelet V, Tsampalas M, Berndt S, et al. Evidence for cross-talk between the LH receptor and LH during implantation in mice. Reproduction, fertility, and development. 2013;25:511-22.
75. Konig TE, van der Houwen LE, Overbeek A, et al. Recombinant LH supplementation to a standard GnRH antagonist protocol in women of 35 years or older undergoing IVF/ICSI: a randomized controlled multicentre study. Hum Reprod. 2013;28:2804-12.
76. Humaidan P, Bungum M, Bungum L, et al. Effects of recombinant LH supplementation in women undergoing assisted reproduction with GnRH agonist down-regulation and stimulation with recombinant FSH: An opening study. Reprod Biomed Online. 2004;8:635-43.
77. Nyboe Andersen A, Humaidan P, Fried G, et al. Recombinant LH supplementation to recombinant FSH during the final days of controlled ovarian stimulation for in vitro fertilization. A multicentre, prospective, randomized, controlled trial. Hum Reprod. 2008;23:427-34.
78. Venetis CA. The Bologna criteria for poor ovarian response: the good, the bad and the way forward. Hum Reprod. 2014;29:1839-41.
79. Alviggi C, Andersen CY, Buehler K, et al. A new more detailed stratification of low responders to ovarian stimulation: from a poor ovarian response to a low prognosis concept. Fertil Steril. 2016;105:1452-3.
80. Papathanasiou A. Implementing the ESHRE 'poor responder' criteria in research studies: methodological implications. Hum Reprod. 2014;29:1835-8.
81. Barrenetxea G, Agirregoikoa JA, Jimenez MR, et al. Ovarian response and pregnancy outcome in poor-responder women: a randomized controlled trial on the effect of luteinizing hormone supplementation on in vitro fertilization cycles. Fertil Steril. 2008;89:546-53.
82. Berkkanoglu M, Isikoglu M, Aydin D, et al. Clinical effects of ovulation induction with recombinant follicle-stimulating hormone supplemented with recombinant luteinizing hormone or low-dose recombinant human chorionic gonadotropin in the midfollicular phase in microdose cycles in poor responders. Fertil Steril. 2007;88:665-9.
83. Ferraretti AP, Gianaroli L, Motrenko T, et al. LH pretreatment as a novel strategy for poor responders. Biomed Res Int. 2014;2014:926172.
84. Bosdou JK, Venetis CA, Kolibianakis EM, et al. The use of androgens or androgen-modulating agents in poor responders undergoing in vitro fertilization: a systematic review and meta-analysis. Hum Reprod Update. 2012;18:127-45.

85. Humaidan P, Chin W, Rogoff D. Abstracts of the 32nd Annual Meeting of the European Society of Human Reproduction and Embryology. Human Reproduction. 2016;31:i1-i513.
86. Alviggi C, Conforti A, Esteves SC. Impact of mutations and polymorphisms of gonadotrophins and their receptors on the outcome of controlled ovarian stimulation. In: Ghumman S (Ed). Principles and Practice of Controlled Ovarian Stimulation in ART. India, New Delh: Springer; 2015. pp. 147-56.
87. Alviggi C, Conforti A, Fabozzi F, et al. Ovarian stimulation for IVF/ICSI cycles: A pharmacogenomic approach. Medecine Therapeutique Medecine de la Reproduction, Gynecologie et Endocrinologie. 2009;11:271-7.
88. Alviggi C, Conforti A, Caprio F, et al. In Estimated Good Prognosis Patients Could Unexpected "Hyporesponse" to Controlled Ovarian Stimulation be Related to Genetic Polymorphisms of FSH Receptor? Reprod Sci. 2016;23:1103-8.
89. Alviggi C, Pettersson K, Longobardi S, et al. A common polymorphic allele of the LH beta-subunit gene is associated with higher exogenous FSH consumption during controlled ovarian stimulation for assisted reproductive technology. Reprod Biol Endocrinol. 2013;11:51.
90. Ferraretti AP, Gianaroli L, Magli MC, et al. Exogenous luteinizing hormone in controlled ovarian hyperstimulation for assisted reproduction techniques. Fertil Steril. 2004;82:1521-6.
91. Yazici Yilmaz F, Gorkemli H, Colakoglu MC, et al. The evaluation of recombinant LH supplementation in patients with suboptimal response to recombinant FSH undergoing IVF treatment with GnRH agonist down-regulation. Gynecol Endocrinol. Official journal of the International Society of Gynecological Endocrinology. 2015;31:141-4.
92. Humaidan P, Bungum L, Bungum M, et al. Ovarian response and pregnancy outcome related to mid-follicular LH levels in women undergoing assisted reproduction with GnRH agonist down-regulation and recombinant FSH stimulation. Hum Reprod. 2002;17:2016-21.
93. Westergaard LG, Laursen SB, Andersen CY. Increased risk of early pregnancy loss by profound suppression of luteinizing hormone during ovarian stimulation in normogonadotrophic women undergoing assisted reproduction. Hum Reprod. 2000;15:1003-8.
94. Fleming R, Rehka P, Deshpande N, et al. Suppression of LH during ovarian stimulation: effects differ in cycles stimulated with purified urinary FSH and recombinant FSH. Hum Reprod. 2000;15:1440-5.
95. Balasch J, Vidal E, Penarrubia J, et al. Suppression of LH during ovarian stimulation: analysing threshold values and effects on ovarian response and the outcome of assisted reproduction in down-regulated women stimulated with recombinant FSH. Hum Reprod. 2001;16:1636-43.
96. Esposito MA, Barnhart KT, Coutifaris C, et al. Role of periovulatory luteinizing hormone concentrations during assisted reproductive technology cycles stimulated exclusively with recombinant follicle-stimulating hormone. Fertil Steril. 2001;75:519-24.
97. Nakagawa K, Ohgi S, Nakashima A, et al. The ratio of late-follicular to mid-follicular phase LH concentrations efficiently predicts ART outcomes in women undergoing ART treatment with GnRH-agonist long protocol and stimulation with recombinant FSH. Journal of assisted reproduction and genetics. 2008;25:359-64.
98. Lisi F, Rinaldi L, Fishel S, et al. Evaluation of two doses of recombinant luteinizing hormone supplementation in an unselected group of women undergoing follicular stimulation for in vitro fertilization. Fertil Steril. 2005;83:309-15.
99. Humaidan P, Quartarolo J, Papanikolaou EG. Preventing ovarian hyperstimulation syndrome: guidance for the clinician. Fertil Steril. 2010;94:389-400.

Chapter 10

Adjuvant Treatments in Low Ovarian Response

Alfredo Guillén

INTRODUCTION

The management of patients with low ovarian reserve is one of the most important challenges in every day practice in the infertility clinic. The percentage of this subgroup of patients is variable among centers and the prevalence in the literature ranges between 9% and 24%.[1] There is a clear tendency to delay the age of the first pregnancy and patients are referred or decide to go to fertility units at more advanced ages. Those are the main reasons why the percentage of patients with a low response to ovarian stimulation is increasing.

Due to the fact that conventional stimulation protocols provide low pregnancy rates, and similar results with no superiority of one over the others, some alternatives have been described.

It is also well known by clinicians that sometimes patients start an active and intense search for different alternatives. Needless to say, that new treatments or procedures have to be performed according the good clinical practice (GCP) guidelines in controlled clinical trials. That would be the only scientific way to provide patients objective data about other treatments to improve their prognosis.

One of the unsolved problems in this matter was the lack of a unique definition for low ovarian response. More than 40 different definitions have been included in the available literature. Fortunately, a consensus definition has been available since 2011. The Bologna Criteria[2] definition can be used in the studies, although it has many critics.

The different treatment options throughout the chapter are summarized in Table 10.1

FOLLICULAR ANDROGENIZATION

Physiological Basis

The creation of a reversible pseudo-polycystic endocrine state with the use of androgens would be the fundamental element of this therapeutic approach. Women with polycystic ovaries often show high responses to ovarian

Table 10.1: Alternatives in low response.

Androgenization
Aromatase inhibitor—letrozole
Dehydroepiandrosterone
Transdermal testosterone
Growth hormone

stimulation that lead to the development of multiple growing follicles. These follicles have been exposed to high androgen levels for a long time, which makes them develop a high sensitivity to follicle-stimulating hormone (FSH) that can lead to a high response.

According to the two cell-two hormones theory, androgens play a critical role in the steroidogenesis process. They act as a substrate for the aromatase in granulosa cells, where are transformed into estrogens.

First data on mice models confirmed that elevated androgen levels induced atresia in developing follicles,[3] nevertheless primate studies have shown an opposite effect.

Androgen receptors are present in granulosa and theca cells in human and primate ovaries. These androgen receptors are highly expressed in granulosa cells in pre-antral and antral follicles. Primate studies have shown that androgens can enhance the ovarian response to gonadotropins.[4]

Other papers have also suggested that androgens have a positive regulatory role in follicular development, since the treatment with testosterone or dehydroepiandrosterone (DHEA) increases FSH receptor expression in granulosa cells.[5,6] It has also been demonstrated that androgens promote the beginning of the development of the primordial follicle, and cause an increase in the number of developing pre-antral and antral follicles.[7]

Another evidence in humans is available. In male-to-woman transsexuals a high exposure to exogenous testosterone is used, and it is associated with polycystic ovary related morphological changes, with a significant increase in the number of antral follicles.

Apart from this evidence in patients with polycystic ovaries a high production of androgens is sometimes present, and there is a positive correlation between the number of follicles and the androgen levels.

In patients with congenital adrenal hyperplasia or with androgen producing tumors (nonovarian hyperandrogenism causes) some similar polycystic ovaries related changes have been described.

All these observations and data suggest that androgens promote follicular development by an indirect amplification of the ovarian response to FSH.

Aromatase Inhibitors

Aromatase inhibitor, letrozole has been used in patients with low ovarian response. For more than a decade letrozole has taken part in different protocols for ovulation induction, insemination and in vitro fertilization (IVF). A Canadian group was the first to publish their experience with letrozole in ovulation induction in 2000. This work was awarded with the prize of the Society for Reproductive Endocrinology and Infertility.[8]

This molecule inhibits the androgen aromatization to estrogens and releases the hypothalamus-pituitary axis from the estrogenic feedback on gonadotropin secretion. The increased gonadotropin concentration would enhance follicular development. There is also a second hypothesis in which a peripheral action would involve an amplified follicular sensitivity to FSH. The temporary accumulation of ovarian androgens would increase the follicular expression of FSH and insulin-like growth factor I (IGF-I) receptors.[9]

From the first papers published by Mitwally and Casper[10] until the latest studies with letrozole[11-16] in patients with low response are summarized in Table 10.2.

Significant differences in clinical outcomes can be found in two publications. Implantation rate is higher in the group that was treated with letrozole in Garcia-Velasco paper[12] and the ongoing pregnancy rate is also better in Schoolcraft[15] work.

Unfortunately, differences in letrozole dose and the variety of stimulation protocols make the comparison and conclusions more difficult. Dose ranged between 2.5 mg/day and 5 mg/day orally during the first 5 days of the gonadotropin administration.

In the case of poor responders letrozole was used in combination with recombinant FSH (rFSH) and highly purified human menopausal gonadotropin (HP-hMG) in antagonist protocol.

Safety issues with letrozole are well-known since 2005. Bijlan et al.[17] showed their data with a 4.7 % malformation rate in 150 babies born after a treatment with letrozole versus a 1.8% malformation rate in a database of 36,050 babies born after spontaneous conception in low risk community hospital. The incidence of cardiac and muscular malformations was significantly higher in the letrozole group. As a result of this data Novartis Pharmaceutical issued a statement to physicians in Canada and a worldwide advising that letrozole in premenopausal women was contraindicated. More recently Tulandiet al.[18] published another study of five centers in Canada with 911 newborns comparing letrozole and clomiphene citrate. Congenital malformations and chromosomal abnormalities were found in 2.4% of babies born after a treatment with letrozole and 4.8% in the clomiphene group. The rate of congenital cardiac malformations was also significantly higher (1.8%) in the clomiphene group compared to the letrozole group (0.2%). During that time letrozole was

Table 10.2: Letrozole in low response.

Study	*Protocol*	*Ovarian Stimulation*	*Case/ Control*	*Dose*	*Pregnancy rate %*	*Implantation rate %*	*Ongoing Pregnancy rate %*
Goswami 2004	Agonist	rFSH + letrozol/rFSH	13/25	2.5 mg/day 5 days	23/24	Unknown	Unknown
Garcia-Velasco 2005	Antagonist	rFSH + hMG + letrozol/ rFSH + hMG	71/76	2.5 mg/day 5 days	22.4/15.2	25/9.4	Unknown
Ozmen 2009	Antagonist	rFSH + Letrozol/rFSH	35/35	5 mg/day 5 days	32.3/24	Unknown	Unknown
Schoolcraft 2008	Antagonist/ agonist microdose flare	rFSH + hMG + letrozol/ rFSH + hMG	179/355	2.5 mg/day 5 days	Unknown	15/21	37/52
Davar 2010	Antagonist/ Agonist	rFSH-hMG + letrozol/rFSH or hMG	45/49	5 mg/day 5 days	5.3/14.3	3.8/7.7	Unknown
Lee 2011	Antagonist	hMG + letrozol/hMG	26/27	2.5 mg/day 5 days	Unknown	21.7/13.9	19.2/7.4

(rFSH: Recombinant follicle-stimulating hormone; hMG: Human menopausal gonadotropin).

also used by our group in ovulation induction, insemination and IVF. Our data were presented in ESHRE meeting in 2006[19] and no significant number of malformations were found in 64 newborns.

Concerns about a teratogenic effect of letrozole are unfunded with the available data.[20] Its short half-life (approximately 45 hours) and its exposition (5 days at the beginning of the stimulation) limit its presence during the time of conception, implantation or organogenesis.

Dehydroepiandrosterone

Dehydroepiandrosterone (DHEA) is an endogenous steroid that is mainly produced in the reticular zone of the adrenal cortex, and in small amounts by the theca cells in the ovary. It is essential in follicular steroidogenesis and increases IGF-I, which facilitates gonadotropic effect.[21]

A first publication of the benefit of DHEA in low response was done in five patients undergoing intrauterine insemination.[22]

Barad and Gleicher have extensively used this molecule later as an adjuvant treatment in low response. Their first case was a 42-year-old patient.[23]

Only some controlled or randomized trials with a small number of patients are available on DHEA. The first meta-analysis on the effect of DHEA in patients with low ovarian reserve was published in 2013.[24] The clinical pregnancy rate was chosen as the main outcome and two studies were included.[25,26] No significant difference was found on the clinical pregnancy rate between patients treated with DHEA or not, however the result was marginally superior in the group treated with DHEA with a relative risk (RR) of 1.87 [95% confidence interval (CI) 0.96–3.64; $p = 0.07$]. This tendency can be explained due to the low number (198) of patients included in both studies. With respect to the number of retrieved oocytes three studies were included,[25-27] and a lower number of oocytes was obtained in the group treated with DHEA.

In 2014 another pilot randomized controlled trial was published[28] including 16 patients in each group. No difference in the ovarian reserve tests (antral follicle count, anti-Müllerian hormone or FSH), ovarian response or IVF outcome was found.

Also a prospective cohort study[29] was published in 2014 with 50 patients. They used DHEA during four months and repeated the same ovarian stimulation protocol previously used (agonist or antagonist). The authors were able to show an increase in the number of oocytes and available embryos after DHEA pretreatment. Main data of DHEA studies are shown in Table 10.3.

The lack of homogeneity in the study populations, the dose and time of DHEA administration are the main limiting factors to obtain solid conclu sions on the role of this molecule in low response. In most of the studies DHEA is used at a dose of 25 mg three times a day during 5–16 weeks. There

Table 10.3: Dehydroepiandrosterone (DHEA) in low response.

Study	*Type*	*Case/Control*	*Intervention*	*Protocol*
Barad et al. 2007	Case-control	89/101	DHEA 25 mg × 3/day during 73 days until pregnancy	Microdose Flare—agonist
Wiser et al. 2010	RCT	17/16	DHEA 75 mg/day at least 6 weeks before stimulation	Long agonist
Gleicher et al. 2010	Case-control	22/44	DHEA 25 mg × 3/days at least 4 weeks before stimulation	Microdose Flare—agonist
Zangmo et al. 2014	Cohorts pro-spective	50	DHEA 25 mg × 3/day during 4 months until the end of stimulation	30 agonist/ 20 antagonist
Yeung et al. 2013	RCT	16/16	DHEA 25 mg × 3/day during 12 weeks	Antagonist
Kara et al. 2013	RCT	104/104	DHEA 25 mg × 3/day during 12 weeks	Microdose Flare—agonist

(RCT: Randomized controlled trial).

is no sufficient evidence to know the optimal duration for the treatment with DHEA, serum or follicular fluid dehydroepiandrosterone sulfate or testosterone levels with different regimens.

Another important factor that could make attractive the use of DHEA is a possible improvement in the oocyte quality with a decrease in the miscarriage rate[30] and lower proportion of aneuploid embryos.[27] The small simple size in these papers makes the results inconclusive.

Another recent paper[31] in an animal model evaluates the effect of DHEA in vivo in the early follicular development. A higher proportion of follicle population in the ovary after DHEA treatment has been found. These data support the general hypothesis that DHEA can be a useful adjuvant treatment in the case of a low ovarian reserve.

Data on the safety of DHEA is limited. Little information is available regarding the side effects of these treatments, although no serious adverse events have been reported on patients or babies.

Transdermal Testosterone

Transdermal testosterone administration in patches or gel has also been used as an adjuvant treatment in patients with low ovarian response with the objective to increase the ovarian androgen concentration.

Table 10.4: Testosterone in low response.

Study	*Type*	*Dose*	*Timing*	*Duration*	*Protocol*	*Stimulation doser*	*Type of study*	*Case/ control*
Massin et al. 2006	Testos-terone gel 1%	10 mg/ day thigh	15–20 days before stimulation	15–20 days before stimula-tion	Mainly long agonist but also short agonist	rFSH/ 300–450 IU	RCT	26/27
Kim et al 2011	Testos-terone gel 1%	12.5 mg/ day arm	6th day of a previous cycle with E2 + P	21 days	Antago-nist	rFSH/ 300 IU	RCT	55/55

(rFSH: Recombinant follicle-stimulating hormone; RCT: Randomized controlled trial).

The application of testosterone gel was first described in two papers.[32,33] The main characteristics of the testosterone gel treatment is summarized in Table 10.4.

In this two studies a total number of 163 patients were included and when data are pooled an increase in 15% in the clinical pregnancy rate and in 11% in the live birth rate is shown in the group of patients treated with testosterone gel.[34]

One of the most cited papers on the use of testosterone patches in the treatment of low response is by Fábregues et al.[35] In this prospective randomized trial 62 patients, with a previous cancellation of a stimulated cycle due to low response, were included. Testosterone patches of 2.5 mg were used daily for 5 days during the gonadotropin-releasing hormone (GnRH) agonist downregulation in a long protocol. In group 1 (with testosterone patches) the ovarian stimulation was done with 400 and 350 IU of rFSH during the first 2 days, followed by 150 IU on stimulation days 3 and 4, and with an individualized dose from day 5 onward. Group 2 (control) was also stimulated with a long agonist protocol with 300 IU of rFSH with 300 IU of HP-hMG on days 1-2, followed by 300 IU of HP-hMG on days 3-4, and with an individualized dose from day 5 onward. It was shown that in the group that was treated with testosterone the proportion of cycles with a low response was lower when compared with the control group (32% vs 71%). A higher number of patients with oocyte retrieval tended to be higher in the group with the testosterone patches (60.6% vs 58.1%), reaching statistical significance in the group of patients with normal basal FSH levels (81.2% vs 41.1%).

A long agonist protocol was used in Fábregues paper, but this is not the most usual protocol in our daily practice. That is the reason why we decided to perform a prospective randomized trial with testosterone patches in an antagonist protocol.[36] Patients from 18 years to 39 years with a low response

(< 5 oocytes and/or a cancellation due to < 5 follicles > 14 mm) in 1–2 previous IVF cycles were included. They were pretreated with an oral contraceptive pill with 30 µg of ethinylestradiol and levonorgestrel for 15–19 days and were randomized before starting the stimulation. Patients on group 1 used a testosterone patch (2.4 mg) 12 hours/day during 5 days from the last pill until the first day of stimulation. Patients on group 2 had no treatment during the 5 days after the pill. The ovarian stimulation was done with a fixed dose of 225 IU of rFSH and 75 IU of hp-hMG. Sixteen patients were included in the group with testosterone and 17 patients in the control group. No significant difference between both groups was shown in the duration, total gonadotropin dose, number of follicles more than 14 mm, endometrial thickness or estradiol level the day of the human chorionic gonadotropin (hCG). There were no differences in the number of retrieved oocytes, number of mature oocytes, fertilization rate or good quality day 3 embryos. No significant difference in the pregnancy rate per embryo transfer (36.3% vs 31.25%) or the implantation rate (29.4% vs 17.8%) was demonstrated.

A recent meta-analysis[37] reviews the role of transdermal testosterone and includes the three papers with the best methodology (Massin, Kim and Fábregues). Pooled data of the studies show that in the groups of patients treated with transdermal testosterone there was a significant increase in the live birth rate when compared with the control groups (RR 1.91, 95% CI 1.01–3.63, $I^2 = 0\%$) and a similar result was shown for the clinical pregnancy rate (RR 2.07, 95% CI 1.13–3.78, $I^2 = 0\%$).

The heterogeneity in the ovarian stimulation protocols and the variation in the duration and exposition to the study drug are the most important limiting factors for the conclusions.

One of the remaining questions of the use of transdermal testosterone is if the duration of the treatment is enough to cause an action in the ovary that led to a clinical significant difference.

No serious side effects of transdermal testosterone have been reported. Although the duration of this alternative is shorter than the duration of the DHEA pretreatment.

GROWTH HORMONE

The last adjuvant treatment used in the low response in this review is the growth hormone (GH). This hormone has a role in early and late follicular development stimulating granulosa cell proliferation and differentiation, and increasing estradiol production in animal and human models.[38,39]

A recent meta-analysis concludes that the use of GH in combination with ovarian stimulation may be beneficial in patients with low response.

The group of patients treated with GH showed a significant increase of the live birth rate of +17% and +16%, respectively in the first[40] and second[41] meta-analysis.

The Cochrane review[42] showed a statistically significant difference in the live birth rate and pregnancy rate using GH as an adjuvant treatment in patients with low response.

Growth hormone is used during the follicular phase with a dose that ranges between 4 IU/day and 24 IU/day. It is started at the beginning of the administration of gonadotropins until the day of the hCG.

The increase of the cost of the GH treatment associated with gonadotropins is an important factor that cannot be forgotten.

Data on security for patients and babies are reassuring although they are limited.

CONCLUSION

The delay in childbearing and the poor ovarian reserve are major disadvantages in our society, and they often come together in the same patient. Although no protocol is known to achieve better results, clinicians (and sometimes patients) seek adjuvant therapies to increase the number of retrieved oocytes. The use of androgenization approaches with letrozol, DHEA, and transdermal testosterone lack of robust data showing an improvement in live birth rates in women with poor ovarian response. Data for the use of transdermal testosterone in a recent meta-analysis showed an increase in live birth rate. The use of growth hormone is conditioned by the cost of this alternative, but a review showed a more favourable result in live birth rate.

REFERENCES

1. Venetis CA, Kolibianakis EM, Tarlatzi TB, et al. Evidence-based management of poor ovarian response. Ann N Y Acad Sci. 2010;1205:199-206.
2. Ferraretti AP, La Marca A, Fauser BC, et al. ESHRE consensus on the definition of "poor response" to ovarian stimulation for in vitro fertilization: the Bologna criteria. Hum Reprod. 2011;26:1616-24.
3. Hillier SG, Ross GT. Effects of exogenous testosterone on ovarian weight, follicular morphology and intraovarian progesterone concentration in estrogen-primed hypophysectomized immature female rats. Biol Reprod. 1979; 20:261-8.
4. Harlow CR, Hillier SG, Hodges JK. Androgen modulation of follicle-stimulating hormone induced granulosa cell steroidogenesis in the primate ovary. Endocrinology. 1986;119:1403-5.
5. Weil S, Vendola K, Zhou J, et al. Androgen and follicle stimulating hormone interactions in primate ovarian follicle development. J Clin Endocrinol Metab. 1999;84:2951-6.
6. Weil SJ, Vendola K, Zhou J, et al. Androgen receptor gene expression in the primate ovary: cellular localization, regulation, and functional correlations. J Clin Endocrinol Metab. 1998;83:2479-85.
7. Vendola KA, Zhou J, Adesanya OO, et al. Androgens stimulate early stages of follicular growth in the primate ovary. J Clin Invest. 1998;101:2622-9.

8. Mitwally MF, Casper RF. The Aromatase Inhibitor, Letrozole: a Promising Alternative for Clomiphene Citrate for Induction of Ovulation. SREI Prize Paper. Fertil Steril. 2000; S35.
9. Casper RF, Mitwally MF. Aromatase inhibitors for ovulation induction. J Clin Endocrinol Metab. 2006;91:760-71.
10. Mitwally MF, Casper RF. Aromatase inhibition improves ovarian response to follicle-stimulating hormone in poor responders. Fertil Steril. 2002;77:776-80.
11. Goswami SK, Das T, Chattopadhyay R, et al. A randomized single-blind controlled trial of letrozole as a low-cost IVF protocol in women with poor ovarian response: a preliminary report. Hum Reprod. 2004;19:2031-5.
12. Garcia-Velasco JA, Moreno L, Pacheco A, et al. The aromatase inhibitor letrozole increases the concentration of intraovarian androgens and improves in vitro fertilization outcome in low responder patients: a pilot study. Fertil Steril. 2005;84:82-7.
13. Ozmen B, Sonmezer M, Atabekoglu CS, et al. Use of aromatase inhibitors in poor-responder patients receiving GnRH antagonist protocols. Reprod Biomed Online. 2009;19:478-85.
14. Davar R, Oskouian H, Ahmadi S, et al. GnRH antagonist/letrozole versus microdose GnRH agonist flare protocol in poor responders undergoing in vitro fertilization. Taiwan J Obstet Gynecol. 2010;49:297-301.
15. Schoolcraft WB, Surrey ES, Minjarez DA, et al. Management of poor responders: can outcomes be improved with a novel gonadotropin-releasing hormone antagonist/letrozole protocol? Fertil Steril. 2008;89:151-6.
16. Chi V, Lee Y, Chi C, et al. Sequential use of letrozole and gonadotropin in women with poor ovarian reserve : a randomized controlled trial. Reprod Biomed Online. 2011;23:380-8.
17. Biljan MM, Hemmings R, Brassard N. The outcome of 150 babies following the treatment with letrozole or letrozole and gonadotropins. Fertil Steril. 2005;84:S64-5.
18. Tulandi T, Martin J, Al-Fadhli R, et al. Congenital malformations among 911 newborns conceived after infertility treatment with letrozole or clomiphene citrate. Fertil Steril. 2006;85:1761-5.
19. Guillén A, Vidal C, Pellicer A, et al. Perinatal outcome in cycles with letrozole: Abstracts of the 22nd Annual Meeting of the ESHRE, Prague, Czech Republic. Hum Reprod. 2006;21(Suppl 1):341.
20. Requena A, Herrero J, Landeras J, et al. Use of letrozole in assisted reproduction: asystematic review and meta-analysis. Hum Reprod Update. 2008; 14:571-82.
21. Casson PR, Santoro N, Elkind-Hirsch K, et al. Postmenopausal dehydroepiandrosterone administration increases free insulin-like growth factor-I and decreases high-density lipoprotein: a six-month trial. Fertil. Steril. 1998;70:107-10.
22. Casson PR, Lindsay MS, Pisarka MD, et al. Dehydroepiandrosterone supplementation augments ovarian stimulation in poor responders: a case series. Hum Reprod. 2000;15:2129-32.
23. Barad D, Gleicher N. Increased oocyte production after treatment with dehydroepiandrosterone. Fertil Steril. 2005;84:756, e1-3.
24. Narkwichean A, Maalouf W, Campbell BK, et al. Efficacy of dehydroepiandrosterone to improve ovarian response in women with diminished ovarian reserve: a meta-analysis. Reprod Biol Endocrinol. 2013;11:44.

25. Wiser A, Gonen O, Ghetler Y, et al. Addition of dehydroepiandrosterone (DHEA) for poor-responder patients before and during IVF treatment improves the pregnancy rate: a randomized prospective study. Hum Reprod. 2010;25: 2496-500.
26. Barad D, Brill H, Gleicher N. Update on the use of dehydroepiandrosterone supplementation among women with diminished ovarian function. J Assist Reprod Genet. 2007;24:629-34.
27. Gleicher N, Weghofer A, Barad DH. Dehydroepiandrosterone (DHEA) reduces embryo aneuploidy: direct evidence from preimplantation genetic screening (PGS). Reprod Biol Endocrinol. 2010;8:140.
28. Yeung TW, Chai J, Li RH, et al. A randomized, controlled, pilot trial on the effect of dehydroepiandrosterone on ovarian response markers, ovarian response, and in vitro fertilization outcomes in poor responders. Fertil Steril. 2014;102:108-15.e1.
29. Zangmo R, Singh N, Kumar S, et al. Role of dehydroepiandrosterone in improving oocyte and embryo quality in IVF cycles. Reprod Biomed Online. 2014;28:743-7.
30. Gleicher N, Ryan E, Weghofer A, et al. Miscarriage rates after dehydroepiandrosterone (DHEA) supplementation in women with diminished ovarian reserve: a case control study. Reprod Biol Endocrinol. 2009;7:108.
31. Narkwichean A, Jayaprakasan K, Maalouf WE, et al. Effects of dehydroepiandrosterone on in vivo ovine follicular development. Hum Reprod. 2014;29: 146-54.
32. Massin N, Cedrin-Durnerin I, Coussieu C, et al. Effects of transdermal testosterone application on the ovarian response to FSH in poor responders undergoing assisted reproduction technique—a prospective, randomized, double-blind study. Hum Reprod. 2006;5:1204-11.
33. Kim CH, Howles CM, Lee HA. The effect of transdermal testosterone gel pretreatment on controlled ovarian stimulation and IVF outcome in low responders. Fertil Steril. 2011;2:679-83.
34. Bosdou JK, Venetis CA, Kolibianakis EM, et al. The use of androgens or androgen-modulating agents in poor responders undergoing in vitro fertilization: a systematic review and meta-analysis. Hum Reprod Update. 2012;18: 127-45.
35. Fábregues F, Penãrrubia J, Creus M, et al. Transdermal testosterone may improve ovarian response to gonadotrophins in low-responder IVF patients: a randomized, clinical trial. Hum Reprod. 2009;24:349-59.
36. Guillén A, Ortega I, Bou C, et al. Testosterona transdérmica con protocolo antagonista en baja respuesta ovárica. Comunicación Oral XXIX Congreso Nacional SEF, Granada 2012 Revista Iberoamericana de Fertilidady Reproducción Humana. 2012;29(Suppl 1):144.
37. González-Comadran M, Durán M, Solà I, et al. Effects of transdermal testosterone in poor responders undergoing IVF: systematic review and meta-analysis. Reprod Biomed Online. 2012;25:450-9.
38. Langhout DJ, Spicer LJ, Geisert RD. Development of a culture system for bovine granulosa cells: effects of growth hormone, estradiol, and gonadotropins on cell proliferation, steroidogenesis, and protein synthesis. J Anim Sci. 1991;69: 3321-34.
39. Lanzone A, Fortini A, Fulghesu AM, et al. Growth hormone enhances estradiol production follicle-stimulating hormone-induced in the early stage of the follicular maturation. Fertil Steril. 1996;66:948-53.

40. Kolibianakis EM, Venetis CA, Diedrich K, et al. Addition of growth hormone to gonadotrophins in ovarian stimulation of poor responders treated by in-vitro fertilization: a systematic review and meta-analysis. Hum Reprod Update. 2009;15:613-22.
41. Kyrou D, Kolibianakis EM, Venetis CA, et al. How to improve the probability of pregnancy in poor responders undergoing in vitro fertilization: a systematic review and meta-analysis. Fertil Steril. 2009;91:749-66.
42. Duffy JM, Ahmad G, Mohiyiddeen L, et al. Growth hormone for in vitro fertilization. Cochrane Database Syst Rev. 2010;1:CD000099.

Chapter 11

Freeze-all in Assisted Reproductive Technology

Natalia Basile, Juan Antonio García-Velasco

INTRODUCTION

There is a new concept in assisted reproductive technology (ART) called "freeze-all". It appears as a consequence of great advancements in the vitrification protocols allowing us to "electively" defer an embryo transfer from a fresh to a frozen cycle. Beyond the most common indications: ovarian hyperstimulation syndrome (OHSS) prevention, high progesterone levels, genetic screening, etc. the freeze-all concept has shifted from a solution when there is an indication to a routine practice in many programs around the world. However, we should analyze when and for who is this freeze-all approach most appropriate. Based on the principle that controlled ovarian stimulation (COS) may cause a less physiological milieu for embryos to implant, the freeze-all concept represents an opportunity to provide a more natural environment for the embryo. However, we must balance this against the possible non-natural changes that we may be causing the embryo as a result from freezing. Physician's treatment choices are influenced by a number of factors, including guidelines, evidence-based medicine, past experience and, to a certain extent, habit.[1] This chapter will go over the different milestones that may have led to the establishment of the freeze-all concept, the critical review of published data, and the conclusion whether the shift should be reverted or not.

FACTORS IN ASSISTED REPRODUCTIVE TECHNOLOGY CONTRIBUTING TO THE FREEZE-ALL POLICY

Introduction of Vitrification: A Safe Technique

Cryopreservation is of crucial importance in reproductive medicine. Advancements in cryopreservation techniques have resulted in similar quality and implantation potential between fresh and frozen embryos.[2,3] Slow freezing was the method of choice for decades for cryopreservation of cleavage stage embryos and blastocysts. In term of oocytes, however, even though a number of pregnancies and births have been reported following the transfer of embryos derived from slow-freezed oocytes;[4-6] survival rates are only close to 50%[7-10] and fertilization rates of frozen-thawed oocytes are low compared to fresh ones (just over 50% overall).[11] Vitrification on the other hand has proven to be more effective than slow freezing in terms of survival rates and clinical outcomes for oocytes and embryos[12-14] representing with no doubt the method of choice in practically every IVF clinic today. Vitrification is a fast cryopreservation method that involves exposure of oocytes/embryos to high concentrations of cryoprotectants and ultra-rapid cooling rates causing an instant solidification (vitrous state) that avoids damages to the cell due to ice crystal formation. It is here where the major advantage with respect to slow freezing relies. Given the excellent results provided by this technique, vitrification can no longer be taken as a complement to IVF treatments but as a fundamental tool for the management of our patients. Low responders, for instance, can benefit from accumulation of oocytes through vitrification allowing them to achieve similar clinical outcomes as normoresponders.[15] Moreover, this strategy is also attractive for patients with advance maternal age (a more difficult group to treat) who, in addition to being low responders, require preimplantation genetic screening (PGS).[16] On the contrary, the vitrification of oocytes (and embryos) has also proven to work with patients at risk of developing OHSS representing a solution when an embryo transfer needs to be delayed.[17,18] Last but not least oocyte vitrification allows women to preserve their fertility today, the so called "social freezing", and clinics to establish egg donor banks with similar results than with fresh oocytes.[19]

In terms of live birth rates a population based cohort study comparing cryopreservation by vitrification or slow freezing in a large data set (over 30,000 cases between the two groups) revealed that vitrified blastocyst transfer cycles resulted in a significantly higher live delivery rate [adjusted relative risk (ARR): 1.41, 95% confidence interval (CI): 1.34–1.49] compared with slow frozen blastocyst transfer cycles, although a limitation of this study is the lack of information available on clinic-specific cryopreservation protocols and processes for slow freezing-thaw and vitrification-warm of blastocysts and the potential impact on outcomes.[20]

Given all these facts it would be plausible to discuss the introduction of freeze-all policies involving the elective vitrification of all the viable embryos from a fresh cycle. The objective of a future transfer of vitrified-warmed embryos would be to place them in a more favorable intrauterine environment, without facing the possible adverse effects of supraphysiologic hormonal levels over the endometrial receptivity.[21]

Implementation of Ovarian Hyperstimulation Syndrome-free Clinics

Ovarian hyperstimulation syndrome represents one of the major complications encountered during COS in IVF. The syndrome has a broad spectrum of clinical manifestations, from mild illness needing only careful observation to severe disease requiring hospitalization and intensive care.[22] It occurs in approximately 1–14% of ART cycles and is related to increased vascular permeability (VP).[23,24] Human chorionic gonadotropin (hCG), either exogenous or endogenous, is the most probable triggering factor of this syndrome.[25] Following the administration of hCG, the expression of vascular endothelial growth factor (VEGF) and VEGF receptor 2 (VEGFR-2) mRNA increases significantly, rising to a maximum level that coincides with peaked VP. These findings suggest that the syndrome can be prevented by inducing ovulation with a gonadotropin-releasing hormone agonist (GnRH) instead of hCG, preventing VEGF overexpression.[26] This strategy would prevent the early, but not the late, onset of OHSS.

For many years GnRH agonists were considered the "gold standard" protocol especially in young normoresponders, but a major drawback of these protocols was the risk of OHSS. The introduction of GnRH antagonists on the other hand seemed to open up a new way toward a more "friendly IVF".[27] Unlike the indirect pituitary suppression induced by GnRH agonists, GnRH antagonists administration causes immediate and dose-related suppression of gonadotropins release by competitive occupancy of the GnRH receptors in the pituitary[28] resulting in a much shorter duration of stimulation and absence of the side-effects caused by profound hypoestrogenemia.[29,30] In addition, COS with antagonists protocols can be combined with complementary measures to avoid even further the risk of OHSS like triggering ovulation induction with GnRH agonist instead of hCG.[31-34] Still, this approach is not 100% safe considering that a few anecdotal cases of severe OHSS following GnRH agonist triggering without any luteal supplementation have been reported.[35-37] Moreover, GnRH agonists triggering has been associated with luteal phase defects presumably due to an excessive negative steroid feedback.[38-40] Two consecutive Cochrane reviews by the same author state that: "GnRH agonist triggering is associated with a lower ongoing pregnancy rate compared with conventional hCG".[34,41,42] This conclusion was qualified as premature and mistaken based on (1) that Cochrane reviews should not be conducted during the research phase when new concepts are being developed and (2) the authors missed the fact that the variable that affects results is the luteal phase support itself and not the use of GnRH agonist trigger for final oocyte maturation.[40] Therefore, if triggering with GnRH agonist (which is the preferred strategy to reduce the risk of OHSS) is associated with luteal phase defects, then a fresh embryo transfer should not take place, the treatment needs to be segmented and the concept of freeze-all becomes attractive.

Rise in Genetic Screening

Preimplantation genetic screening is increasingly being used to improve implantation rates after IVF. The European Society of Human Reproduction and Embryology (ESHRE) preimplantation genetic diagnosis (PGD) consortium collects PGD data from a number of clinics worldwide and according to the last report 52% of the PGD cycles in 2010 were used as PGS. The most common indications for PGS in IVF include patients with advanced maternal age (AMA), repeated implantation failure (RIF), recurrent pregnancy loss (RPL) and, to a lesser extent, patients with partners with male factor infertility[43,44] and egg donors.[45] From a technical point of view genetic screening has evolved from the early fluorescence in situ hybridization (FISH) years to the use of array comparative genomic hybridization (CGH) and next generation sequencing (NGS). Moreover, the stage in which embryos are being biopsied has also changed from biopsies of the oocyte's first and second polar bodies[46,47] to biopsies on cleavage stage embryos and blastocysts. The first clinical studies with biopsies on cleavage-stage embryos showed higher implantation and ongoing pregnancy rates as well as lower abortion rates.[48,49] The initial thinking about day 3 biopsy was that it gave the laboratory plenty of time to do the actual testing and still be able to do a fresh embryo transfer on day 5; however, there were several drawbacks including mosaicism and embryo damage due to removal of a large percentage of the embryo´s cells.[50] Fortunately, advancements in culture media formulations allowed embryologists to culture embryos to later stages of development and the first cases of trophectoderm biopsy took place in 2005.[51] Today, trophectoderm biopsy is the method of choice not only due to a decreased likelihood of mosaicism but also to an increase in the amount of DNA available for testing and less damage to the embryo. The use of comprehensive chromosome screening (CCS) in blastocyst stage with elective single embryo transfer (eSET) has been proposed as effective as double-embryo transfer of unscreened embryos with the advantage of dramatically reducing the risk of twins.[52] However, it is unclear if the screened embryo transfer results in better outcomes when performed in fresh or frozen embryo transfer (FET) cycles.

From a practical point of view we should consider that not all the programs are able to obtain a 24 hour turn around and perform a fresh embryo transfer following a thophectoderm biopsy. In addition, those embryos requiring a day 6 biopsy may not be eligible for fresh transfer due to an asynchrony between the embryo and the endometrium. It is within this context that the idea of freeze-all plays a role overcoming time restraints and allowing us to biopsy the embryos at later stages of development, vitrify them immediately after, send the cells to be tested, wait for the results to come back and schedule the transfer of a normal embryo in a subsequent cycle. Needless to say that a good vitrification program is mandatory and that the logistics of an IVF laboratory will change the more genetic screening we offer to our patients, not only due to the biopsy process but due to a significant increase in the percentage of patients being vitrified.

Concern on Perinatal and Obstetric Outcomes

There is a growing body of evidence highlighting concerns regarding perinatal and obstetric outcomes after ART, and in particular following fresh transfers.

Different studies have shown that children born after assisted reproductive techniques (ART) have poorer outcomes in terms of preterm birth (PTB), low birthweight (LBW), small for gestational age (SGA) and perinatal mortality when compared with newborns of natural conceptions.[53-55] Within those undergoing IVF, results between fresh and FETs in terms of obstetric perinatal outcome are still unclear.[56-58] A systematic review and meta-analysis based on 11 observational studies concluded that singleton pregnancies after the transfer of frozen thawed embryos resulted in lower risk of antepartum hemorrhage [relative risk (RR) = 0.67, 95% CI 0.55–0.81], PTB (RR = 0.84, 95% CI 0.78–0.90), SGA (RR = 0.45, 95% CI 0.30–0.66), LBW (RR = 0.69, 95% CI 0.62–0.76), and perinatal mortality (RR = 0.68, 95% CI 0.48–0.96) than with fresh embryos.[59] A Scandinavian study including three different countries.[57] corroborated some of these findings but also observed that frozen-thawed embryos had a higher risk of post-term birth [adjusted odds ratio (aOR) 1.40, 95% CI 1.27–1.55], large for gestational age (LGA) (aOR 1.45, 95% CI 1.27–1.64), macrosomia (aOR 1.58, 95% CI 1.39–1.80) and perinatal mortality (aOR 1.49, 95% CI 1.07–2.07) which was in line with other large-population-based studies.[60,61] More recent evidence from another large observational study in Australia[62] confirmed that embryo transfers of vitrified-warmed blastocysts yield equivalent live birth rates than fresh blastocysts but significantly improved neonatal outcomes in terms of gestational age, being on average 0.3 weeks longer, and for live birth weight with babies born on average 145 g heavier as compared with fresh transfers, however we may ask ourselves what is the clinical relevance of this. Finally, this year a report from a group in Brussels analyzed 1,072 singletons and twins born after embryo vitrification on day 3 and day 5 concluding that neonatal health parameters, including the prevalence of congenital malformations were similar to or slightly better than after fresh embryo transfer.[63] It should be acknowledged that the majority of these studies are observational and that vitrified embryos are always second choice for transfer. We could assume that elective FET with first choice embryos could yield even better results but these studies are yet to be performed. Therefore, the published data suggest that it is still unclear if perinatal and obstetric outcomes are better with FETs compared to fresh ones (Table 11.1).

EVIDENCE IN FAVOR OF FREEZE-ALL

There is not much evidence backing up the freeze-all policy. A recent meta-analysis[64] concluded that: "the use of FET, compared with fresh embryo

Table 11.1: Perinatal and obstetric outcomes of frozen embryo transfers.

Reduced risks in FET	*Increased risks with FET*	*Unclear*
LBW (<2,500 g)	Macrosomia (>4,500 g)	Ectopic pregnancy
SGA (<10%)	Large for GA	Preeclampsia
Placental abruption	Placenta accreta	Congenital abnormalities
Placenta previa	C-section delivery	NICU
Antepartum hemorrhage		VLBW (<1,500 g)
Perinatal mortality		VPTB (<32 weeks)

(FET: Frozen embryo transfer; LBW: Low birth weight; SGA: Small for gestational age; GA: Gestational age; NICU: Neonatal intensive care unit; VLBW: Very low birth weight; VPTB: Very preterm birth).

transfer, significantly improves clinical and ongoing pregnancy rates in patients submitted to ART". However, this conclusion is highly questionable due to different factors:

- *First,* the meta-analysis includes only three small studies. A proper meta-analysis should involve at least 3–4 RCTs with no less than 1,000 participants.[65] This was not met in this review considering that the total number of patients included was only 633. In addition, one of the studies,[66] in fact, the largest one was retracted at the request of the editor and the ASRM Publications Committee, due to serious methodological flaws, diminishing even more the total number to backup such conclusion.
- *Second,* the three studies are very heterogeneous in terms of the types of patients included (normo and high responders) as well as some technical aspects. Normo and high responders represent two different entities in terms of clinical approach, management and IVF outcomes, not to mention safety issues, which are very different from one group of patients to the other. In addition, the cryopreservation technique and the stage of development at which the embryos were cryopreserved were different. Both studies by Shapiro et al.[67,68] performed slow freezing of 2PNs whereas Aflatoonian et al. did vitrification on day 2 of development.
- *Third,* the study by Shapiro et al.[68] including normo-responders was underpowered (the required sample size was 411 patients and the study randomized only 67 patients for fresh transfer and 70 for FET), involved co-interventions such as dual trigger for final oocyte maturation and led to pregnancy rates in the FET group of 84% which were far higher than those reported from European or American registries.
- *Fourth,* none of these RCTs were able to provide data on live birth rates, cost-effectiveness and acceptability from the patient.

In our opinion, there is no doubt that patients at risk of OHSS are good candidates for this approach. For this type of patients, the combination of the right stimulation protocol plus the vitrification of oocytes/embryos has transformed what was a high-risk situation into an anecdotic one.[69,70] As described by Devroey et al.,[71] the strategy to obtain an OHSS-free clinic is closely related to the concept of segmentation. It consists of: Segment A, stimulation with GnRH antagonist and triggering with GnRH agonist; Segment B, optimum cryopreservation of oocytes or embryos through vitrification; and Segment C, embryo replacement into a receptive, non-stimulated endometrium in a natural cycle or with artificial endometrial preparation. With respect to Segment B a common question is whether if we should vitrify oocytes or embryos. According to a prospective comparison by Herrero et al., both approaches are safe since they result in similar ongoing pregnancy rates and live births after three transfers.[17] Therefore, the decision to do one or the other will most likely depend on the individual patient's preferences as well as ethical and cultural issues and not on clinical outcomes. A trial regarding the expectations and perceptions of frozen embryo holders revealed that many couples are concerned about frozen embryo disposition for ethical reasons.[72] Given these concerns, in the end, oocyte vitrification may be a more attractive and realistic alternative for certain groups of society.[73] With respect to segment C, there is little consensus on the most effective method of endometrium preparation prior to FET. A systematic review and meta-analysis published in 2013 compared clinical and ongoing pregnancy rates as well as live birth rates in (a) true natural cycle FET (NC-FET), (b) modified NC-FET with hCG, (c) artificial cycle FET (AC-FET), and (d) AC-FET supplemented with GnRH agonists. The study revealed no significant advantage of one specific approach to prepare the endometrium for FET in terms of clinical pregnancy rates or live birth rates.[74] Results were in line with the previous systematic review published in 2008.[75] Either way and independently of the particular characteristics of segment B and C, there is no doubt that the segmentation approach for patients with OHSS works[69,70,76,77] and the freeze-all policy is without controversy in this situation.

On the other side, controversy does exist when it comes to normoresponders. The benefits of the freeze-all policy on patients at risk of OHSS cannot be extrapolated to safe normoresponders. A recent study by our group[78] revealed no difference in terms of ongoing pregnancy and live birth rates between normoresponder patients that underwent fresh and deferred embryo transfers. This was a retrospective study including 882 patients aged 20–44 undergoing their first or second IVF/ICSI (intracytoplasmic sperm injection) cycle, in which a normal oocyte yield (4–20) was obtained. Patients were divided in two groups: 364 (41.3%) had a fresh embryo transfer and 518 (58.7%) were submitted to freeze-all according to the doctor's preference. No differences were observed between both patients groups in terms of demographic characteristics and ovarian stimulation parameters. The raw analysis showed that ongoing pregnancy (36.2% vs 33.8%, p = 0.51) and live birth (33.2% vs 32.9%, p = 0.94) rates for freeze-all versus fresh cycles respectively were similar. When adjustments were made for patient age and other variables likely to affect results, there was still no evidence of any impact of freezing. All the patients in the study were considered "normal responders" and were thus representative of a routine IVF patient population. Opposite to these results, a different study by Roque et al.[79] did find better ongoing pregnancy rates using freeze-all policy in patients with progesterone levels less than or equal to 1.5 ng/mL on the day of triggering. However, the sample size was lower than our study (total 530 patients: 351 in fresh group and 179 in FET group). In addition, the retrospective design of this study does not allow us to understand if poor responders were transferred and normo and high responders were frozen, which would have biased the results.

It should be acknowledged that a normal response per se is not exclusive of freeze-all. Normoresponders can face situations where this policy may apply like those undergoing genetic screening, presenting high progesterone levels, impaired endometrium, etc. But, out of an indication, the question whether freeze-all represents a benefit for the general IVF population still remains and further well-designed prospective studies will answer this question. This is the case of an ongoing randomized controlled trial taking place in UK (E-FREEZE trial). In this multicentric study, 1,086 women (543 in each arm) will be randomized in a period of 2 years to show (or not) an absolute difference in the primary outcome of at least 9% (with 90% power and a two-sided 5% level of statistical significance). The primary outcome has been defined as, "a live singleton baby born at term with an appropriate weight for gestation (AGA)". A composite primary outcome has been chosen to reflect safety (single, term and AGA) and effectiveness (live birth) as the goal of modern IVF is accepted to be a healthy baby and a healthy mother (with no OHSS), for details visit website at http://www.nets.nihr.ac.uk/projects/hta/1311582.

What about Costs?

Regardless of the evidence in favor or against the freeze-all policy, a not minor issue to take in consideration is the additional cost that this policy entails. Unfortunately there are no studies evaluating the cost-effectiveness of elective FET when compared to fresh embryo transfer. It is necessary to conduct these studies to determine whether a change in policy (performing elective FET instead of fresh embryo transfer) is cost-effective taking in consideration (a) the cryopreservation costs, (b) the costs associated with endometrial priming, and (c) the emotional cost associated to the distress arising in patients not undergoing a fresh ET.

CONCLUSION

Freeze-all, Freeze-none or Freeze-some?

A change in practice should be based on good evidence and sufficiently powered studies. As of today, the benefits of the freeze-all policy are based mainly on high responder patients and they cannot be extrapolated to the general IVF population. An interesting opinion paper published last year performed a SWOT (strengths, weaknesses, opportunities and threats) analysis of the freeze-all policy shedding light to the different aspects of this strategy. The authors concluded that although the major advantage or strength of a freeze-all strategy is the potential for eliminating OHSS, several other factors also support a move toward this approach including: enhanced cycle scheduling and improved organization of the IVF unit. However, potential threats were also presented including: costs and outcomes (LGA).[80]

We are entering the era of individualized treatments in IVF, not only from a clinical point of view but also from the laboratory technologies that we are offering our patients. Why would the freeze-all policy be exempt from this individualization, especially since there is not enough data to justify it?

Clear indications should be specified (Box 11.1). In our center, indications for freeze-all are not only restricted for patients at risk of OHSS but also for any type of patient with a clear indication: patients seeking for genetic screening; patients with an altered endocrine and cardiovascular profile at the moment of transfer (elevated progesterone, hypertension, etc.); patients with inadequate uterine cavity for embryo transfer (i.e. fluid in cavity), and low-responders seeking for a strategy to accumulate oocytes or embryos. In addition, in some areas around the world, especially Latin America, the endemic situation of the Zica virus is causing patients to either postpone or

Box 11.1: Indications for frozen embryo transfers.
FET indications
OHSS
Elevated progesterone
Genetic screening
Low responders
Inadequate uterine cavity
Hypertension
Zica virus (areas affected)

(FET: Frozen embryo transfer; OHSS: Ovarian hyperstimulation syndrome).

interrupt their IVF treatments to avoid infection during pregnancy. However, postponing is not a choice for some of our patients since they are already fighting with their biological clock, therefore initiating the treatment and freezing all the embryos represents a solution.

The importance of a good laboratory should be emphasized. Implementation of the freeze-all policy will not work unless high survival rates for oocytes and embryos are guaranteed. This aspect is not minor and it is the essence for this policy to work. Any embryologist would agree that vitrification is a laborious process, requiring a lot of focus and it is inevitably affected by a long learning curve. In this context, perhaps the introduction of automatic systems may help in the standardization of results and the easier implementation of freeze-all policies. Finally, we should consider the following: would IVF patients accept this shift? Are we ready to handle their expectations? A study evaluating patients attitudes toward eSET clearly showed that even though informed patients are sufficiently concerned about the adverse outcomes of multiple pregnancies they become less risk concerned when faced with multiple IVF failures and economic burden.[72] Then the question is—"why would elective freezing be any different than eSET?"

Enough questions still need to be answered and more well-designed trials are still necessary to confirm the clinical benefits of this policy and to justify a shift in current ART practice. Therefore, we believe that the freeze-all policy should only be implemented when there is a real indication for it.

REFERENCES

1. Lode H, Torres A, Cockle A. What drives our choices? Evidence, guidelines or habit? Int J Antimicrob Agents. 2007;29:S17-22.
2. Cobo A, de los Santos MJ, Castello D, et al. Outcomes of vitrified early cleavage-stage and blastocyst-stage embryos in a cryopreservation program: evaluation of 3,150 warming cycles. Fertil Steril. 2012;98:1138,46.e1.
3. Herrero L, Martinez M, Garcia-Velasco JA. Current status of human oocyte and embryo cryopreservation. Curr Opin Obstet Gynecol. 2011;23:245-50.
4. Tucker MJ, Wright G, Morton PC, et al. Birth after cryopreservation of immature oocytes with subsequent in vitro maturation. Fertil Steril. 1998;70:578-9.
5. Borini A, Bonu MA, Coticchio G, et al. Pregnancies and births after oocyte cryopreservation. Fertil Steril. 2004;82:601-5.
6. De Santis L, Cino I, Rabellotti E, et al. Oocyte cryopreservation: clinical outcome of slow-cooling protocols differing in sucrose concentration. Reprod Biomed Online. 2007;14:57-63.
7. Porcu E, Fabbri R, Seracchioli R, et al. Birth of a healthy female after intracytoplasmic sperm injection of cryopreserved human oocytes. Fertil Steril. 1997;68:724-6.
8. Chia CM, Chan WB, Quah E, et al. Triploid pregnancy after ICSI of frozen testicular spermatozoa into cryopreserved human oocytes: case report. Hum Reprod. 2000;15:1962-4.
9. Miller KA, Elkind-Hirsch K, Levy B, et al. Pregnancy after cryopreservation of donor oocytes and preimplantation genetic diagnosis of embryos in a patient with ovarian failure. Fertil Steril. 2004;82:211-4.

10. Greco E, Iacobelli M, Rienzi L, et al. Birth of a healthy boy after fertilization of cryopreserved oocytes with cryopreserved testicular spermatozoa from a man with nonmosaic Klinefelter syndrome. Fertil Steril. 2008;89:991.e5, 991.e7.
11. Gook DA, Edgar DH. Human oocyte cryopreservation. Hum Reprod Update. 2007;13:591-605.
12. Rezazadeh Valojerdi M, Eftekhari-Yazdi P, Karimian L, et al. Vitrification versus slow freezing gives excellent survival, post warming embryo morphology and pregnancy outcomes for human cleaved embryos. J Assist Reprod Genet. 2009;26:347-54.
13. Stehlik E, Stehlik J, Katayama KP, et al. Vitrification demonstrates significant improvement versus slow freezing of human blastocysts. Reprod Biomed Online. 2005;11:53-7.
14. Cobo A, Perez S, De los Santos MJ, et al. Effect of different cryopreservation protocols on the metaphase II spindle in human oocytes. Reprod Biomed Online. 2008;17:350-9.
15. Cobo A, Garrido N, Crespo J, et al. Accumulation of oocytes: a new strategy for managing low-responder patients. Reprod Biomed Online. 2012;24:424-32.
16. Milan M, Cobo AC, Rodrigo L, et al. Redefining advanced maternal age as an indication for preimplantation genetic screening. Reprod Biomed Online. 2010;21:649-57.
17. Herrero L, Pareja S, Aragones M, et al. Oocyte versus embryo vitrification for delayed embryo transfer: an observational study. Reprod Biomed Online. 2014;29:567-72.
18. Herrero L, Pareja S, Losada C, et al. Avoiding the use of human chorionic gonadotropin combined with oocyte vitrification and GnRH agonist triggering versus coasting: a new strategy to avoid ovarian hyperstimulation syndrome. Fertil Steril. 2011;95:1137-40.
19. Cobo A, Kuwayama M, Perez S, et al. Comparison of concomitant outcome achieved with fresh and cryopreserved donor oocytes vitrified by the Cryotop method. Fertil Steril. 2008;89:1657-64.
20. Li Z, Wang YA, Ledger W, et al. Clinical outcomes following cryopreservation of blastocysts by vitrification or slow freezing: a population-based cohort study. Hum Reprod. 2014;29:2794-801.
21. Shapiro BS, Daneshmand ST, Garner FC, et al. High ongoing pregnancy rates after deferred transfer through bipronuclear oocyte cryopreservation and post-thaw extended culture. Fertil Steril. 2009;92:1594-9.
22. Practice Committee of American Society for Reproductive Medicine. Ovarian hyperstimulation syndrome. Fertil Steril. 2008;90:S188-93.
23. Nastri CO, Ferriani RA, Rocha IA, et al. Ovarian hyperstimulation syndrome: pathophysiology and prevention. J Assist Reprod Genet. 2010;27:121-8.
24. Youssef MA, van Wely M, Hassan MA, et al. Can dopamine agonists reduce the incidence and severity of OHSS in IVF/ICSI treatment cycles? A systematic review and meta-analysis. Hum Reprod Update 2010;16:459-66.
25. Humaidan P, Quartarolo J, Papanikolaou EG. Preventing ovarian hyperstimulation syndrome: guidance for the clinician. Fertil Steril. 2010;94:389-400.
26. Gomez R, Soares SR, Busso C, et al. Physiology and pathology of ovarian hyperstimulation syndrome. Semin Reprod Med. 2010;28:448-57.
27. Olivennes F, Frydman R. Friendly IVF: the way of the future? Hum Reprod. 1998;13:1121-4.
28. Huirne JA, Homburg R, Lambalk CB. Are GnRH antagonists comparable to agonists for use in IVF? Hum Reprod. 2007;22:2805-13.

29. Borm G, Mannaerts B. Treatment with the gonadotrophin-releasing hormone antagonist ganirelix in women undergoing ovarian stimulation with recombinant follicle stimulating hormone is effective, safe and convenient: results of a controlled, randomized, multicentre trial. The European Orgalutran Study Group. Hum Reprod. 2000;15:1490-8.
30. Fluker M, Grifo J, Leader A, et al. Efficacy and safety of ganirelix acetate versus leuprolide acetate in women undergoing controlled ovarian hyperstimulation. Fertil Steril. 2001;75:38-45.
31. Kolibianakis EM, Schultze-Mosgau A, Schroer A, et al. A lower ongoing pregnancy rate can be expected when GnRH agonist is used for triggering final oocyte maturation instead of HCG in patients undergoing IVF with GnRH antagonists. Hum Reprod. 2005;20:2887-92.
32. Kolibianakis EM, Tarlatzis B, Devroey P. GnRH antagonists in IVF. Reprod Biomed Online. 2005;10:705-12.
33. Griesinger G, Diedrich K, Devroey P, et al. GnRH agonist for triggering final oocyte maturation in the GnRH antagonist ovarian hyperstimulation protocol: a systematic review and meta-analysis. Hum Reprod Update. 2006;12:159-68.
34. Youssef MA, Van der Veen F, Al-Inany HG, et al. Gonadotropin-releasing hormone agonist versus HCG for oocyte triggering in antagonist-assisted reproductive technology. Cochrane Database Syst Rev. 2014;10:CD008046.
35. Fatemi HM, Popovic-Todorovic B, Humaidan P, et al. Severe ovarian hyperstimulation syndrome after gonadotropin-releasing hormone (GnRH) agonist trigger and "freeze-all" approach in GnRH antagonist protocol. Fertil Steril. 2014;101:1008-11.
36. Gurbuz AS, Gode F, Ozcimen N, et al. Gonadotrophin-releasing hormone agonist trigger and freeze-all strategy does not prevent severe ovarian hyperstimulation syndrome: a report of three cases. Reprod Biomed Online. 2014;29:541-4.
37. Santos-Ribeiro S, Polyzos NP, Stouffs K, et al. Ovarian hyperstimulation syndrome after gonadotropin-releasing hormone agonist triggering and "freeze-all": in-depth analysis of genetic predisposition. J Assist Reprod Genet. 2015;32:1063-8.
38. Segal S, Casper RF. Progesterone supplementation increases luteal phase endometrial thickness and oestradiol levels in in-vitro fertilization. Hum Reprod. 1992;7:1210-3.
39. Casper RF. Introduction: Gonadotropin-releasing hormone agonist triggering of final follicular maturation for in vitro fertilization. Fertil Steril. 2015;103:865-6.
40. Kol S, Humaidan P, Alsbjerg B, et al. The updated Cochrane review 2014 on GnRH agonist trigger: repeating the same errors. Reprod Biomed Online. 2015;30:563-5.
41. Hamamah S, Matha V, Berthenet C, et al. Comparative protein expression profiling in human cumulus cells in relation to oocyte fertilization and ovarian stimulation protocol. Reprod Biomed Online. 2006;13:807-14.
42. Huirne JA, Lambalk CB, van Loenen AC, et al. Contemporary pharmacological manipulation in assisted reproduction. Drugs. 2004;64:297-322.
43. Silber S, Escudero T, Lenahan K, et al. Chromosomal abnormalities in embryos derived from testicular sperm extraction. Fertil Steril. 2003;79:30-8.
44. Platteau P, Staessen C, Michiels A, et al. Comparison of the aneuploidy frequency in embryos derived from testicular sperm extraction in obstructive and non-obstructive azoospermic men. Hum Reprod. 2004;19:1570-4.
45. Munne S, Fischer J, Warner A, et al. Preimplantation genetic diagnosis significantly reduces pregnancy loss in infertile couples: a multicenter study. Fertil Steril. 2006;85:326-32.

46. Munne S, Dailey T, Sultan KM, et al. The use of first polar bodies for preimplantation diagnosis of aneuploidy. Hum Reprod. 1995;10:1014-20.
47. Verlinsky Y, Kuliev A. Preimplantation polar body diagnosis. Biochem Mol Med. 1996;58:13-7.
48. Munne S, Chen S, Fischer J, et al. Preimplantation genetic diagnosis reduces pregnancy loss in women aged 35 years and older with a history of recurrent miscarriages. Fertil Steril. 2005;84:331-5.
49. Gianaroli L, Magli MC, Ferraretti AP, et al. Preimplantation diagnosis for aneuploidies in patients undergoing in vitro fertilization with a poor prognosis: identification of the categories for which it should be proposed. Fertil Steril. 1999;72:837-44.
50. Cohen J, Wells D, Munne S. Removal of 2 cells from cleavage stage embryos is likely to reduce the efficacy of chromosomal tests that are used to enhance implantation rates. Fertil Steril. 2007;87:496-503.
51. McArthur SJ, Leigh D, Marshall JT, et al. Pregnancies and live births after trophectoderm biopsy and preimplantation genetic testing of human blastocysts. Fertil Steril. 2005;84:1628-36.
52. Forman EJ, Hong KH, Ferry KM, et al. In vitro fertilization with single euploid blastocyst transfer: a randomized controlled trial. Fertil Steril. 2013;100:100,7.e1.
53. Helmerhorst FM, Perquin DA, Donker D, et al. Perinatal outcome of singletons and twins after assisted conception: a systematic review of controlled studies. BMJ. 2004;328:261.
54. Henningsen AK, Pinborg A, Lidegaard O, et al. Perinatal outcome of singleton siblings born after assisted reproductive technology and spontaneous conception: Danish national sibling-cohort study. Fertil Steril. 2011;95:959-63.
55. Bloise E, Feuer SK, Rinaudo PF. Comparative intrauterine development and placental function of ART concepti: implications for human reproductive medicine and animal breeding. Hum Reprod Update. 2014;20:822-39.
56. Pelkonen S, Koivunen R, Gissler M, et al. Perinatal outcome of children born after frozen and fresh embryo transfer: the Finnish cohort study 1995-2006. Hum Reprod. 2010;25:914-23.
57. Wennerholm UB, Henningsen AK, Romundstad LB, et al. Perinatal outcomes of children born after frozen-thawed embryo transfer: a Nordic cohort study from the CoNARTaS group. Hum Reprod. 2013;28:2545-53.
58. Ishihara O, Araki R, Kuwahara A, et al. Impact of frozen-thawed single-blastocyst transfer on maternal and neonatal outcome: an analysis of 277,042 single-embryo transfer cycles from 2008 to 2010 in Japan. Fertil Steril. 2014;101:128-33.
59. Maheshwari A, Pandey S, Shetty A, et al. Obstetric and perinatal outcomes in singleton pregnancies resulting from the transfer of frozen thawed versus fresh embryos generated through in vitro fertilization treatment: a systematic review and meta-analysis. Fertil Steril. 2012;98:368-77. e1-9.
60. Pinborg A, Loft A, Aaris Henningsen AK, et al. Infant outcome of 957 singletons born after frozen embryo replacement: the Danish National Cohort Study 1995-2006. Fertil Steril. 2010;94:1320-7.
61. Sazonova A, Kallen K, Thurin-Kjellberg A, et al. Obstetric outcome in singletons after in vitro fertilization with cryopreserved/thawed embryos. Hum Reprod. 2012;27(5):1343-50.
62. Roy TK, Bradley CK, Bowman MC, et al. Single-embryo transfer of vitrified-warmed blastocysts yields equivalent live-birth rates and improved neonatal outcomes compared with fresh transfers. Fertil Steril. 2014;101:1294-301.
63. Belva F, Bonduelle M, Roelants M, et al. Neonatal health including congenital malformation risk of 1072 children born after vitrified embryo transfer. Hum Reprod. 2016;31:1610-20.

64. Roque M, Lattes K, Serra S, et al. Fresh embryo transfer versus frozen embryo transfer in in vitro fertilization cycles: a systematic review and meta-analysis. Fertil Steril. 2013;99:156-62.
65. Humaidan P, Polyzos NP. (Meta)analyze this: systematic reviews might lose credibility. Nat Med. 2012;18:1321.
66. Aflatoonian A, Oskouian H, Ahmadi S, et al Can fresh embryo transfers be replaced by cryopreserved-thawed embryo transfers in assisted reproductive cycles? A randomized controlled trial. J Assist Reprod Genet. 2010;27:357-63.
67. Shapiro BS, Daneshmand ST, Garner FC, et al. Evidence of impaired endometrial receptivity after ovarian stimulation for in vitro fertilization: a prospective randomized trial comparing fresh and frozen-thawed embryo transfers in high responders. Fertil Steril. 2011;96:516-8.
68. Shapiro BS, Daneshmand ST, Garner FC, et al. Evidence of impaired endometrial receptivity after ovarian stimulation for in vitro fertilization: a prospective randomized trial comparing fresh and frozen-thawed embryo transfer in normal responders. Fertil Steril. 2011;96:344-8.
69. Griesinger G, Kolibianakis EM, Papanikolaou EG, et al. Triggering of final oocyte maturation with gonadotropin-releasing hormone agonist or human chorionic gonadotropin. Live birth after frozen-thawed embryo replacement cycles. Fertil Steril. 2007;88:616-21.
70. Griesinger G, Schultz L, Bauer T, et al. Ovarian hyperstimulation syndrome prevention by gonadotropin-releasing hormone agonist triggering of final oocyte maturation in a gonadotropin-releasing hormone antagonist protocol in combination with a "freeze-all" strategy: a prospective multicentric study. Fertil Steril. 2011;95:2029,33, 2033.e1.
71. Devroey P, Polyzos NP, Blockeel C. An OHSS-Free Clinic by segmentation of IVF treatment. Hum Reprod. 2011;26:2593-7.
72. Nachtigall RD, Mac Dougall K, Lee M, et al. What do patients want? Expectations and perceptions of IVF clinic information and support regarding frozen embryo disposition. Fertil Steril. 2010;94:2069-72.
73. Heng BC. Oocyte cryopreservation as alternative to embryo cryopreservation—some pertinent ethical concerns. Reprod Biomed Online. 2007;14:402-3.
74. Groenewoud ER, Cantineau AE, Kollen BJ, et al. What is the optimal means of preparing the endometrium in frozen-thawed embryo transfer cycles? A systematic review and meta-analysis. Hum Reprod Update. 2013;19:458-70.
75. Ghobara T, Vandekerckhove P. Cycle regimens for frozen-thawed embryo transfer. Cochrane Database Syst Rev. 2008;1:CD003414.
76. Atkinson P, Koch J, Ledger WL. GnRH agonist trigger and a freeze-all strategy to prevent ovarian hyperstimulation syndrome: a retrospective study of OHSS risk and pregnancy rates. Aust N Z J Obstet Gynaecol. 2014;54:581-5.
77. Borges E Jr, Braga DP, Setti AS, et al. Strategies for the management of OHSS: Results from freezing-all cycles. JBRA Assist Reprod. 2016;20:8-12.
78. Celada P, Bosch E, De los Santos MJ, et al. Elective frozen embryo transfer does not improve reproductive outcome in normo-responder patients. Hum Reprod. 2015;30:i112.
79. Roque M, Valle M, Guimaraes F, et al. Freeze-all policy: fresh vs. frozen-thawed embryo transfer. Fertil Steril. 2015;103:1190-3.
80. Blockeel C, Drakopoulos P, Santos-Ribeiro S, et al. A fresh look at the freeze-all protocol: a SWOT analysis. Hum Reprod. 2016;31:491-7.

Chapter 12

Ideal Protocol for Egg Donors

Pilar Alamá Faubel, Diana Collado Muñoz

INTRODUCTION

Selecting the best stimulation protocol is essential for adequate ovarian response. In egg donation program the stimulation protocol besides being cost-effective should be short and safe. In egg donors the best stimulation protocol is chosen based on: body mass index, antral follicle count (AFC) and experience in another stimulation cycles. The AFC is the most important control to choose the starting dose of gonadotropin to the stimulation in egg donors.

At present, the optimal protocol for donors is a protocol with gonadotropin-releasing hormone (GnRH) antagonist. This protocol has been shown to offer an advantage over standard long agonist protocol in terms of decreasing incidence of ovarian hyperstimulation syndrome (OHSS), short duration of treatment, lower cost, lesser doses of gonadotropins required and being more patient friendly. There are no differences in term of ovarian response and outcomes depending on the type of gonadotropins used. In GnRH antagonist, GnRH analogs are used for triggering in all cases, avoiding OHSS in these patients. Frequently contraceptives can be used to avoid weekend retrievals and to distribute the oocyte retrievals during the week.

The ovarian stimulation protocol is very important in order to obtain a good ovarian response. Although the number of oocytes is important, it is equally important the quality of oocytes. The main goal of assisted reproductive technology (ART) is live birth.

The choice of the best ovarian stimulation protocol depends on the cause of sterility, age of the patient, ovarian reserve, body mass index (BMI), response to stimulation in previous cycles and experience of the specialist.

In egg donor population we take into account: ovarian reserve, age, BMI and response to stimulation in previous cycles. Egg donors are young people, most of them have their own fertility, who undergo voluntary stimulation treatment, to give all the oocytes obtained in the pickup, to other couple.

For this reason in egg donation program, we need to consider the efficiency of the protocol (good ovarian response and good ovarian quality), as well as, short and safe protocols in order to achieve greater adherence of women to stimulation treatments.

OVARIAN STIMULATION DRUGS FOR EGG DONOR PROGRAM

Four different types of drugs are needed to perform an ovarian stimulation: (1) pretreatment in luteal phase, (2) pituitary desensitization, (3) gonadotropins for ovarian stimulation, and finally (4) drugs for ovarian triggering.

Pretreatment

Gonadotropin-releasing hormone agonists were introduced in assisted reproductive treatments in the 1980s, to reversibly block pituitary function and prevent a luteinizing hormone surge.

The major benefits of the Gonadotropin-releasing hormone agonists include decreased cancellation rate through prevention of premature luteinizing hormone (LH) surge and luteinization, enhancement of follicular recruitment, allowing the recovery of a larger number of oocytes, and the improvement in routine patient treatment schedule. The long protocol, starting Gonadotropin-releasing hormone agonists (GnRH agonists) in the midluteal phase of the preceding cycle had been considered the gold standard protocol in young normogonadotropic women.

Gonadotropin-releasing hormone agonists long protocol induces profound suppression of endogenous release of gonadotropins during the early follicular phase, allowing the early antral follicles to grow coordinately in response to exogenous gonadotropins to accomplish simultaneous maturation. This leads to an extended widening of the follicle-stimulating hormone (FSH) window, an increased number of recruited mature follicles and a higher number of retrieved oocytes and pregnancy rates and take home baby rates.

The introduction of GnRH antagonists in ART to prevent LH surge, seemed to open up a new way toward a more "friendly in vitro fertilization (IVF)": The GnRH antagonist offers a viable alternative to the long agonists, providing a shorter duration of treatment with fewer injections and with less frequent occurrence of side effects (e.g. hot flushes, headache, bleeding, and cyst development) during the desensitization period.

In the GnRH antagonists protocol, the gonadotropins are started on day 2–3 of the cycle. This fact makes it difficult to schedule the clinic's activity to avoid weekend oocyte retrievals.

Some authors have proposed to advance or delay the triggering date according classical criteria to pick-up to avoid weekend oocyte retrievals, but this strategy was not useful.[2]

There are different strategies for planning the start of the stimulation cycle. The most used are combined oral contraceptive (OC) and estradiol valerate pretreatment in luteal phase. Both are based on suppressing the rise of FSH that takes place during the transition of the luteal phase and the initial proliferative phase, to achieve a synchronization of the follicular cohort, and thus to obtain a more synchronized response.

In egg donor population, the best strategy to make easier the planning of the stimulation cycle is the used of OC. All of them are young women of childbearing age and in many cases already use OC as a contraceptive method.

According to a survey conducted in 2009 on contraceptive habits in Spain, 24% of women of child-bearing age used hormonal contraceptives in any of their routes of administration. It is also estimated that about three millions women use OCs not only for contraceptive protection but also for their additional benefits to regulate the menstrual cycle.[3]

There are several published studies on the use of OCs before a stimulation cycle with GnRH antagonists. Early retrospectives studies showed that pretreatment with OC had no effect on the results of the stimulation. In 2008, Griesinger et al.[4] published a meta-analysis showing that gonadotropins doses, days of stimulation, as well as cycle outcomes (pregnancy and implantation rate) were worse with pretreatment with OCs. This publication generated a great debate in the scientific population, due to the results it showed, but when studying the review in detail, there was a great heterogeneity in the included studies, so caution should be exercised when interpreting the results. The reason for which pregnancy rates were supposed to decrease with OCs pretreatment was related to deleterious effect on the endometrial implantation.

A subsequent study by Bermejo in egg donors found no difference in the expressive pattern of the genes involved in endometrial receptivity depending on whether or not they used ACOs in the previous cycle.[5]

Another fact to emphasize is the days that pass between the last pill of COs and the start of the stimulation. Starting the stimulation early or late after the stop of COs may have an impact on the outcome of the stimulation. At the present time the studies defend to start the stimulation at the 5th day after stopping the last pill of COs[6] since it is the period necessary for the normalization of the hormonal previously inhibited values by the use of COs.

A recent study in IVI group compared estradiol valerate pretreatment with COs in cycles with GnRH antagonists in patients 18–38 years of age, finding no significant difference in cycle parameters and clinical outcomes. The only significant difference found was the duration of treatment in favor of estrogens.[7]

We can conclude that in egg donors we can use the COs to be able to assure a better planning of the cycle, without that has impact in the results of the cycle.

Gonadotropin-releasing Hormone Analog for Pituitary Desensitization

Through the early 1980s, GnRH agonist was applied to prevent the LH surge during ovarian stimulation. By the end of the decade, the so-called long downregulation protocol with GnRH agonist was established IVF practice, significantly reducing the rate of cycle cancellation, improving outcomes and enabling some flexibility to schedule oocyte retrieval.[1] Two decades later, GnRH antagonists have been introduced into IVF and have emerged as an alternative in preventing premature LH surges. There are a number advantages of GnRH antagonists versus GnRH agonists: (a) less FSH dosage required for ovarian stimulation;[8] (b) fewer secondary effects due to hypoestrogenism; (c) less stimulation days; (d) less consumption of gonadotropins with the subsequent relation with the cost of the cycle; (e) reduction in a 50% of the OHSS.

For all these reasons, it was evident a change in the stimulation protocols in favor of the usage of the GnRH antagonists. Nevertheless, a review published in 2006 by Al-Inany et al.[9] showed worst rates on live births on cycles with GnRH antagonists than those ones with agonists. Some authors consider that the initial results difference was due to the learning curve of the GnRH antagonist usage, and also due to the usage of GnRH antagonist with patients of advanced age, low response and worst diagnosis.

Nevertheless, on the last review published by Cochrane in 2011 about the use of GnRH agonists and antagonists concludes that there are not significant differences in the live birth rate rates between both protocols; and there is a relevant decrease of the incidence of the OHSS in cycles with GnRH antagonists.[10]

In the oocyte donor population, in addition to the advantages described above in this text, GnRH antagonists allow to trigger the ovulation with GnRH agonists, keeping in mind that the OHSS can almost be completely let aside.

As far as the introduction of the GnRH antagonists[10] in a fixed or flexible protocol is concerned, different trials have shown that the introduction of a flexible protocol with 13–14 mm follicles could improve the performance of the stimulation cycles, since it helps to reduce the dosage of gonadotropins used, as well as the number of antagonist vials.[11]

Induction of the Multiple Follicle Development in Oocyte Donors

Taking the previous criteria into account, during the election of the suitable stimulation protocol for donors we will evaluate:

- Initial FSH dosage
- Controversy respect to recombinant and urinary gonadotropins.

Initial FSH Dosage

The initial FSH dosage is decided in a personalized way by the specialist dealing with the patient, depending on her age, body mass index, ovarian response in previous cycles and ovarian reserve previous to the stimulation—including, at least, the AFC.[12]

This initial evaluation has a vital importance when it is time to reach adequate results in the oocyte donation program in order to reduce the number of cancellations due to high or low response.

We should not forget that we are dealing with young patients, healthy, normoresponders and without fertility problems. One study published by Melo et al. in 2009 established the cut-off point in AFC to predict a bad response to the stimulation in 12 antral follicles in both ovaries. Under this AFC the possibility of a cancellation of an ovarian stimulation cycle could reach up to a 40%, depending on the criteria of the cancellation of the cycle.[13]

That is the reason why the initial dosage of gonadotropins usually ranges:

- When the AFC more than 20 in both ovaries: 150 IU of FSH or 187/225 of highly purified human menopausal gonadotropin (HP-hMG).
- When the AFC is between 12 and 20 in both ovaries: Between 200 and 225 IU of FSH or 150 IU of FSH/75 IU of HP-hMG. In the case of using corifollitropin alfa, the election dosage will vary depending on the weight of the patient: When more than 60 kg, 150 µg of corifollitropin alfa; when the weight is less than 60 kg: 100 µg of corifollitropin alfa.

In the case of using medication with urinary origin, in both FSH and HP-hMG, the starting dosages use to be slightly higher.

Controversy Respect to Recombinant and Urinary Gonadotropins

In relation to the controversial question about the usage of recombinant or urinary gonadotropins, there are many reviews and all of them conclude that there are not differences in the gonadotropin to be used.

In 2011 the last Cochrane review was published, where Van Wely et al.[14] compared recombinant and urinary gonadotropins in normoresponder patients under 35, including 42 trials with 9,606 couples and clearly similar results as far as effectiveness and security are concerned. One exception arises when it has been compared the group with hMG/HP-hMG and the recombinant FSH one, where results show a 3% higher number of live birth than the hMG group.

Another study performed by Melo et al. [20] in our group compared, in donor women, rFSH versus HP-hMG + rFSH and protocols with HP-hMG in a protocol with GnRH agonists. No differences were found in those three protocols in the ovarian stimulation parameters, or in the clinical outcomes. Nevertheless, the protocols where HP-hMG was used were more cost-efficient than the rest.

It is also relevant to mention a recent study performed by our group in the oocyte donor population where it was compared the use of corifollitropin alfa with rFSH daily dosage. Although there were no differences between the number of retrieved oocytes and the final results, it is true that those women stimulated with corifollitropin alfa, preferred in a 75% the same protocol, while just a 25% rFSH[15] wanted so.

Therefore, as a conclusion, choose the best gonadotropin for ovarian stimulation protocol for oocyte donors must depend on the availability, convenience and cost of the treatment.

Ovulation Induction: Final Oocyte Maturation with GnRH Agonists

The introduction of GnRH antagonists in stimulation protocols was a key factor to open the option to use a single GnRH agonist bolus as the trigger to the oocyte maturation at the end of the stimulation.

The LH[16] surge that goes with the *flare* effect after the GnRH agonist administration promotes the periovulatory changes that lead to the oocyte maturation and the ovulation triggering.

Advantages in the use of GnRH agonist:

- The amount of gonadotropins released during the surge promoted by the GnRH agonist is reduced drastically when it is compared to the ones released during the natural cycle.[17]
- Triggering with GnRH agonist, compared to the use of hCG, is responsible for FSH wave compared to the one of a spontaneous cycle. Some studies have remarked a greater number of mature oocytes retrieved when the final maturation is completed with GnRH agonist; and a possible explanation for that would be the change which produced, is more physiologic and natural since it includes the FSH wave along with the LH[16] surge.
- But no doubt about this, its main advantage is the great reduction of a potentially dangerous situation such as OHSS[18-19] and it will not harm neither the ovarian quality nor the pregnancy rates in recipient patients.
- The luteal phase defect linked to this oocyte maturation option does not present an inconvenience, but it brings another advantage in the oocyte donors, since the menstruation will take place 3–5 days after the follicle pick up.

CONCLUSION

In the daily practice in our clinics, all the patients included in the donation program are stimulated with a protocol with daily dosage antagonists with the different options of available gonadotropins in the market.

In most of the cases, donors will use contraceptive pills (COs) in the previous month to the stimulation start which, in our case, will take place from Friday to Sunday since the goal is to redistribute pick ups throughout the week.

The final oocyte maturation will happen when the follicles reach diameters around 17–22 mm, which is a range that allows—in most of the cases—to program the pick up in those days where the clinics have more activity, avoiding to have pick ups during the weekend and additional workloads for the IVF laboratory—improving, therefore, its performance.

We carry out the oocyte maturation with triptorelina 0.2 mg in a single dosage under skin, programming the ovarian pick up 36 hours after its administration.

REFERENCES

1. Tarlatzis BC, Kolibianakis EM. GnRH agonists vs antagonists. Best Pract Res Clin Obstet Gynaecol. 2007;21:57-65.
2. Tremellen K, Lane M. Avoidance of weekend oocyte retrievals during GnRH antagonist treatment by simple advancement or delay of hCG administration does not adversely affect IVF live births outcomes. Hum Reprod. 2010;25: 1219-24.
3. De la Cuesta Benjumea R, Franco Tejeda C, Iglesias Goy E. Actualización en anticoncepción hormonal. del Sistema Nacional de Salud. Volumen 35, No 3/2011. pp. 75-87.
4. Griesinger G, Venetis CA, Marx T, et al. Oral contraceptive pill pretreatment in ovarian stimulation with GnRH antagonists for IVF: a systematic review and meta-analysis. Fertil Steril. 2008;90:1055-63.
5. Bermejo A, Iglesias C, Ruiz-Alonso M, et al. The impact of using the combined oral contraceptive pill for cycle scheduling on gene expression related to endometrial receptivity. Hum Reprod. 2014;29:1271-8.
6. Cédrin-Durnerin I, Bständig B, Parneix I, et al. Effects of oral contraceptive, synthetic progestogen or natural estrogen pre-treatments on the hormonal profile and the antral follicle cohort before GnRH antagonist protocol. Hum Reprod. 2007;22:109-16.
7. Hauzman EE, Zapata A, Bermejo A, et al. Cycle scheduling for in vitro fertilization with oral contraceptive pills versus oral estradiol valerate: a randomized, controlled trial. Reprod Biol Endocrinol. 2013;11:96.
8. Borm G, Mannaerts B. Treatment with the gonadotrophin-releasing hormone antagonist ganirelix in women undergoing ovarian stimulation with recombinant follicle stimulating hormone is effective, safe and convenient: results of a controlled, randomized, multicentre trial. The European Orgalutran Study Group. Hum Reprod. 2000;15:1490-8.
9. Al-Inany HG, Abou-Setta AM, Aboulghar M. Gonadotrophin-releasing hormone antagonists for assisted conception. Cochrane Database Syst Rev. 2006;3:CD001750.
10. Al-Inany HG, Youssef MA, Aboulghar M, et al. Gonadotrophin releasing hormone antagonists for assisted reproductive technology. Cochrane Database Syst Rev. 2011;5:CD001750.
11. Ludwig M, Katalinic A, Banz C, et al. Tailoring the GnRH antagonist cetrorelix acetate to individual patients' needs in ovarian stimulation for IVF: results of a prospective, randomized study. Hum Reprod. 2002;17:2842-5.
12. Broekmans FJ, de Ziegler D, Howles CM, et al. The antral follicle count: practical recommendations for better standardization. Fertil Steril. 2010;94:1044-51.
13. Melo MA, Garrido N, Álvarez C, et al. Antral follicle count (AFC) can be used in the prediction of ovarian response but cannot predict the oocyte/embryo quality in the IVF outcome in a egg donation programme. Fertil Steril. 2009;91: 148-56.

14. van Wely M, Kwan I, Burt AL, et al. Recombinant versus urinary gonadotrophin for ovarian stimulation in assisted reproductive technology cycles. Cochrane Database Syst Rev. 2011;2:CD005354.
15. Requena A, Cruz M, Collado D, et al. Evaluation of the degree of satisfaction in oocyte donors using sustained-release FSH corifollitropina α. Reprod Biomed Online. 2013;26:253-9.
16. Humaidan P, Bredkjaer HE, Bungum L, et al. GnRh agonist (buserelin) or hCG for ovulation induction in GnRH antagonist IVF/ICSI cycles: a prospective randomized study. Hum Reprod. 2005;20:1213-20.
17. Aboulghar MA, Mansour RT, Serour GI, et al. Oocyte quality in patients with severe ovarian hyperstimulation syndrome. Fertil Steril. 1997;68:1017-21.
18. Bodri D, Guillen JJ, Trullenque M, et al. Early ovarian hyperstimulation syndrome is completely prevented by gonadotropin releasing-hormone agonist triggering in high-risk oocyte donor cycles: a prospective, luteal-phase follow-up study. Fertil Steril. 2010;93:2418-20.
19. Melo M, Busso CE, Bellver J, et al. GnRH agonist versus recombinant HCG in an oocyte donation programme: a randomized, prospective, controlled, assessor-blind study. Reprod Biomed Online. 2009;19:486-92.
20. Melo M, Bellver J, Garrido N, et al. A prospective, randomized, controlled trial comparing three different gonadotropin regimens in oocyte donors: ovarian response, in vitro fertilization outcome, and analysis of cost minimization. Fertil Steril. 2010;94:958-64.

Chapter 13

Protocols for Thaw Embryo Transfer

Krithika Devi J

INTRODUCTION

Cryopreservation heralded a new era in assisted reproductive technology. Trounson and Mohr in 1983 reported the first live birth following frozen embryo transfer (FET). Despite the growing importance of FET in the treatment of subfertility, there is little consensus on the best method for endometrial preparation.[1] Different in vitro fertilization (IVF) clinics have different protocols for giving these medications, and there is no definite consensus over an ideal protocol.

Key Points for a Successful Frozen Embryo Transfer

- Selecting proper embryos
- Accurate synchronization of endometrium and embryos
- Luteal support.

The various available options for endometrial preparation for a FET cycle are described in Table 13.1.

NATURAL CYCLE FROZEN EMBRYO TRANSFER

In patients with predictable menstrual cycles, we can carefully monitor the cycle to determine the precise timing of ovulation. Once the precise date of ovulation is set, then the uterine lining should be receptive to embryo transfer 3/5 days later depending on the day it was frozen. In this way, the embryos can

Table 13.1: Protocols for a thaw embryo transfer cycle.

S No	*Protocols*	*Drugs*
1.	Natural cycle	No drugs
2.	Modified natural cycle	hCG trigger ± progesterone
3.	Stimulation cycle	Clomiphene citrate /hMG/FSH
4.	Hormone replacement cycle	Estrogens and progesterones/GnRH analogs

(hCG: Human chorionic gonadotropin; hMG: Human menopausal gonadotropin; FSH: Follicle-stimulating hormone; GnRH: Gonadotropin-releasing hormone).

be replaced at approximately the time when they would normally be arriving in the uterus. Pregnancy rates in natural cycle frozen embryo transfer (NC-FET) are closely dependent on the timely identification of ovulation and calculation of the likely subsequent period of optimal endometrial receptivity.[2,3]

Natural cycle frozen embryo transfer poses the risk of unobserved ovulation. If ovulation occurs without notice, accurate planning of embryo thawing and transfer is not possible, which results in cycle cancellation (7–12%).[4]

Natural cycle frozen embryo transfer involves frequent monitoring of urine and/or blood luteinizing hormone (LH) levels, early luteal serum progesterone levels, and ultrasound monitoring of the developing dominant follicle. For optimal FET results precise identification of the LH surge and adequate natural corpus lutein function are required which may be difficult for logistic reasons.

The advantages and disadvantages of the natural cycle thaw embryo transfer are shown in Figure 13.1.

Luteinizing Hormone Monitoring—Practical Challenges in a Natural Cycle

- Possible only in women with perfect ovulatory cycles
- Luteinizing hormone surges in urine lag up to 21 hours behind the appearance of the surge in blood, and this should be taken into consideration when interpreting urinary measurements[5-8]
- Variation in timing of LH surge occurrence between cycles and between patients[9]
- Luteinizing hormone levels needs to be assessed daily and preferably twice a day around ovulatory period. LH urine kits have a large variation in thresholds, which involve the risk of up to 30% of false-negative testing.[8,10,11]

Drawbacks of Natural Cycle Frozen Embryo Transfer

- Planning NC-FET carries the risk of unexpected ovulation and difficulty in ensuring timely thawing and transfer of the embryo
- It demands frequent monitoring around the time of ovulation
- The optimal time for implantation may fall at an unpredictable time during the laboratory work schedule, so some clinics choose not to offer NC-FET.

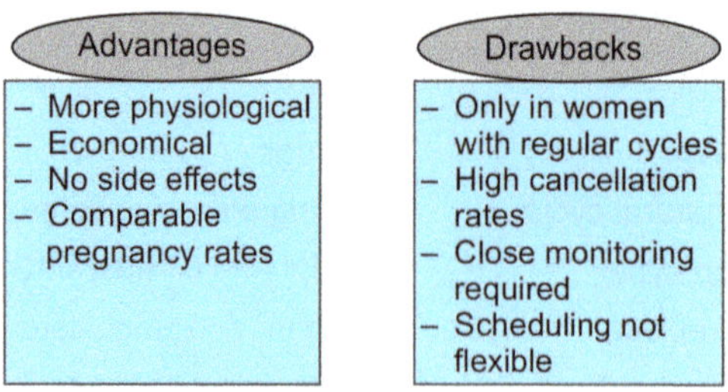

Fig. 13.1: Natural cycle—Thaw embryo transfer.

MODIFIED NATURAL CYCLE FROZEN EMBRYO TRANSFER

To overcome the disadvantages of LH monitoring, human chorionic gonadotropin (hCG) triggering of ovulation is often employed in NC-FET in what is termed "modified NC-FET". Modified natural cycles do not require LH monitoring, but regular ultrasound evaluation of the dominant follicle is required to ensure appropriate timing of hCG administration.

Ultrasound measurements of the endometrial stripe and monitoring of serum hormone levels is also done. As soon as the dominant follicle is of sufficient size (17–18 mm), hCG is administered as a surrogate to the endogenous LH surge to trigger final oocyte maturation and ovulation, which takes place approximately 36–38 hours later.[5]

This approach allows for precise definition of the ovulation trigger for scheduling FET, and also provides luteal support in the form of hCG in case of possible luteal dysfunction.

True Natural Cycle versus Modified Natural Cycle Using hCG

It is important to make a distinction between natural and modified natural FET protocols because of the inherent additional luteal phase support provided by hCG injection in the modified NC protocols. In both true and modified NC cycles, thawing and transfer of the embryo should be performed 3–5 days after ovulation depending on the stage of the embryo when frozen.[12,13] The advantages of modified NC-FET are its simplicity with no injections (besides the hCG trigger shot) and minimal additional medications with an overall cost savings compared with a medicated FET.

Five studies, representing 1,965 cycles, were identified comparing true NC-FET with modified NC-FET.[4,14-16] The pooled result of all studies analyses showed no significant difference with regard to clinical pregnancy [odds ratio (OR) 0.91, 95% confidence interval (CI) 0.74–1.1], ongoing pregnancy (OR 1.0, 95% CI 0.66–1.6) and live birth (OR 1.0, 95% CI 0.63–1.6).

Role of Luteal Phase Progesterones in Natural Cycles

In fertility proven women, endogenous production of progesterone from the corpus luteum is sufficient to support the embryo implantation in a natural ovulatory cycle. However, the women undergoing FET are often subfertile or infertile, and their corpus luteal progesterone production may be insufficient during their natural cycles in some women. Inadequate progesterone production during the luteal phase or early pregnancy period can result in implantation failure or spontaneous abortion.

In the prospective randomized controlled trial (RCT) by Bjuresten et al.[17] and in other studies,[18,19] progesterone supplementation showed higher live birth rates and reduced miscarriage rates in patients undergoing NC-FET with luteal support. However, there are few studies published regarding luteal phase support in NC-FET including Kyrou et al.,[20] Eftekhar et al.[21] who showed in their analysis no benefit of luteal phase support in patients undergoing modified NC-FET.

Based on the conflicting results of the studies it can be concluded that currently there is too little evidence supporting a positive effect of luteal phase support in patients undergoing NC-FET.

STIMULATED CYCLE FROZEN EMBRYO TRANSFER

Stimulated cycle is where fertility drugs such as gonadotropin injection is usually recommended for women who did not ovulate regularly and did not respond to hormone replacement treatment (HRT) in a previous cycle.

Stimulated FET cycles consist of the administration of human menopausal gonadotropins (hMG) or follicle-stimulating hormone (FSH) in low doses 50 or 75 IU/day from cycle day 2 or day 3. Sizes of follicles are monitored with ultrasound, and ovulation is induced with exogenous hCG administration when the dominant follicle reaches more than 17–18 mm in diameter and estradiol levels exceed 300 pg/mL. Embryo transfer is undertaken when these criteria are met. Progesterone is provided for luteal support (Fig. 13.2).[22]

Cochrane review on treatment regimes in FET concluded that current evidence does not demonstrate a significant difference in pregnancy rates between these methods of endometrial preparation.[23]

HORMONE REPLACEMENT FROZEN EMBRYO TRANSFER CYCLE

Hormone replacement cycle (HRT) allows the couple to avoid some of the pitfalls associated with a NC-FET. Medicated FETs do allow for advance scheduling, which both patients and physicians find attractive. The patient and medical team can focus on preparing the uterine lining and will thaw the embryos when the patient's lining is most likely to allow for implantation.

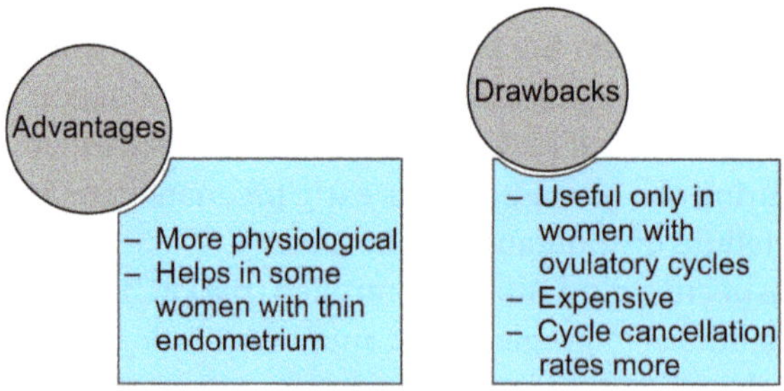

Fig. 13.2: Stimulation cycle for thaw embryo transfer.

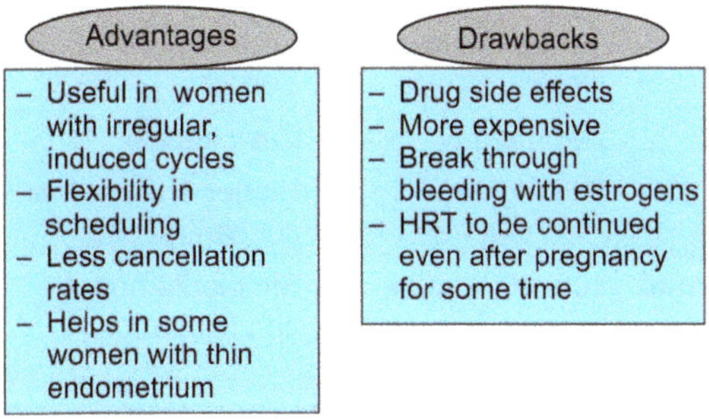

Fig. 13.3: HRT cycle for thaw embryo transfer.
(HRT: Hormone replacement treatment).

The HRT carries some advantages over natural cycles. By using HRT, fewer times of visits were needed during the cycles—which considerably benefit the patients. The day of embryos thawing and transfer can be scheduled in advance. Treatment cancellation rate are limited in HRT, due to the programed exogenous hormone replacement and suppression of ovulation. HRT constitutes a more suitable option for some specific patients, such as women with more than 40 years old, premature ovarian failure, and oligomenorrhea (Fig. 13.3).

In programed FET, estrogen and progesterone are administered in a sequential regimen, which aims to mimic the endocrine exposure of the endometrium in the normal cycle. Initially, estradiol is given in order to cause proliferation of the endometrium, while suppressing the development of the dominant follicle. This is continued until the endometrium is observed to be 7–9 mm thick on ultrasound, at which time progesterone assay is done and after ascertaining it is low (preferred cut off—less than 0.5 ng/mL) progesterone is added to initiate secretory changes.[24] The physiological mid-cycle shift from estrogen to progesterone is thus emulated.[25,26] The day progesterone is started is considered ovulation/OPU day and the time of thaw/transfer is planned accordingly.

When to Start and Stop Estrogen

The moment of commencing estrogen (E2) supplementation can differ, but all studies are suggesting to start before the fourth day of the cycle. Timely starting of E2 reduces the chance of unwanted follicular development and thus ovulation. In artificial endometrial preparation cycles without GnRH agonist use, it is better to start estrogens early at day 1–2 of menstrual cycle, after this time the inhibition of spontaneous ovulation is questionable.

If the pregnancy test is positive estrogen supplementation is maintained until 10–12 weeks of pregnancy. The dose can be reduced, tapered and stopped around that time.

Table 13.2: Estrogen administration.

S No	Route	Dose	Benefits	Drawbacks
1.	Oral	2–8 mg/day	Easy intake	Multiple doses
2.	Vaginal	2–8 mg/day	Higher endometrial concentrations	Inconvenient
3.	Transdermal	100–400 µg/24 hours	Simple/24 hours administration	Expensive

Estrogen Administration

In patients who are unable to tolerate oral route, vaginal and transdermal route seemed to be an equally effective alternative (Table 13.2).

Zhihong Niu et al.[27] suggested step-up protocol estradiol instead of fixed high dose estrogen because the former protocol is more similar to physiologic pattern and it is more suitable for endometrial maturation and then embryo implantation. Navot et al.[28] reported that shorter (5-10 days) and lower dosage protocols of estradiol priming of the endometrium could result in higher abortion rates. Borini et al.[29] also found a proliferative phase of less than 10 days is related to a higher abortion rate. This indicates an optimal endometrial proliferation, which is necessary to enable optimal development of progesterone receptors and subsequent transformation into an endometrium receptive to the transferred embryo. Devroey and Pados[30] presumed that an adequate period of estrogen administration is necessary in order to achieve a subsequent normal secretory endometrium.

HORMONE REPLACEMENT CYCLE WITH GnRH AGONIST

In some women GnRH agonists may be given in addition to hormone replacement to suppress any hormone production by the ovaries, which may interfere with the treatment.

The administration of estrogen and progesterone does not guarantee complete pituitary suppression, and a dominant follicle may therefore occur. If the follicle undergoes spontaneous lutenization, it may cause premature exposture of the endometrium to progesterone's and affect the synchrony between the endometrium and the embryo implantation. For this reason GnRH agonist co-treatment may be used to downregulate the pituitary and prevent follicular growth. However, it remains unclear whether any one of these approaches is superior to another with regard to ongoing pregnancy rate and patients preference.

The aim of pretreatment with GnRH agonist is to avoid spontaneous ovulation, but it is costly and there is a risk of hypoestrogenic side effect that would lengthen the preparation. Many published studies compared the two artificial protocols and showed the similar clinical outcome.[24,31,32] Van de Vijver et al.[33] in his study retrospectively analyzed 1,129 frozen transfer cycles and concluded that live birth rates after cryopreserved embryo transfer in artificial cycles did not increase when a GnRH agonist was administered.[34]

Givens et al.[35] observed no difference in pregnancy rates between NC-FET and HRT-FET. Pregnancy rates did not differ significantly between both groups.

HRT-FET with or without GnRH: Both require medication and are therefore less "physiological", but the cycles are easier to plan making it popular among many patients and their doctors.

ROLE OF PROGESTERONE ASSAY IN HORMONE REPLACEMENT FROZEN EMBRYO TRANSFER CYCLES

Since programed FET does not guarantee complete downregulation, luteinization may occur in 5% of the cases and can affect the pregnancy rates.[24] Doing a progesterone assay before the start of progesterone in the cycle helps in identifying premature luteinization and cycle cancellation is recommended if the value is more than 0.5 ng/mL.

In cases where progesterone hormone levels are too high, the delicate synchronization of the embryo and the uterine lining (a.k.a. endometrium) are disturbed. Increased levels of progesterone can result in "advancement" of the uterine lining, such that the uterus is no longer optimally receptive when the embryo is ready to implant. From a cost-efficiency perspective, this aspect is of great importance and should be taken into account.

Whether an ovulatory HRT cycle should be cancelled constitutes a dilemma in practice of FET treatment. The unsuppressed follicle development and ovulation may alter the hormone profile, and thus impair the endometrial receptivity and pregnancy. Studies have found decreased implantation rates and pregnancy rates in ovulatory patients. This finding has clinical implication that the HRT cycle with unsuppressed ovulation may need to be cancelled.

OPTIMAL ENDOMETRIAL THICKNESS/ENDOMETRIAL PATTERN

Endometrial thickness and pattern still remain the most researched parameters for their predictive value in IVF. An endometrial thickness of less than 7 mm at the time of embryo implantation is considered suboptimal in ART.

Kumbak et al.[37] looked at the cycle characteristics and outcomes of 175 patients with an endometrial thickness of less than 7 mm on the day of oocyte retrieval. Patients were stratified according to three endometrial thickness groups ≥4 mm and <5 mm, ≥5 mm and <6 mm, and ≥6 mm and <7 mm. Pregnancy rate and implantation rate did not show a statistically significant difference among the three groups though an increasing trend in values was observed as endometrial thickness increased.

A contrary view was given by Kasius et al.,[36] based on a systematic review and meta-analysis of 1,170 studies. Their review suggests that endometrial thickness cannot be used as a parameter to decide on cycle cancelation, freezing of all embryos or discontinuing IVF treatment. One can conclude from this review that *endometrial thickness can give us probability but cannot be predictive of pregnancy*.

In all studies, the start of progesterone was determined based on the endometrium thickness (7–8 mm). This is in-line with the fact that not duration of estrogen supplementation but the endometrium thickness should be the leading factor in determining the start of progesterone.[12,38]

Endometrial thickness was not significantly associated with clinical outcomes of euploid embryos. A type 3-endometrial pattern at trigger day suggests a prematurely closed window of implantation.[39]

EXTENDED ESTROGEN SUPPORT

Endometrial thickness can be improved by extending the estrogen administration for 14–60 days, in HRT-FET cycles. A receptive endometrium should reach a thickness of at least 7–8 mm. Above this threshold, the endometrium can maintain its receptivity for up to 40–60 days, as has been shown by oocyte donation programs.[40]

IS ASSESSMENT OF FUNCTIONALITY IMPORTANT?

As suggested by various case reports and studies—thin endometrium is not necessarily nonreceptive. The endometrium receptivity array (ERA) test is a molecular test that defines the window of endometrial receptivity. This test can be used to confirm the receptivity of a thin endometrium before planning FET. In case of a changed window of receptivity, a personalized embryo transfer can be performed. A study done on patients with thin endometrium less than or equal to 6 mm patients revealed that ERA was nonreceptive in 23% (3/13) and receptive in 77% (10/13). The proportion of receptive to nonreceptive endometrium was not different from patients with endometrial thickness more than 6 mm. The overall pregnancy rate in the thin endometrium group—who underwent embryo transfer after ERA was 33.3% (6/9).[41]

The burning question regarding treatment of thin refractory endometrium remains unanswered. A number of treatments have been tried. Intrauterine insertion of granulocyte-colony stimulating factor (G-CSF), sildenafil, tocopherol, aspirin, and L-arginine have been used to improve endometrial vascularity but none validated so far.

Thin endometrium may not necessarily be secondary to a disease process. It can result from individual uterine architecture or the intrinsic properties of endometrium that affect its growth.[42]

MONITORING THE FROZEN EMBRYO TRANSFER CYCLE

Involves a baseline ultrasound for all the patients irrespective of the protocol used. Baseline hormone profile to exclude cysts in selective cases after scan. In HRT cycles estrogen valerate is started at a dose of 4 mg a day, and stepped-up to 6 mg/day. An ultrasound assessment of the endometrial lining is made between the 9th day and 11th day and estradiol dose can be increased up to 8–10 mg/day if required. A trilaminar pattern with a thickness of 7–9 mm or above is indicative of good proliferation. A blood test for serum progesterone is done, and vaginal progesterone is started. Embryo transfer is carried out 3/5 days later depending on the day it was frozen.

WHEN TO STOP PROGESTERONES?

The available data have been insufficient to determine the optimal duration of therapy, and prolonged progesterone protocols have been the rule, with most clinicians following the dictum, "better safe than sorry". A growing body of evidence, however, has challenged this concept and adds to the increasing concern that progesterone supplementation of early pregnancy after IVF/ICSI might be unnecessary.

Frozen embryo transfer cycles with HRT and donor oocyte recipient cycles are different from stimulated IVF cycles in that there is no endogenous progesterone production, and therefore instead of luteal phase supplementation, there is a need for luteal phase "creation" or replacement.

Vaginal progesterone supplementation is equally effective and better tolerated by patients than intramuscular preparations. Sufficient evidence of efficacy and tolerability to make vaginal supplementation the main route of progesterone support in stimulated IVF cycles exists. Food and Drug Administration (FDA) has approved vaginal gel for supplementation at once daily dose and for replacement at twice daily dose.

Once daily vaginal gel, or twice or thrice daily micronized progesterone 200 mg thrice a day are optimal doses of vaginal progesterone for luteal phase support in IVF. Patients should have a choice about which preparation to use based on convenience and cost considerations.

CONCLUSION

A properly powered RCT is much needed to establish the best endometrial preparation protocol for FET cycles. Until then, based on the limited prospective data and conflicting retrospective results, it can be concluded that as further given points.

- Natural FET cycles are most appropriate for patients with regular ovulatory cycles who are able to comply with strict regimen of frequent urine and blood hormonal measurements. Luteal phase support with progesterone does not appear to increase pregnancy rates
- Modified natural FET cycles require ultrasound monitoring and blood hormonal measurements for optimal timing of hCG trigger. Because of the luteotrophic effect of hCG progesterone support after embryo transfer could be optional and should use the most convenient and cost-effective preparation
- Programed FET cycles are the most convenient with respect to limited monitoring requirements and ease and flexibility of scheduling. However, they have not been shown to be superior to properly timed natural or modified natural FET protocols.

Based on the current literature including the ANTARCTICA trial study with large numbers, it is not possible to identify one method of endometrium preparation in FET as being more effective than another.[43,44] Therefore, patients' individual patient factor and convenience, as well as costs should be considered when choosing the method of endometrial preparation.

REFERENCES

1. Ghobara T, Vandekerckhove P. Cycle regimens for frozen-thawed embryo transfer. Cochrane Database Syst Rev. 2008;1:CD003414.
2. Harper MJ. The implantation window. Baillieres Clin Obstet Gynaecol. 1992;6:351-71.
3. Tabibzadeh S, Shea W, Lessey BA, et al. From endometrial receptivity to infertility. J Semin Reprod Endocrinol. 1999;17:197-203.
4. Fatemi HM, Kyrou D, Bourgain C, et al. Cryopreserved-thawed human embryo transfer: spontaneous natural cycle is superior to human chorionic gonadotropin-induced natural cycle. Fertil Steril. 2010;94:2054-8.
5. Andersen AG, Als-Nielsen B, Hornnes PJ, et al. Time interval from human chorionic gonadotropin (hCG) injection to follicular rupture. Hum Reprod. 1995;10:3202-5.
6. Hoff JD, Quigley ME, Yen SS. Hormonal dynamics at midcycle: a reevaluation. J Clin Endocrinol Metab. 1983;57:792-6.
7. Frydman R, Testart J, Feinstein MC, et al. Interrelationship of plasma and urinary luteinizing hormone preovulatory surge. J Steroid Biochem. 1984;20:617-9.
8. Miller PB, Soules MR. The usefulness of a urinary LH kit for ovulation prediction during menstrual cycles of normal women. Obstet Gynecol. 1996;87:13-7.
9. Park SJ, Goldsmith LT, Skurnick JH, et al. Characteristics of the urinary luteinizing hormone surge in young ovulatory women. Fertil Steril. 2007;88:684-90.
10. Guermandi E, Vegetti W, Bianchi MM, et al. Reliability of ovulation tests in infertile women. Obstet Gynecol. 2001;97:92-6.
11. O'Connor KA, Brindle E, Miller RC, et al. Ovulation detection methods for urinary hormones: precision, daily and intermittent sampling and a combined hierarchical method. Hum Reprod. 2006;21:1442-52.
12. Nawroth F, Ludwig M. What is the 'ideal' duration of progesterone supplementation before the transfer of cryopreserved-thawed embryos in estrogen/progesterone replacement protocols? Hum Reprod. 2005;20:1127-34.

13. Paulson RJ Hormonal induction of endometrial receptivity. Fertil Steril. 2011;96:530-5.
14. Weissman A, Horowitz E, Ravhon A, et al. Spontaneous ovulation versus HCG triggering for timing natural-cycle frozenthawed embryo transfer: a randomized study. Reprod Biomed Online. 2011;23:484-9.
15. Chang EM, Han JE, Kim YS, et al. Use of the natural cycle and vitrification thawed blastocyst transfer results in better in-vitro fertilization outcomes: cycle regimens of vitrification thawed blastocyst transfer. J Assist Reprod Genet. 2011;28:369-74.
16. Tomax C, Alsbjerg B, Martikainen H, et al. Pregnancy loss after frozen-embryo transfer—a comparison of three protocols. Fertil Steril. 2012;98:1165-9.
17. Bjuresten K, Landgren BM, Hovatta O, et al. Luteal phase progesterone increases live birth rate after frozen embryo transfer. Fertil Steril. 2011;95:534-7.
18. You-Jeong Lee, Kyung-Hee Lee, Su-Kyung Kwon, et al.The effect of luteal phase progesterone supplementation on natural frozen-thawed embryo transfer cycles. Obstet Gynecol Sci. 2014;57:291-6.
19. Bjuresten K, Landgren BM, Hovatta O, et al. Luteal phase progesterone increases live birth rate after frozen embryo transfer. Fertil Steril. 2011;95:534-7.
20. Kyrou D, Fatemi HM, Popovic-Todorovic B, et al. Vaginal progesterone supplementation has no effect on ongoing pregnancy rate in hCG-induced natural frozen-thawed embryo transfer cycles. Eur J Obstet Gynecol Reprod Biol. 2010;150:175-9.
21. Eftekhar M, Rahsepar M, Rahmani E. Effect of progesterone supplementation on natural frozen-thawed embryo transfer cycles: a randomized controlled trial. Int J Fertil Steril. 2013;7:13-20.
22. Karen P, Couck I, Debrock S, et al. Frozen-thawed embryo transfer in a natural or mildly hormonally stimulated cycle in women with regular ovulatory cycles: a RCT. Hum Reprod. 2015;30:2552-62.
23. Dal PL, Borini A. Best protocol for frozen-thawed embryo transfer-cost benefit analysis needed. Fertil Steril. 2006;86:1554-5.
24. El-Toukhy T, Taylor A, Khalaf Y, et al. Pituitary suppression in ultrasound-monitored frozen embryo replacement cycles. A randomized study. Hum Reprod. 2004;19:874-9.
25. Dor J, Rudak E, Davidson A, et al. Endocrine and biological factors influencing implantation of human embryos following cryopreservation. Gynecol Endocrinol. 1991;5:203-11.
26. Jaroudi KA, Hamilton CJ, Willemsen WN, et al. Artificial endometrial stimulation for frozen embryo replacement. Fertil Steril. 1991;55:835-7.
27. Niu Z, Feng Y, Sun Y, et al. Estrogen level monitoring in artificial frozen-thawed embryo transfer cycles using step-up regime without pituitary suppression: is it necessary? J Exp Clin Assist Reprod. 2008;5:4.
28. Navot D, Bergh PA, Williams M, et al. An insight into early reproductive processes through the in vivo model of ovum donation. J Clin Endocrinol Metab. 1991;72:408-14.
29. Borini A, Dal Prato L, Bianchi L, et al. Effect of duration of estradiol replacement on the outcome of oocyte donation. J Assist Reprod Genet. 2001;18:187-92.
30. Devroey P, Pados G. Preparation of endometrium for egg donation. Hum Reprod Update. 1998;4:856-61.
31. Hill MJ, Miller KA, Frattarelli JL. A GnRH agonist and exogenous hormone stimulation protocol has a higher live-birth rate than a natural endogenous hormone protocol for frozen-thawed blastocyst-stage embryo transfer cycles: an analysis of 1391 cycles. Fertil Steril. 2010;93:416-22.

32. Azimi Nekoo E, Chamani M, Shahrokh Tehrani E, et al. Artificial endometrial preparation for frozen-thawed embryo transfer with or without pretreatment with depot gonadotropin releasing hormone agonist in women with regular menses. J Family Reprod Health. 2015;9(1):1-4.
33. van de Vijver A, Polyzos NP, Van Landuyt L, et al. Cryopreserved embryo transfer in an artificial cycle: is GnRH agonist down-regulation necessary? Reprod BioMed Online. 2014;29:588-94.
34. Trounson A, Mohr L. Human pregnancy following cryopreservation, thawing and transfer of an eight-cell embryo. Nature. 1983;305:707-9.
35. Givens CR, Markun LC, Ryan IP, et al. Outcomes of natural cycles versus programmed cycles for 1677 frozen-thawed embryo transfers. Reprod Biomed Online. 2009;19:380-4.
36. Kasius A, Smit JG, Torrance HL, et al. Endometrial thickness and pregnancy rates after IVF: a systematic review and meta-analysis. Hum Reprod Update. 2014;20:530-41.
37. Kumbak B, Erden HF, Tosun S, et al. Outcome of assisted reproduction treatment in patients with endometrial thickness less than 7 mm. Reprod Biomed Online. 2009;18:79-84.
38. ElToukhy T, Coomarasamy A, Khairy M, et al. The relationship between endometrial thickness and outcome of medicated frozen embryo replacement cycles. Fertil Steril. 2008;89:832-9.
39. Gingold JA, Lee JA, Rodriguez-Purata J, et al. Endometrial pattern, but not endometrial thickness, affects implantation rates in euploid embryo transfers. Fertil Steril. 2015;104:620-8.e5.
40. Chen MJ, Yang JH, Peng FH, et al. Extended estrogen administration for women with thin endometrium in frozen-thawed in-vitro fertilization programs. J Assist Reprod Genet. 2006;23:337-42.
41. Mahajan N. Endometrial receptivity array: Clinical application. J Hum Reprod Sci. 2015;8:121-9.
42. Scioscia M, Lamanna G, Lorusso F, et al. Characterization of endometrial growth in proliferative and early luteal phase in IVF cycles. Reprod Biomed Online. 2009;18:73-8.
43. Groenewoud ER, Cohlen BJ, Al-Oraiby A, et al. A randomized controlled, non-inferiority trial of modified natural versus artificial cycle for cryo-thawed embryo transfer. Hum Reprod. 2016;31:1483-92.
44. Groenewoud ER, Macklon NS, Cohlen BJ, et al. Cryo-thawed embryo transfer: natural versus artificial cycle. A non-inferiority trial (ANTARCTICA trial). BMC Womens Health. 2012;12:27.

Chapter 14

Ovarian Stimulation Protocols in Fertility Preservation

Puneet R Arora

CANCER AND FERTILITY

Improvement in cancer therapies has led to improvement in cancer survival rates. This has not only led to increase in life expectancy but also highlighted issues affecting long-term survivors. The toxic effects of some of the chemotherapeutic agents like alkylating agents (e.g. cyclophosphamide, busulfan, and ifosfamide), which are common components of chemotherapy for breast cancer, lymphomas, leukemia, and sarcomas are well documented. Pelvic radiation therapy is also known to cause follicular destruction, and exposure to 5–10 Gy pelvic radiation appears to be toxic to oocytes, resulting in premature ovarian insufficiency in many women. These effects are dependent on age of the women at the time of treatment and the baseline ovarian reserve prior to starting the treatment for cancer. The potential adverse effect of the disease process itself remains unknown.

Oncofertility, a new sub-specialty bridging oncology care with reproductive medicine addresses essential part of comprehensive reproductive patient care prior to cancer therapy.

OPTIONS OF FERTILITY PRESERVATION IN CANCER PATIENTS

There is importance of reproduction for many cancer patients especially those who are young. In a survey conducted on young women affected by breast cancer,[1] more than half of respondents were concerned with infertility as side effect. As a part of cancer care and counseling, patient should be made aware of the possible long-term consequences of cancer therapy in the form of impairment of fertility. Available fertility preservation options should be discussed as a part of cancer counseling. The discussion with regard to fertility preservation at the time of diagnosis of cancer might not be taken that well and can pose a challenge. This should be done in a best possible way jointly with treating oncologist. Embryo cryopreservation and oocyte cryopreservation are the standard options available at present. Embryo cryopreservation and oocyte cryopreservation both need ovarian stimulation prior to oocyte recovery. Other options such as cortical tissue cryopreservation, in vitro maturation of the immature oocytes and ovarian cryopreservation are very promising but at this stage are experimental and need further trials. Use of medical therapies like gonadotropin-releasing hormone (GnRH) agonist is controversial and need further robust randomized controlled trials. The time interval available between the diagnosis and the initiation of the cancer therapy is an important aspect as to which available option to be utilized prior to starting cancer treatment.

EFFECT OF CANCER ON OVARIAN STIMULATION

Controlled ovarian hyperstimulation (COH) is essential for embryo and oocyte cryopreservation. This can be achieved with either conventional methods of ovarian stimulation or with random start ovarian stimulation protocols (ROS). Recent studies[2,3] have demonstrated no significant change in ovarian reserve or response to gonadotropins in patients with different cancers who are undergoing in vitro fertilization (IVF) treatment. By contrast others[4,5] have found a decline in ovarian response in cancer patients who are undergoing ovarian stimulation protocols to preserve their fertility prior to cancer therapy. A recent meta-analysis[6] found a reduced number of oocytes in patients with malignancies undergoing COH for fertility preservation. One of the theories behind this varied response to ovarian stimulation is put down to fact that cancer is typically a catabolic state increasing stress hormone levels and altering the hypothalamic pituitary axis thereby impairing reproductive capacity. Many patients also experience weight loss that could also affect hypothalamic pituitary axis. Stress can lead to increase in prolactin and endogenous opioids, which could also affect ovary and its responsiveness. Another study[7] to evaluate COH in women with cancer compared with healthy women found no significant differences in the number of oocytes retrieved, number of mature oocytes retrieved and the number of oocytes fertilized. However, the patients with cancer had longer duration of stimulation and higher total dose of gonadotropin, which could be explained by some element of hypothalamic dysfunction. There is also varied stimulation response seen in cancer patients positive for BRCA mutations. Mutations in BRCA genes are associated with an increased risk of breast and ovarian cancers. A low response to ovarian stimulation in BRCA mutation positive breast cancer patients was seen in another study.[8]

OVARIAN STIMULATION PROTOCOLS IN CANCER PATIENTS

Proper understanding of the reproductive endocrinology is essential when planning ovarian stimulation protocols for such group of women as they may present in any part of their menstrual cycle and patients are not advises to delay the start of preservation. At the same time achieving optimal reproductive outcome is of paramount importance in such group of women as well as they may not get another chance of considering their reproductive potential. Protocols for ovarian stimulation can be broadly divided into:

1. Conventional protocols of ovarian stimulation (COS)
2. Random start ovarian stimulation protocols.

Conventional methods of ovarian stimulation are related with onset of menstrual cycle. It involves initiation of the gonadotropins for ovarian stimulation in the follicular phase of the menstrual cycle for approximately 10–14 days to achieve multi-follicular development. The suppression of luteinizing hormone (LH) surge for spontaneous ovulation has been successfully achieved either with GnRH agonist started in the preceding luteal phase or with GnRH antagonist started when the dominant follicle has attained diameter of 14 mm or on day 6 of ovarian stimulation. GnRH antagonist protocols may offer advantage in ovarian stimulation for cancer patients by shortening the time frame from patient presentation to embryo/oocyte cryopreservation, but this protocol still requires onset of menses before initiating ovarian stimulation. Waiting for onset of menstrual cycle prior to starting ovarian stimulation for fertility preservation prior to initiation of cancer treatment can increase the stress and anxiety of patient and treating oncologist with regards to outcome of cancer therapies and hence prevent patients from forgoing fertility preservation treatment. This has been overcome by random start ovarian stimulation protocol (ROS).

With better understanding of the reproductive physiology, endocrinology and ovarian folliculogenesis, ROS have been developed to minimize the time interval needed for initiation of ovarian stimulation and hence with a hope to increase the uptake of these fertility preserving strategies. It is no longer felt that there is a single wave of folliculogenesis initiating in the follicular phase but there are two to three waves in one interovulatory cycle. Studies on changes in ovarian follicular dynamics during the human menstrual cycle have now well documented that there are wave like changes in follicle number rather than a single cohort of antral follicles occurring only during the follicular phase of menstrual cycle. This concept has been used in providing ovarian stimulation in any part of menstrual cycle and has been extrapolated to providing ovarian stimulation prior to cancer therapies' as this subgroup of women can present in any part of menstrual cycle. The rest of the pattern of stimulation with regards to dose and type of gonadotropins is very much similar as in conventional protocols.

Depending on the timing of presentation in relation to menstrual cycle, random start protocols can be divided into starting controlled ovarian stimulation in early follicular phase, late follicular phase, early luteal phase, and late luteal phase (Figs. 14.1A to E).[9] Early follicular phase is defined as presentation within first 7 days of onset of menstruation. Late follicular phase is primarily defined as presentation after 7 days of onset of menstrual cycle, or presence of dominant follicle of more than 12 mm diameter or

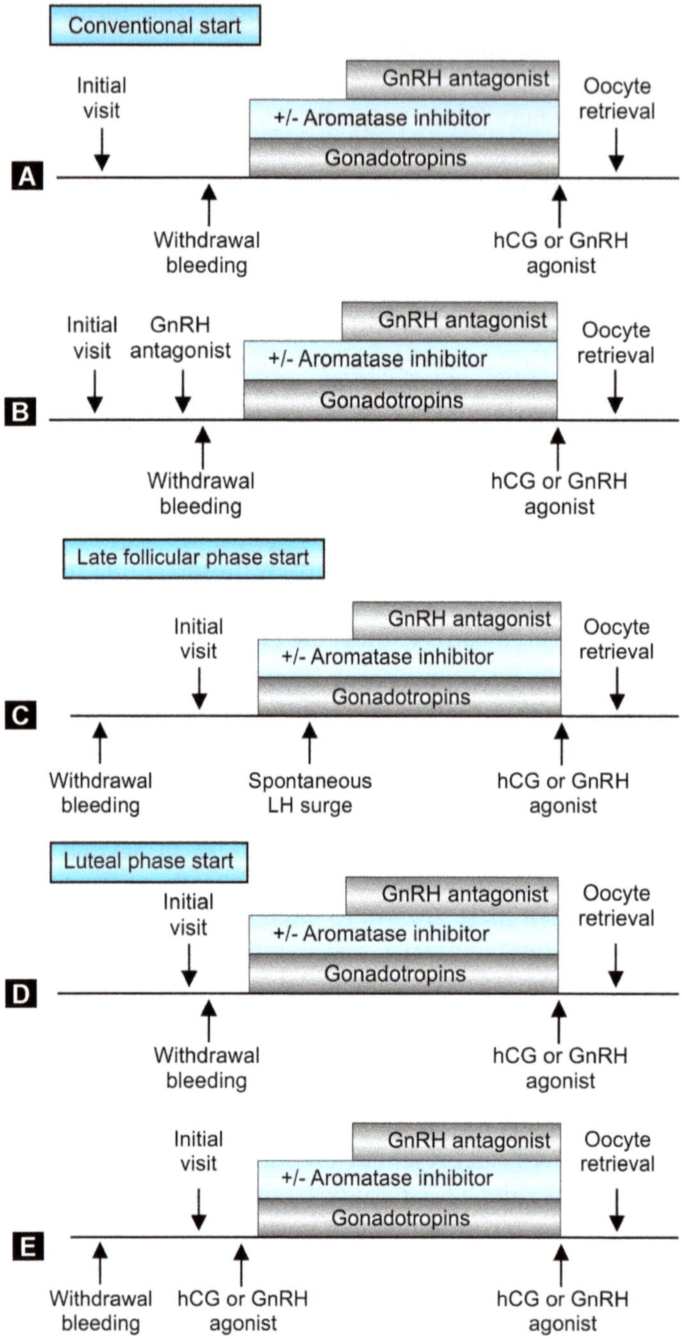

Figs. 14.1A to E: Conventional and random-start antagonist in vitro fertilization (IVF) protocols for cancer patients undergoing fertility preservation.[9] (A) COS can be started with spontaneous menses; (B) or with menses following luteolysis induced by gonadotropin-releasing hormone (GnRH) antagonist; (C) COS can also be initiated in the late follicular; (D) or luteal phase following spontaneous luteinizing hormone (LH) surge; (E) or after ovulation induction with human chorionic gonadotropin (hCG) or GnRH agonist.

progesterone level less than 2 ng/mL. Early luteal phase is defined as presentation within first 7 days after ovulation. Late luteal phase is presentation within last 7 days of the last menstrual cycle. Late follicular phase and early luteal phase are the most challenging time for random start ovarian stimulation protocol.

Presentation in early follicular phase can very similarly be treated like convention stimulation regimens with GnRH antagonist protocol provided there is no dominant follicle more than 12 mm. If there is already dominant follicle more than 12 mm, it can then be treated as being in late follicular phase, which will be discussed subsequently.

Late follicular ovarian stimulation involves assessment of the ovaries for the presence or absence of dominant follicles. If the ovary contains dominant follicle more than 12 mm, further management would involve leutolysis of the dominant follicle with either GnRH antagonist or progesterone followed by stimulation for the rest of the follicles. Prior to leutolysis, stimulation of the follicle with minimal dose of follicle-stimulating hormone (FSH) until the follicle reaches 18 mm followed by triggering and aspiration of the follicle and preserving it if viable. GnRH antagonist is then administered for 4–5 days depending on the ovarian reserve of the patient, ovarian stimulation can then be started by appropriate gonadotropins based on age, ovarian reserve parameters [anti-Müllerian hormone (AMH), antral follicular count (AFC)].

Early luteal phase is defined as the completion of spontaneous luteinizing hormone (LH) surge and presence of corpus luteum in the ovaries. Early and late luteal phase can be essentially treated in the same way. Leutolysis of the corpus luteum can be achieved by GnRH antagonist 3 mg stat or in multiple doses of 0.25 mg for 4–5 days. The objective of antagonist is to achieve estradiol levels below 60 pg/mL and not to delay the stimulation cycle until the start of new menstrual cycle. This can be followed by gonadotropin stimulation in conventional way preferably with recombinant FSH avoiding exogenous LH activity, which might prevent leutolysis. Pituitary suppression for LH surge by GnRH antagonist can be initiated in usual way when the dominant follicle reaches 14 mm and use of either human chorionic gonadotropin (hCG) or GnRH agonist for trigger of the final maturation of the oocyte.

The dose of gonadotropin should be individualized depending on age, ovarian reserve, and weight of the patient. Using higher doses of gonadotropins can be one of the strategies to increase the embryo and oocyte yield per cycle. In a study comparing a low-dose antagonist IVF protocol (150 IU FSH) and a higher-dose antagonist IVF protocol (> 150 IU) in cancer patients, although the number of follicles more than 17 mm was greater in the higher-dose group, there was no difference in numbers of oocytes generated between the two groups.[10] That study suggests that the use of higher doses of gonadotropins may not necessarily result in higher oocyte/embryo yield consistent with the theory that higher doses of gonadotropins may stimulate the recruitment of chromosomally abnormal or incompetent oocytes.[11] However, in patients with decreased ovarian reserve as assessed with the use of AFC and/or AMH, higher doses of gonadotropins may be required.

The studies have suggested that these protocols have been able to provide reasonable number of mature eggs able to fertilize but the exact implantation potential and subsequent pregnancy rates of embryos and oocytes retrieved through these protocols is still unanswered. Being relatively new and being tried mainly in cases in cancer patients, these have been reported in very few studies.

Controlled ovarian stimulation leads to elevation of the serum estradiol levels up to 10–15 times higher than physiological levels. In women with estrogen sensitive breast tumors, to avoid this elevation, addition of aromatase inhibitors (letrozole) and tamoxifem is recommended. The peak of estradiol in the protocols of ovarian stimulation with tamoxifem or with letrozole is slightly higher than the levels achieved in natural cycle around 300–350 pg/mL. Letrozole (5 mg/day) or tamoxifem (20–40 mg/day) is usually administered 2–3 days prior to starting gonadotropins. Study by Oktay et al.[12] concluded that stimulation protocols using letrozole alongside with gonadotropins are currently preferred over tamoxifem protocols as treatment with letrozole results in a higher number of oocytes obtained and fertilized when compared to tamoxifem protocols.

There has been case report by Reichmann et al.[13] of using these ovarian stimulation protocols for oocyte vitrification in prepubertal girls diagnosed with cancer that have not yet attained menarche and hence got no gonadotropin recruitable follicles. This has been reported as having successful ovarian stimulation and oocyte retrieval. This approach needs further robust evidence before it can be widely applicable to such group of cancer affected females.

The goal of superovulation for this group of patients represents a compromise between obtaining a relatively large number of oocytes for vitrification, to maximize chances of later pregnancy, and the absolute need for avoidance of ovarian hyperstimulation in a patient who will shortly begin chemotherapy.

The patients referred for fertility preservation may not necessarily represent the typical population of subfertile patients treated in IVF units. Cancer may affect multiple tissues throughout the body and can result in variety of complications during ovarian stimulation. Cancer may induce hypercoagulable state and when combined with increased serum estradiol levels may put cancer patients undergoing controlled ovarian stimulation are at increased risk of thromboembolic events. Therefore, consideration should be given for commencement of anticoagulation therapy around the time of ovarian stimulation. The other strategy of preventing thromboembolic events is to use letrozole during ovarian stimulation as in women undergoing ovarian stimulation with estrogen sensitive malignancies to keep estradiol levels close to less than 500 pg/mL. Letrozole or GnRH antagonist should be continued even after oocyte retrieval for up to a week depending on the estradiol levels at the time of ovulation induction.

Some blood-borne malignancies may alter the hemostatic function and may create a tendency toward bleeding during oocyte retrieval owing to thrombocytopenia, platelet dysfunction, or defective coagulation factor synthesis. Collaborative team approach involving hematologist, anesthetist should be preferred to prevent complication of bleeding in these patients. Pelvic infection after oocyte retrieval can be a problem especially in neutropenic patients. In the case of neutropenia, consultation from the patient's oncologist for the use of granulocyte colony-stimulating factor to increase the neutrophil count should be obtained, and prophylactic antibiotics should be given before oocyte retrieval to decrease the risk of infection. Cancers involving tracheal compression, or large pleural effusion, may preclude safe administration of anesthesia for oocyte pick up. This should be discussed with anesthetists prior to starting ovarian stimulation.

Another aspect of ovarian stimulation, which needs further consideration, is the fact that success in vitrification has been seen in nonmalignant healthy infertile population and little information is obtained about vitrification in cancer patients though studies have shown no difference in oocytes and embryos derived from patients with cancer and in nonmalignant conditions.

Successful implementation of fertility preservation services requires establishing liaisons with reproductive specialists, oncology colleagues. Whilst survival is clearly the most important issue facing a young woman with cancer, it is clear that future fertility is also important. A rapid and efficient referral system with minimal delay can bring good results and this can be established in close collaboration and effective communication with colleagues in medical, surgical and radiation oncology.

In cancer patients, antagonist protocols should be preferred and where possible trigger for final maturation to be planned with GnRH agonist to prevent the risk of ovarian hyperstimulation syndrome (OHSS). The impact of OHSS can be profound and all measures should be taken to prevent it. In cancer patients, its effect can be more profound as it may result in delaying or complicating planned life-saving cancer therapy.

REFERENCES

1. Partridge AH, Gilbert S, Peppercorn J, et al. Web-based survey of fertility issues in young women with breast cancer. J Clin Oncol. 2004;22:4174-83.
2. Van Casteren NJ, Boellaard WP, Romijn JC, et al. Gonadal dysfunction in male cancer patients before cytotoxic treatment. Int J Androl. 2010;33:73-9.
3. Knopman JM, Noyes N, Talebian S, et al. Women with cancer undergoing ART for fertility preservation: a cohort study of their response to exogenous gonadotropins. Fertil Steril. 2009;91:1476-8.

4. Pal L, Leykin L, Schifren JL, et al. Malignancy may adversely influence the quality and behavior of oocytes. Hum Reprod. 1998;13:1837-40.
5. Quintero RB, Helmer A, Huang JQ, et al. Ovarian stimulation for fertility preservation in patients with cancer. Fertil Steril. 2010;93:865-8.
6. Friedler S, Koc O, Gidoni Y, et al. Ovarian response to stimulation for fertility preservation in women with malignant disease: a systematic review and meta-analysis. Fertil Steril. 2012;97:125-33.
7. Das M, Shehata F, Moria A, et al. Ovarian reserve, response to gonadotropins, and oocyte maturity in women with malignancy. Fertil Steril. 2011;96:122-5.
8. Oktay K, Kim JY, Barad D, et al. Association of BRCA1 mutations with occult primary ovarian insufficiency: a possible explanation for the link between infertility and breast/ovarian cancer risks. J Clin Oncol. 2010;28:240-4.
9. Cakmak H, Rosen MP. Ovarian stimulation in cancer patients. Fertil Steril. 2013;99:1476-84.
10. Lee S, Oktay K. Does higher starting dose of FSH stimulation with letrozole improve fertility preservation outcomes in women with breast cancer? Fertil Steril. 2012;98:961-4.e1.
11. Baart EB, Martini E, Eijkemans MJ, et al. Milder ovarian stimulation for in-vitro fertilization reduces aneuploidy in the human preimplantation embryo: a randomized controlled trial. Hum Reprod. 2007;22:980-8.
12. Oktay K, Buyuk E, Libertella N, et al. Fertility preservation in breast cancer patients: a prospective controlled comparison of ovarian stimulation with tamoxifen and letrozole for embryo cryopreservation. J Clin Oncol. 2005;23:4347-53.
13. Reichmann DE, Davis OK, Zaninovic N, et al. Fertility preservation utilizing controlled ovarian hyper-stimulation and oocyte cryo-preservation in a pre-menarcheal female with myelodysplastic syndrome. Fertil Steril. 2012;98:1225-8.

Chapter 15

Complications of Ovarian Stimulation: Prevention and Management

Julia K Bosdou, Stratis Kolibianakis

INTRODUCTION

The goal of ovarian stimulation is to induce development of multiple follicles and in the case of in vitro fertilization (IVF) to enable the retrieval of several oocytes. This approach has led to increased pregnancy rates[1,2] in infertile couples, however, it might be accompanied by complications. The most serious complications of ovarian stimulation are ovarian hyperstimulation syndrome (OHSS)[3] and multiple pregnancy.[4] In addition, ovarian stimulation has also been associated with adnexal torsion[5] and thromboembolic events.[6]

Clinicians should be familiar with these complications and understand the underlying pathophysiological mechanisms, in order to be able to adequately prevent, recognize and manage them. Although this is true for any medical intervention, it is especially important in assisted reproductive technologies (ART), since ovarian stimulation is applied to otherwise healthy women longing for parenthood.

OVARIAN HYPERSTIMULATION SYNDROME

Ovarian hyperstimulation syndrome is the most serious iatrogenic complication of ovarian stimulation that is triggered by exogenous administration of human chorionic gonadotropin (hCG), used for induction of final oocyte maturation and/or by its endogenous production in cases of pregnancy. OHSS can be early or late, based on the time of its onset. Early OHSS occurs in the early luteal phase, within 10 days from oocyte retrieval,[7] while late OHSS occurs in the late luteal phase, more than or equal to 10 days from oocyte retrieval and usually in cycles leading to pregnancy.[8]

Ovarian hyperstimulation syndrome has traditionally been classified as mild, moderate, severe or critical[9,10] (Fig. 15.1). Mild and moderate OHSS do not require specific treatment and patients can be treated symptomatically on an outpatient basis. On the other hand, severe OHSS requires patient hospitalization.

Although most OHSS cases will occur during ovarian stimulation for IVF, this is also possible, albeit less frequently, in patients undergoing ovulation induction or enhancement of ovulation.

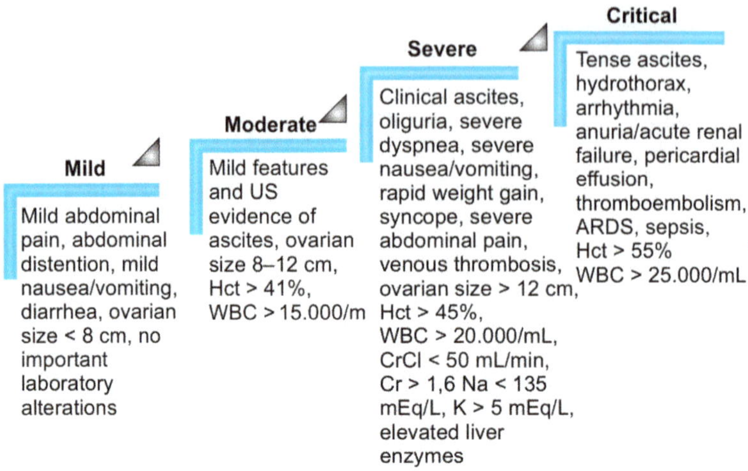

Fig. 15.1: Classification of ovarian hyperstimulation syndrome (OHSS): clinical symptoms and laboratory features.
(Hct: Hematocrit; WBC: White blood cell; CrCl: Creatinine clearance; Cr: Creatinine; ARDS: Acute respiratory distress syndrome).
Source: Adapted from Navot D, Bergh PA, Laufer N. Ovarian hyperstimulation syndrome in novel reproductive technologies: prevention and treatment. Fertil Steril. 1992;58:249-61. Mathur R, Jenkins J. Towards a clinically useful classification of OHSS. Reprod Biomed Online. 2009;19:434.

Ovarian Hyperstimulation Syndrome after Ovulation Induction/ Enhancement of Ovulation

In anovulatory women, such as those with polycystic ovarian syndrome (PCOS), the goal of ovarian stimulation is to induce monofollicular growth.[2] For this purpose, several approaches have been proposed, the most commonly used being clomiphene citrate (CC), aromatase inhibitors or low-dose gonadotropins.

Clomiphene citrate, the standard first-line treatment for ovulation induction, acts as an estrogen receptor blocker, leading to elevation of endogenous follicle-stimulating hormone (FSH) production, which in turn stimulates follicular development.[11] This inexpensive, simple and widely used approach is considered quite efficient since it may lead to ovulation in about 75% of patients.[12]

Letrozole is an aromatase inhibitor which has been introduced as an alternative treatment to CC for ovulation induction in women with PCOS. Even though it is still an off-label drug in many countries, it is considered an efficient treatment for ovulation induction, by inhibiting the aromatase activity and thus inducing an hypoestrogenic state that stimulates the release of FSH.[13]

Clomiphene citrate and letrozole usually lead to induction of monofollicular development [CC: 54.85%, 95% confidence interval (CI): 40.3–68.9;

letrozole: 79.49%, 95% CI: 65.3–88.9].[14] Not unexpectedly, the incidence of OHSS with the use of both CC and letrozole is very rare. In a meta-analysis of randomized controlled trials (RCTs), comparing aromatase inhibitors with CC for ovulation induction in subfertile women with PCOS, no OHSS cases were reported in 1,809 patients, while no difference was present in the incidence of OHSS when letrozole was compared with CC [risk difference (RD): 0.00, 95% CI: –0.01 to 0.00][15] (Figs. 15.2A and B).

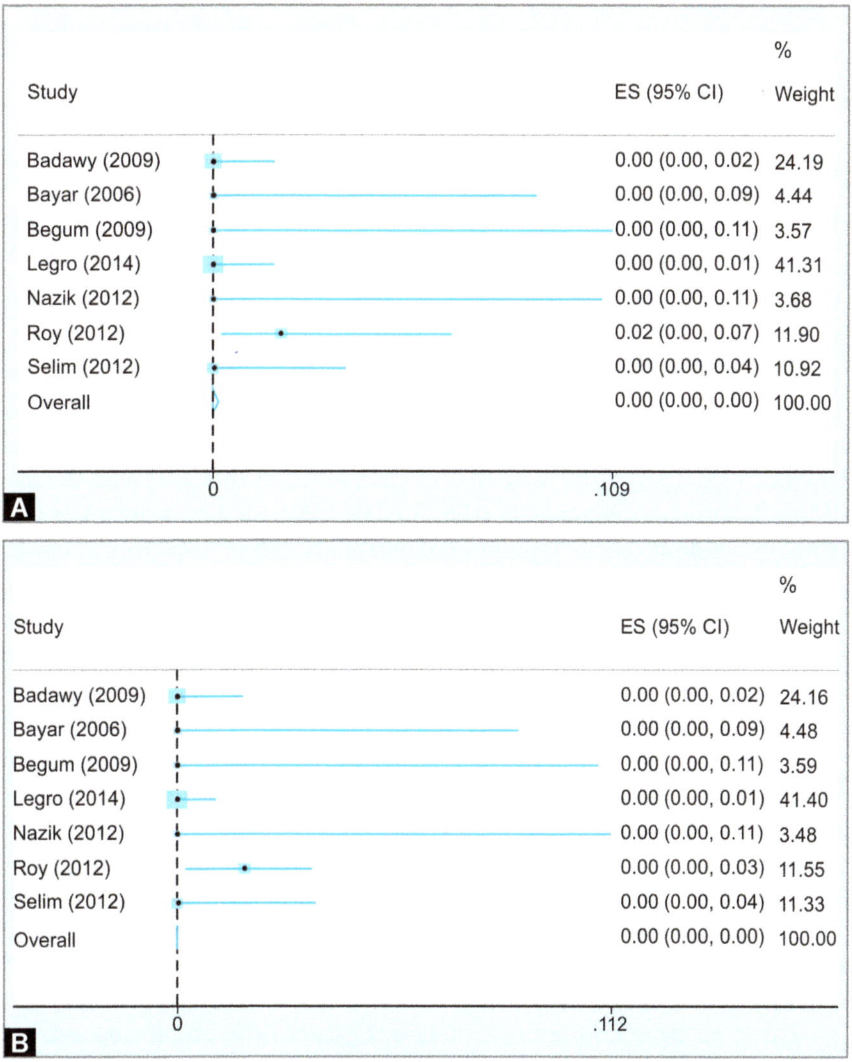

Figs. 15.2A and B: (A) Incidence of ovarian hyperstimulation syndrome (OHSS) with the use of clomiphene citrate (CC) in polycystic ovarian syndrome (PCOS) patients; (B) Incidence of OHSS with the use of letrozole in PCOS patients.
(ES: Estimate; CI: Confidence interval).

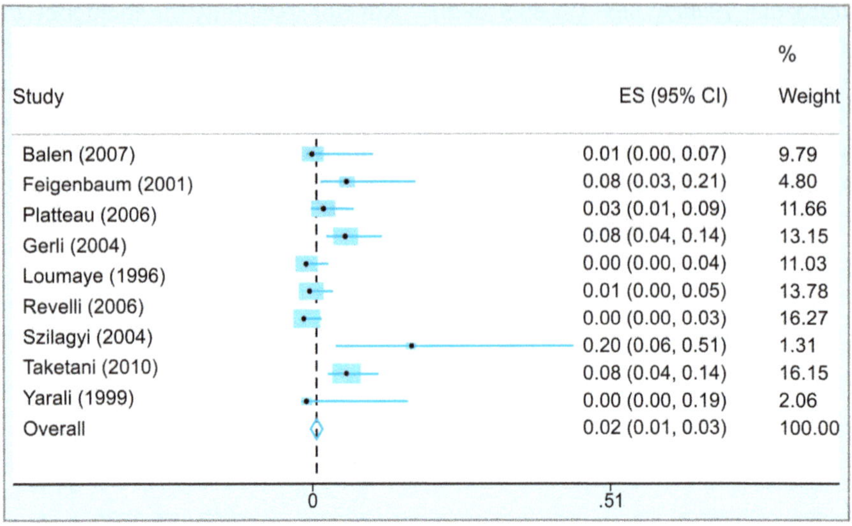

Fig. 15.3: Incidence of ovarian hyperstimulation syndrome (OHSS) with the use of low-dose recombinant follicle-stimulating hormone (FSH) in polycystic ovarian syndrome (PCOS) patients.
(ES: Estimate; CI: Confidence interval).

An alternative treatment of infertility in anovulatory women with PCOS involves the use of low-dose gonadotropins.[16] Based on the meta-analysis by Weiss et al. (2015), the incidence of OHSS in PCOS patients with the use of low-dose recombinant FSH (rFSH) is 2% (95% CI: 1–3) (Fig. 15.3) and is not dependent on the type of gonadotropins used.[17] However, it has to be noted that in the majority of the RCTs included in that meta-analysis, either no definition of OHSS was given or the definition was variable, while hCG was not administered in case of excessive response using variable criteria.

Clomiphene citrate, letrozole as well as low-dose gonadotropins have also been used for enhancement of ovulation in women with unexplained infertility. However, since in these patients, the target of ovarian stimulation is to allow development of two to three follicles, in order to increase the probability of conception, CC and letrozole, whose administration is associated usually with monofollicular development, are less frequently used. No cases of OHSS after CC administration for unexplained fertility were reported in meta-analyses of relevant RCTs comparing CC with letrozole[18] (Figs. 15.4A and B).

Based on data reported in a meta-analysis of RCTs employing ovarian stimulation with the use of low dose gonadotropins for the treatment of women with unexplained infertility, male infertility or mild endometriosis, the incidence of OHSS (for which, however, no definition was given) was 2% (95% CI: 0–3)[19] (Fig. 15.5).

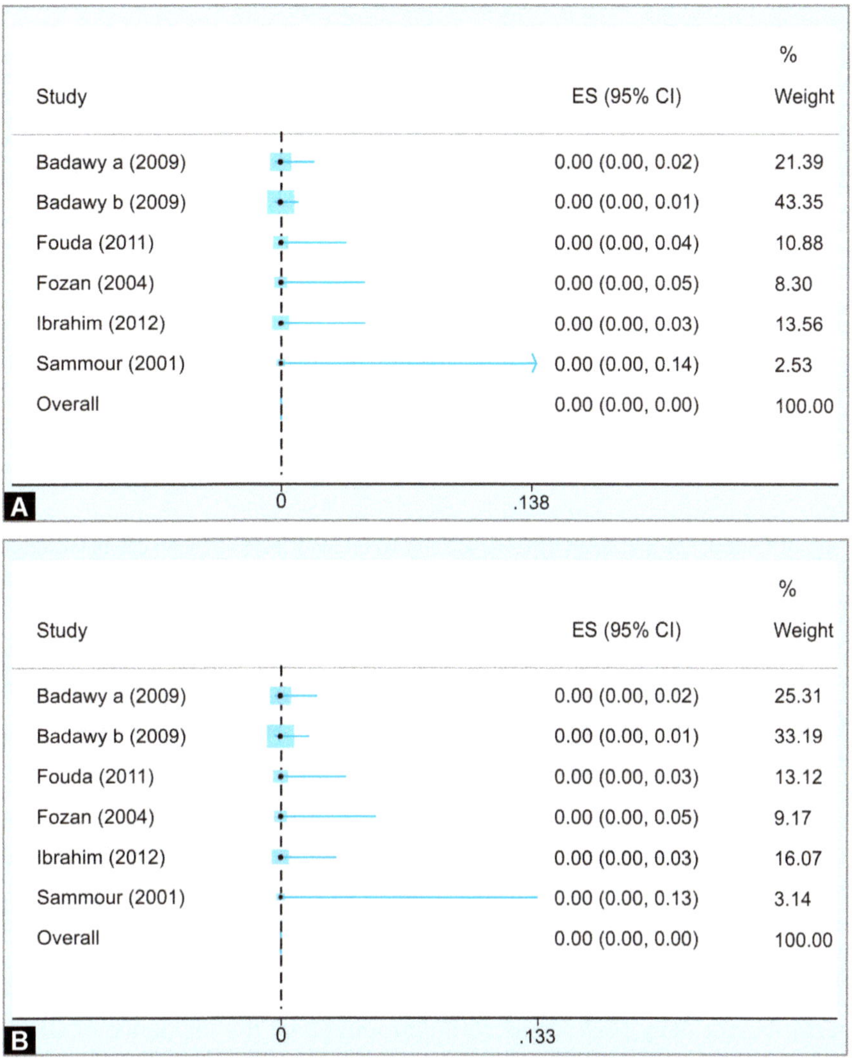

Figs. 15.4A and B: (A) Incidence of ovarian hyperstimulation syndrome (OHSS) with the use of clomiphene citrate (CC) in patients with unexplained fertility; (B) Incidence of OHSS with the use of letrozole in patients with unexplained fertility.
(ES: Estimate; CI: Confidence interval).

In an attempt to reduce the risk of OHSS when an excessive follicle number has developed following ovulation induction or enhancement of ovulation, cycle cancellation by withholding hCG or conversion of the cycle to IVF/embryo transfer have been proposed. In this way, the occurrence of OHSS is largely prevented,[20-23] although it can still occur. However, it should be noted that cycle cancellation has been associated with patient's disappointment and dissatisfaction, whereas conversion to IVF might not be acceptable by the patient due to financial constraints.[22]

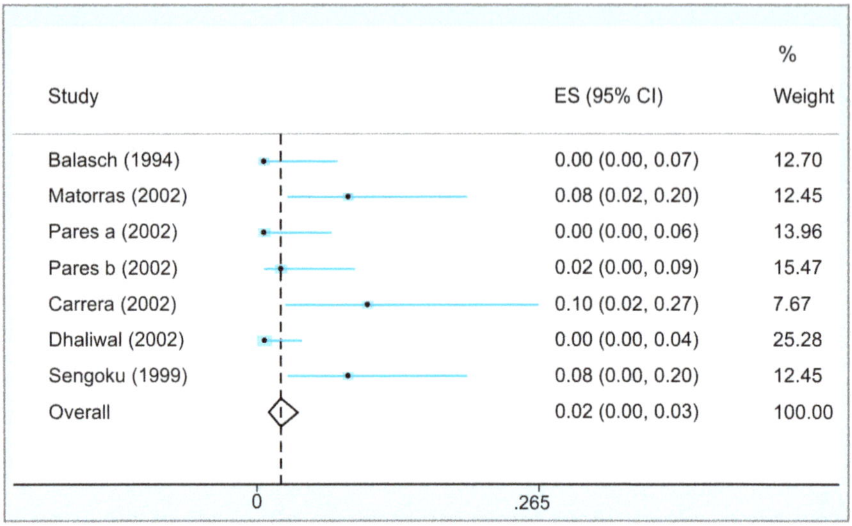

Fig. 15.5: Incidence of ovarian hyperstimulation syndrome (OHSS) with the use of low-dose recombinant follicle-stimulating hormone (FSH) in patients with unexplained fertility, male infertility or mild endometriosis.
(ES: Estimate; CI: Confidence interval).

Ovarian Hyperstimulation Syndrome after Multi-follicular Development for In Vitro Fertilization

Based on data provided by the European IVF-monitoring Consortium, the incidence of OHSS (for which, however, no definition was given) in Europe, is estimated to be 0.78% (95% CI: 0.74–0.82) of all stimulated IVF cycles.[1] Moreover, data from the USA show that the incidence of severe OHSS is 0.28% (95% CI: 0.25–0.31).[24] Based on published meta-analyses of RCTs comparing gonadotropin-releasing hormone (GnRH) agonists with antagonists[25] and recombinant daily FSH versus corifollitropin alfa,[26] the incidence of OHSS varies from 1.3% to 20.3% according to the characteristics of the patients treated and the type of IVF protocol used (Table 15.1).

Prevention of Ovarian Hyperstimulation Syndrome

Although a substantial decrease in the incidence of severe OHSS has been observed following the introduction of GnRH antagonists, severe OHSS is still possible, especially in high risk patients, such as those with PCOS.

Prevention of OHSS can be attempted at different time points and preferably before the initiation of ovarian stimulation. This is feasible by identifying known risk factors for OHSS and classifying patients accordingly. For this purpose, important variables to consider include history of OHSS, assessment of the antral follicle count (AFC) and of anti-Müllerian hormone (AMH) levels. Following assessment of OHSS risk, selection of

Table 15.1: Incidence of ovarian hyperstimulation syndrome (OHSS) according to the characteristics of the patients treated and the type of in vitro fertilization (IVF) protocol used in published meta-analyses of randomized controlled trials (RCTs) comparing gonadotropin-releasing hormone (GnRH) agonists with antagonists and recombinant daily follicle-stimulating hormone (FSH) versus corifollitropin alfa.

Protocol	*Population*	*Source*	*Incidence %*	*95% CI*
GnRH agonists	All women	Al-Inany, 2011	9	7.7–10.5
GnRH agonists	PCOS	Al-Inany, 2011	20.3	16–25.5
GnRH antagonists	All women	Al-Inany, 2011	3.2	2.6–4
GnRH antagonists	PCOS	Al-Inany, 2011	4.8	2.9–7.9
Corifollitropin alfa	Normal responders	Tarlatzis, 2012	1.8	1.1–2.8
rFSH	Normal responders	Tarlatzis, 2012	1.3	0.7–2.2

(GnRH: Gonadotropin-releasing hormone; PCOS: Polycystic ovarian syndrome; rFSH: Recombinant follicle-stimulating hormone).
Source: Adapted from Al-Inany HG, Youssef MA, Aboulghar M, et al. Gonadotrophin-releasing hormone antagonists for assisted reproductive technology. Cochrane Database Syst Rev. 2011;5:CD001750.
Tarlatzis BC, Griesinger G, Leader A, et al. Comparative incidence of ovarian hyperstimulation syndrome following ovarian stimulation with corifollitropin alfa or recombinant FSH. Reprod Biomed Online. 2012;24:410-9.

appropriate stimulation protocols, dose individualization and tight monitoring of ovarian stimulation are essential. Alarming signals for the occurrence of OHSS during ovarian stimulation are a rapid rise of estradiol (E2) levels, very high E2 levels or an excessive number of developing follicles. In an attempt to predict high-risk patients for developing severe OHSS, a cut-off value for more than or equal to 19 follicles of more than or equal to 11 mm on the day of hCG has been proposed, yielding a sensitivity of 74.3% and a specificity of 75.3%.[27]

Several strategies have been suggested to minimize the risk of severe OHSS after hCG administration, including co-administration of dopamine agonists, intravenous administration of albumin, hydroxyethyl starch (HES), low-dose aspirin, ketoconazole, corticosteroids, metformin, "coasting", continuation of GnRH agonist administration after hCG combined with embryo cryopreservation or reduction of the hCG dose used to trigger final oocyte maturation. However, the use of these strategies can only decrease the incidence of severe OHSS but not result in its elimination.[28]

The use of GnRH antagonists for suppressing premature luteinizing hormone (LH) surge has made feasible the substitution of hCG for final oocyte maturation with GnRH agonists. This has changed dramatically clinical practice in ART, resulting in the virtual elimination of severe OHSS, increasing in this way the safety of ovarian stimulation to the benefit of infertile couples.[29] The replacement of hCG with a GnRH agonist for triggering final oocyte maturation avoids the sustained hCG stimulation of corpora lutea for 10 days. With the use of GnRH agonist triggering, the endogenously elicited LH lasts only 24–36 hours, decreasing in this way the occurrence of severe OHSS as compared to hCG. However, the absence of corpora lutea stimulation results in low steroids levels and is associated with a decreased probability of pregnancy after fresh embryo transfer.[30]

In an effort to enhance the endogenous sex steroid production and restore the deficient luteal phase after triggering with GnRH agonist, hCG supplementation in the luteal phase has been proposed. However, severe OHSS is still present with this strategy.[31] Other alternative approaches include the luteal supplementation with recLH after triggering with GnRH agonist,[32] the dual triggering of final oocyte maturation with the combination of GnRH agonist and hCG,[33] the stimulation of endogenous LH levels with repeated GnRH agonist administration,[34] the intensive luteal phase steroid supplementation after GnRH agonist triggering[35] and the administration of GnRH antagonist in the luteal phase and cryopreservation of all embryos.[36,37] Although no severe OHSS cases were observed following these approaches, no firm conclusions regarding the incidence of severe OHSS can be drawn, due to the small number of studies performed and the participants included.[30]

A simpler approach to the problem of low pregnancy rates, due to a defective luteal phase after GnRH agonist triggering, is to avoid any attempt of enhancing either LH activity or steroid levels and instead defer embryo transfer in a subsequent cycle. In this way, embryo transfer takes place in a normally developed endometrium with optimal chances to support implantation. This is the basis for the "freeze all" approach after GnRH agonist triggering.[38] By synthesizing the results from all available studies until November 2015, prospective and retrospective,[39-50] in which GnRH agonist was used for triggering final oocyte maturation and no luteal phase support was administered,[30] the incidence of severe OHSS was 0% (95% CI: 0–0) (Fig. 15.6).

Management of Ovarian Hyperstimulation Syndrome

The management of OHSS depends on its severity and the presence or absence of pregnancy. The basic principles for evaluating, monitoring and managing severe OHSS are shown in Figure 15.7.[51,52]

Outpatient Management of Ovarian Hyperstimulation Syndrome

Women undergoing outpatient management of OHSS should be appropriately counseled and provided with information regarding fluid intake and output monitoring.

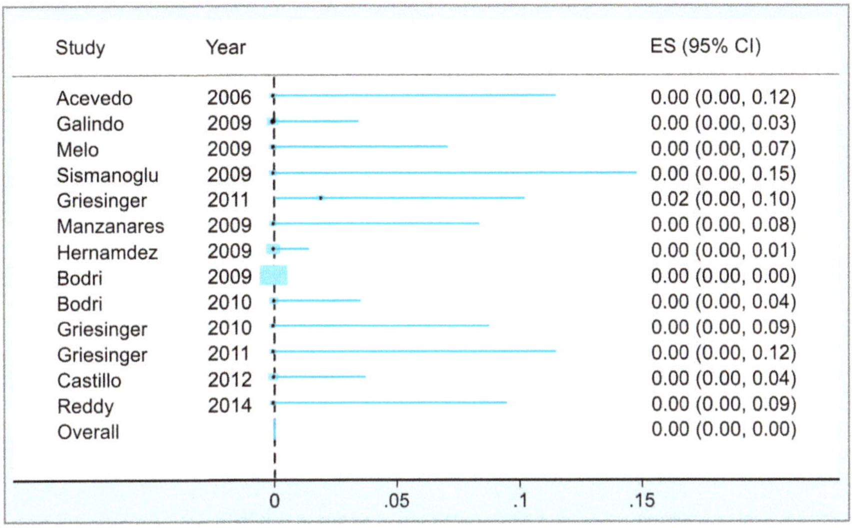

Fig. 15.6: Estimated probability of severe ovarian hyperstimulation syndrome (OHSS) in patients triggered by gonadotropin-releasing hormone (GnRH) agonist.
(ES: Estimate; CI: Confidence interval).
Source: Adapted from Tarlatzis B, Bosdou J, Kolibianakis E. Elimination of OHSS by GnRH Agonist and Freezing Embryos. In: Rizk B, Gerris J (Eds). Complications and Outcomes of Assisted Reproduction. United Kingdom: Cambridge University Press; 2017. pp. 149-63. (In Press).

Nonsteroidal anti-inflammatory agents should be avoided, as they may compromise renal function. Women with severe OHSS being managed on an outpatient basis should receive thromboprophylaxis. In patients with severe OHSS, outpatient ultrasound-guided paracentesis has been suggested as a safe alternative to hospitalization for the management of OHSS in an outpatient setting.[51,52]

Hospitalization

Assessment of severity usually involves physical examination, recording of vital signs, body weight, abdominal circumference, ultrasound examination and laboratory tests such as hemoglobin, hematocrit, serum creatinine, electrolytes, liver enzymes and coagulation.[10] Since symptomatic moderate or severe OHSS is a hypovolemic state, the mainstay of treatment involves fluid resuscitation, supportive care, paracentesis and prophylactic anticoagulation.[52]

There are no trials on the optimum method for maintaining fluid balance in women with severe OHSS.[10] Women with hemoconcentration and dehydration may need more intensive initial rehydration and may benefit from colloids such as human albumin, HES, dextran or mannitol.

Paracentesis under ultrasound guidance should be carried out for patients with severe discomfort, abdominal pain, respiratory distress or oliguria due

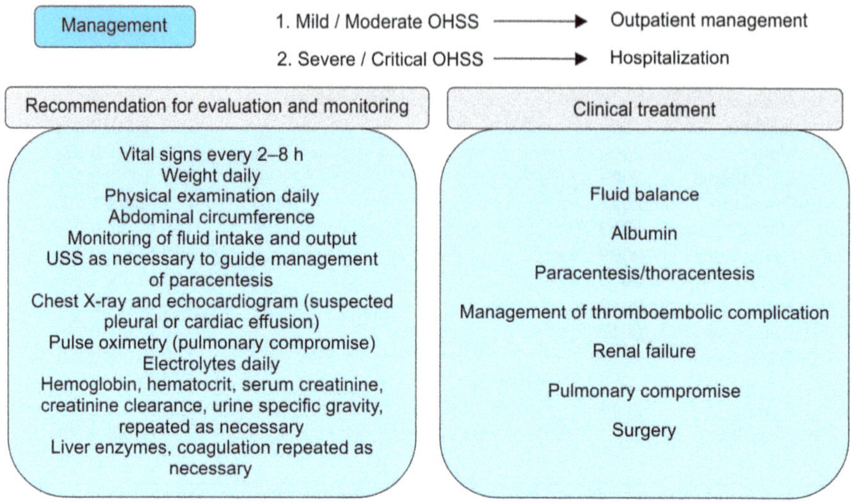

Fig. 15.7: Management of ovarian hyperstimulation syndrome (OHSS).

to the large amount of ascites.[52] Symptomatic hydrothorax persisting despite abdominal paracentesis may be drained directly.[10]

All patients hospitalized with OHSS should be provided with prophylactic anticoagulation to avoid the potentially serious effects of thromboembolism. The duration of thromboprophylaxis should be individualized according to patient risk factors and outcome of treatment.[51,52]

Since the risk of adnexal torsion or ovarian rupture appears to be increased in women with OHSS, particularly in the presence of pregnancy, surgery is indicated as a treatment option in these patients.[51,52]

Multiple Pregnancy

The increased incidence of maternal and neonatal complications associated with multiple pregnancies has been well recognized.[53,54] Thus, one of the main challenges in ART is to avoid multiples while maintaining at the same time the probability of live birth. This principle has led to significant changes in embryo transfer policies and the establishment of relevant legislations in several European countries. Moreover, it has led to more conservative approaches to ovulation induction and enhancement of ovulation which are responsible for the majority of multiple pregnancies in infertility treatment.[55-57]

Ovulation Induction/Enhancement of Ovulation

As it has already been mentioned, both the use of letrozole and CC lead to monofollicular development in the majority of women treated. Thus, the expected incidence of multiple pregnancy with their use is low. Indeed, based on data reported in the meta-analysis by Franik et al. (2014), comparing aromatase inhibitors with CC for ovulation induction in patients with PCOS, the incidence of multiple pregnancy per patient treated with the use of aromatase inhibitors was 0% (95% CI: 0–1), while that with the use of CC was 1% (95% CI: 0–2) (Figs. 15.8A and B). The incidence of multiple pregnancy per pregnancy achieved with the use of aromatase inhibitors was 0% (95% CI: 0–1), while that with the use of CC was 3% (95% CI: 1–6) (Figs. 15.9A and B). The difference in the incidence of multiple pregnancy per woman treated

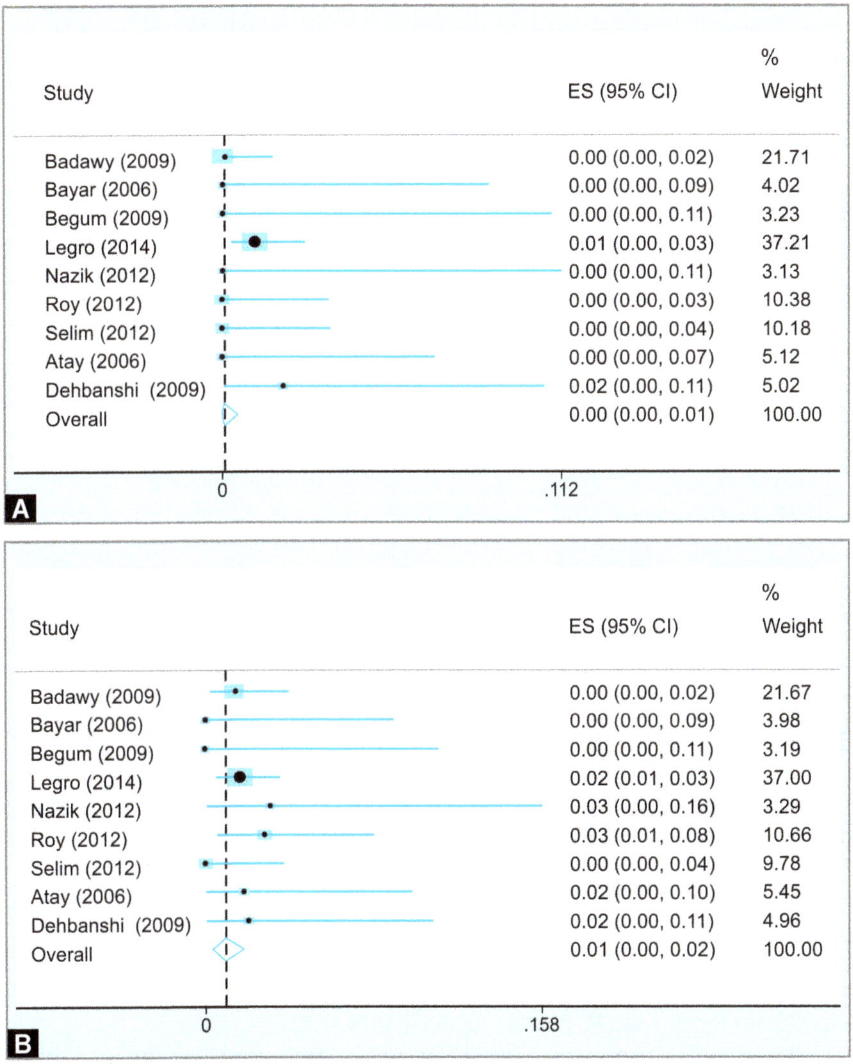

Figs. 15.8A and B: (A) Incidence of multiple pregnancy per patient treated with the use of aromatase inhibitors for ovulation induction in women with polycystic ovarian syndrome (PCOS); (B) Incidence of multiple pregnancy per patient treated with the use of clomiphene citrate (CC) for ovulation induction in women with PCOS.
(ES: Estimate; CI: Confidence interval).

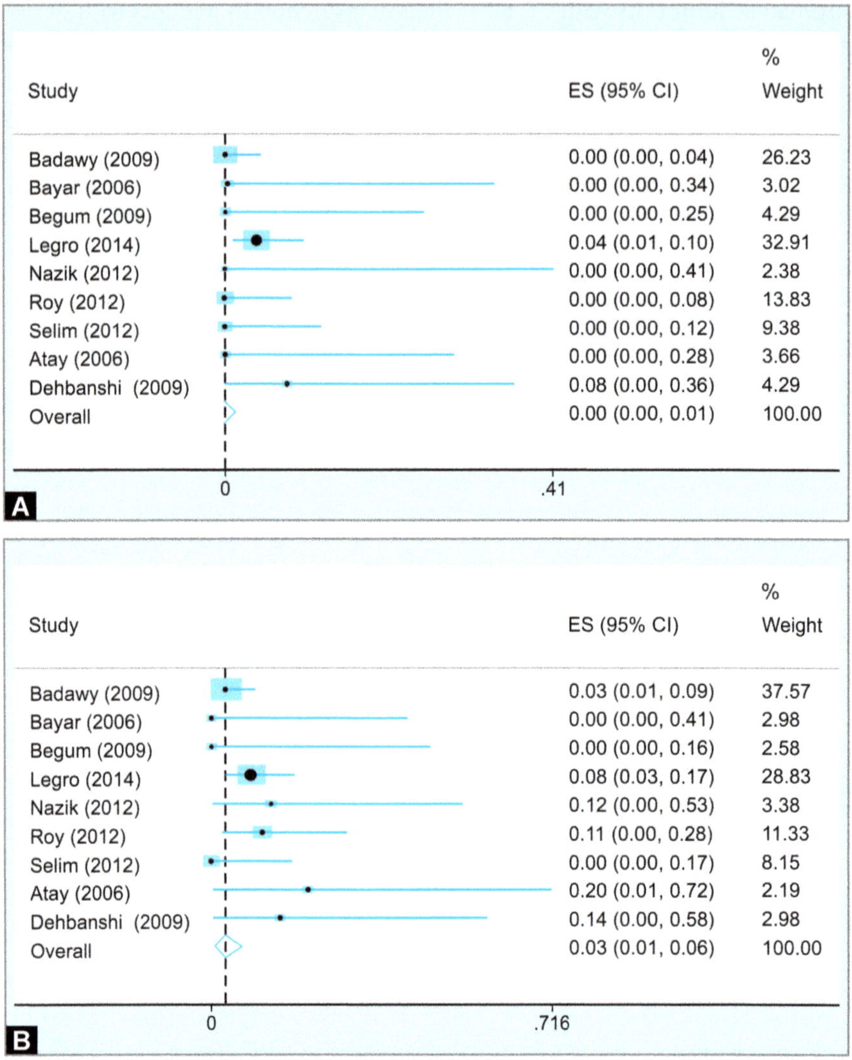

Figs. 15.9A and B: (A) Incidence of multiple pregnancy per pregnancy achieved with the use of aromatase inhibitors for ovulation induction in women with polycystic ovarian syndrome (PCOS); (B) Incidence of multiple pregnancy per pregnancy achieved with the use of clomiphene citrate (CC) for ovulation induction in women with PCOS.
(ES: Estimate; CI: Confidence interval).

between these two agents used for ovulation induction was not statistically significant [odds ratio (OR): 0.41, 95% CI: 0.17–1.01].[15]

Based on data reported in the meta-analysis by Weiss et al. (2015), comparing various types of gonadotropins for ovulation induction in women with PCOS and CC resistance or CC failure, the incidence of multiple pregnancy per woman treated with low-dose rFSH was 2% (95% CI: 1–3),[17] while that per pregnancy was 7% (95% CI: 3–12), (Figs. 15.10A and B). In addition,

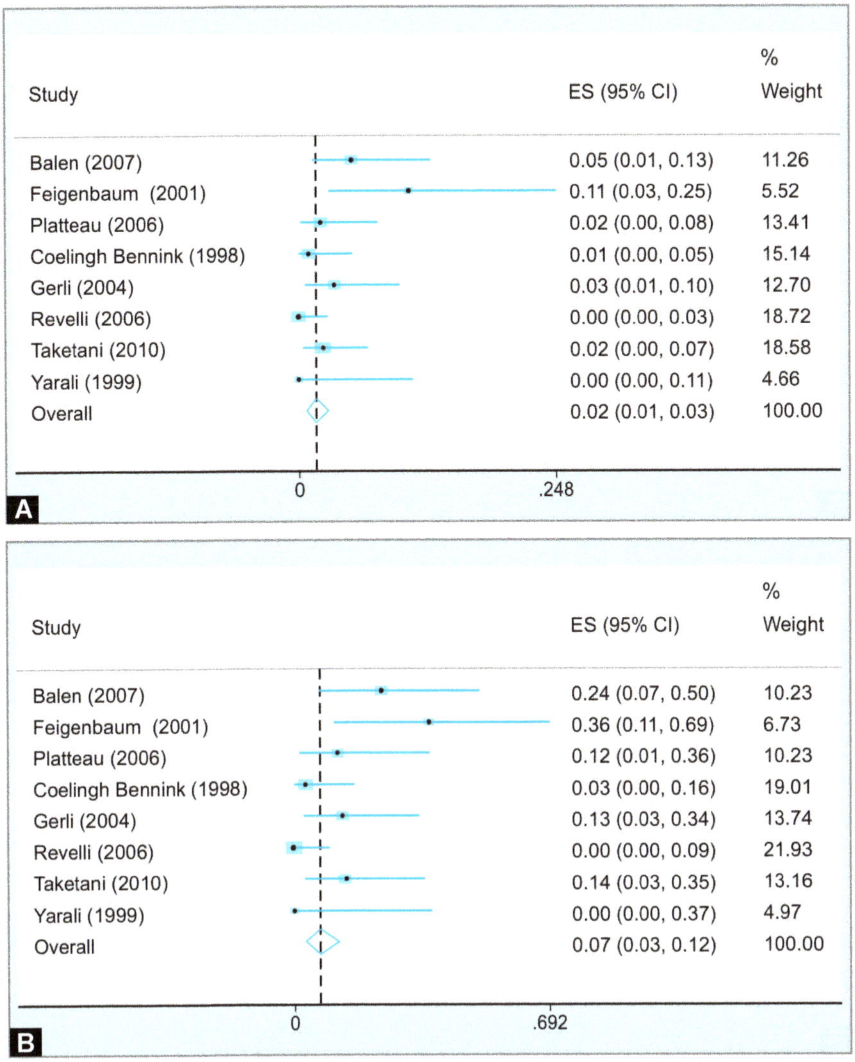

Figs. 15.10A and B: (A) Incidence of multiple pregnancy per woman treated with low-dose recombinant follicle-stimulating hormone (FSH) for ovulation induction in women with polycystic ovarian syndrome (PCOS); (B) Incidence of multiple pregnancy per pregnancy achieved with low-dose recombinant FSH for ovulation induction in women with PCOS. (ES: Estimate; CI: Confidence interval).

the incidence of multiple pregnancy per woman treated with urinary FSH was 2% (95% CI: 1–3),[17] while that per pregnancy was 9% (95% CI: 4–15) (Figs. 15.11A and B). No evidence of a difference in multiple pregnancy either per woman treated (OR: 0.86, 95% CI: 0.44–1.65) or per pregnancy (OR: 0.69, 95% CI: 0.33–1.43) was present between rFSH and urinary FSH.[17]

Based on data reported in a meta-analysis of RCTs comparing aromatase inhibitors with CC for enhancement of ovulation in women with unexplained

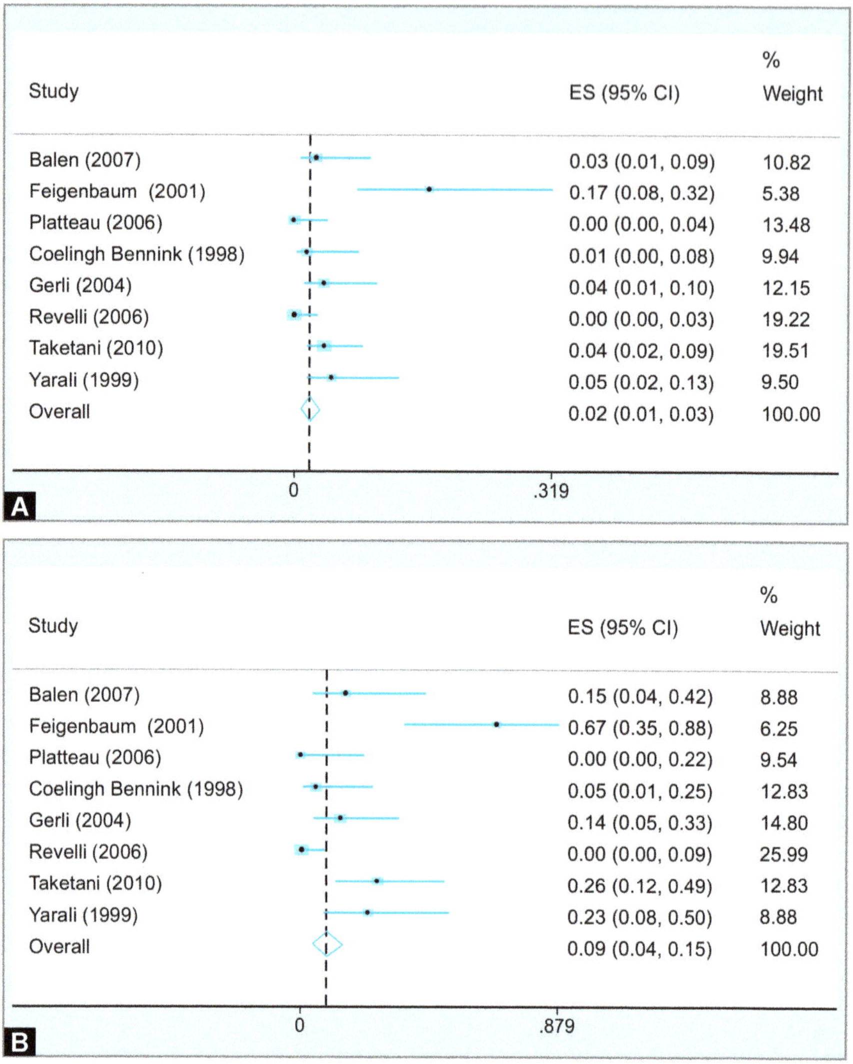

Figs. 15.11A and B: (A) Incidence of multiple pregnancy per woman treated with urinary follicle-stimulating hormone (FSH) for ovulation induction in women with polycystic ovarian syndrome (PCOS); (B) Incidence of multiple pregnancy per pregnancy achieved with urinary FSH for ovulation induction in women with PCOS.
(ES: Estimate; CI: Confidence interval).

infertility, the incidence of multiple pregnancy per woman treated with aromatase inhibitors was 1% (95% CI: 0–1) and that per pregnancy achieved was 2% (95% CI: 0–5) (Figs. 15.12A and B). The incidence of multiple pregnancy per woman treated with CC was 2% (95% CI: 1–3) and per pregnancy achieved 6% (95% CI: 3–11) (Figs. 15.13A and B).[18]

Based on data reported in a meta-analysis of RCTs employing ovarian stimulation with the use of gonadotropins for the treatment of women with

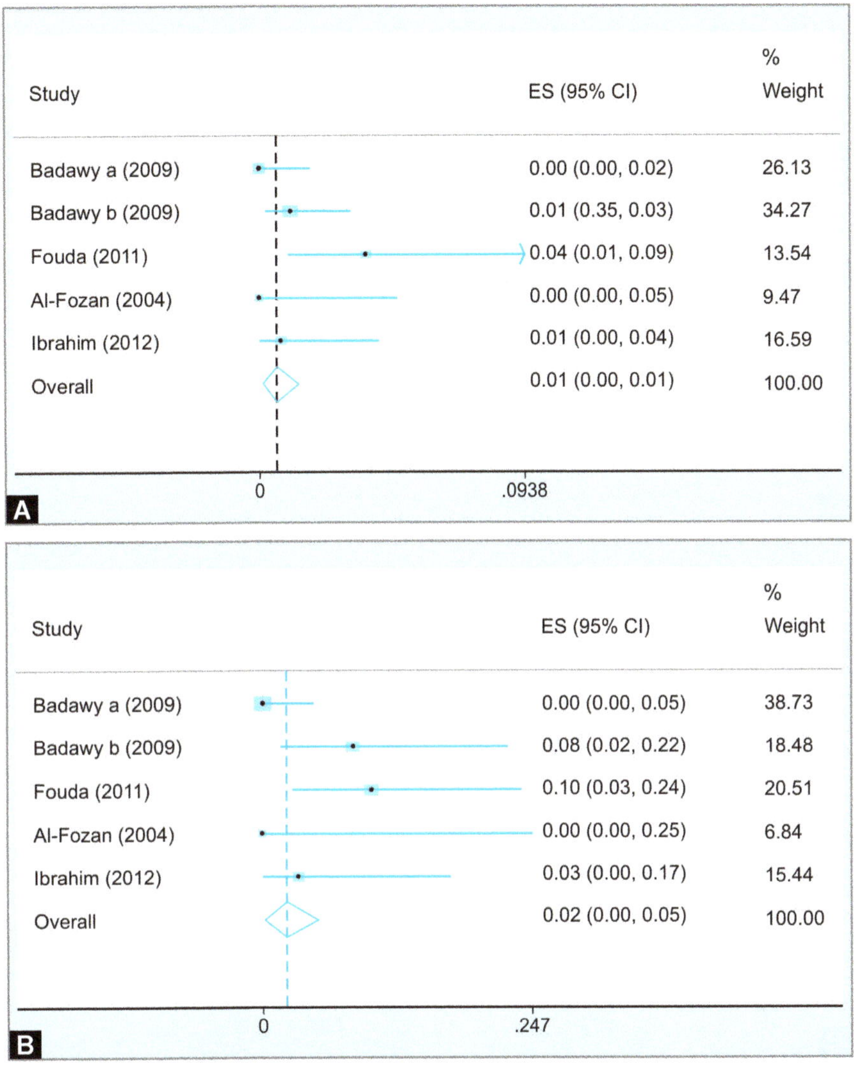

Figs. 15.12A and B: (A) Incidence of multiple pregnancy per woman treated with aromatase inhibitors for enhancement of ovulation in women with unexplained infertility; (B) Incidence of multiple pregnancy per pregnancy achieved with aromatase inhibitors for enhancement of ovulation in women with unexplained infertility.
(ES: Estimate; CI: Confidence interval).

unexplained infertility, male infertility or mild endometriosis, the incidence of multiple pregnancy was 4% (95% CI: 3–5) per women treated and 15% (95% CI: 11–19) per pregnancy achieved[19] (Figs. 15.14A and B). In the above studies, the estimated incidence of multiple pregnancy per woman treated without the use of GnRH analogs was 4% (95% CI: 3–6), while that per pregnancy achieved without the use of GnRH analogs was 13% (95% CI: 9–18) (Figs. 15.15A and B). In addition, the estimated incidence of multiple pregnancy per woman treated

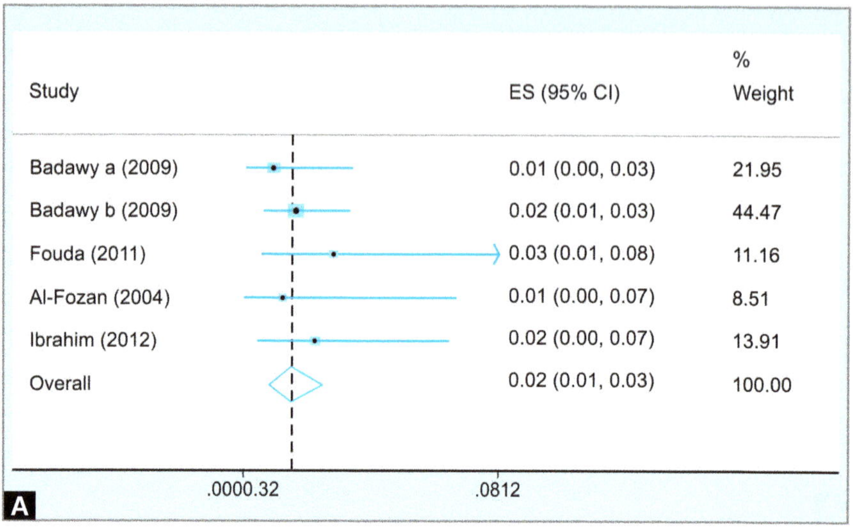

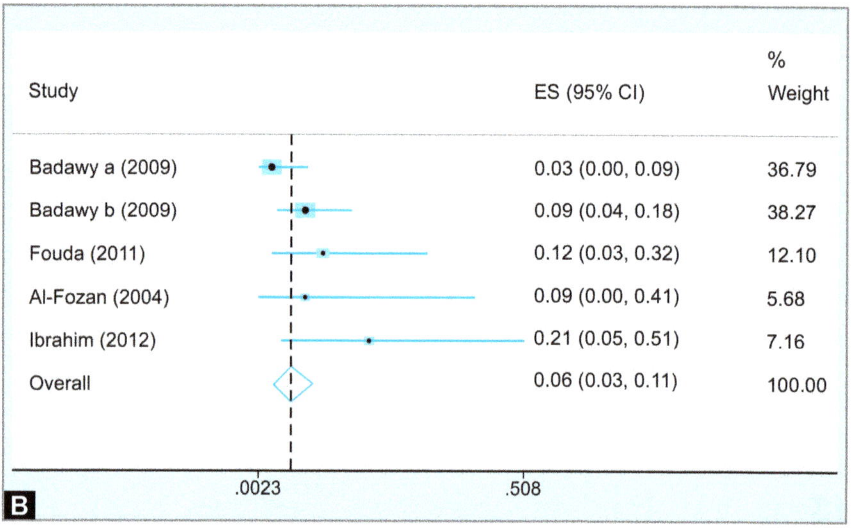

Figs. 15.13A and B: (A) Incidence of multiple pregnancy per woman treated with clomiphene citrate (CC) for enhancement of ovulation in women with unexplained infertility; (B) Incidence of multiple pregnancy per pregnancy achieved with CC for enhancement of ovulation in women with unexplained infertility.
(ES: Estimate; CI: Confidence interval).

with the use of GnRH agonist for inhibition of premature LH surge was 8% (95% CI: 4–12), while that per pregnancy achieved was 40% (95% CI: 25–55) (Figs. 15.15A and B). The estimated incidence of multiple pregnancy per woman treated with the use of GnRH antagonist was 1% (95% CI: 0–7), while that per pregnancy achieved was 7% (95% CI: 0–22) (Figs. 15.15A and B).

In order to reduce the risk of multiple births when high E2 levels and/or an excessive follicle number has developed following ovulation induction or enhancement of ovulation, cycle cancellation by withholding hCG or conversion of the cycle to IVF/embryo transfer should be considered. High E2 levels and numbers of follicles (E2 ≥1,500 pg/mL or >3 mature follicles) have been considered as warning signals for multiple gestation and could be used as indications for cycle cancellation or conversion to IVF.[23,58,59]

Multiple Pregnancy after Multi-follicular Development for In Vitro Fertilization

The chance of multiple pregnancy after IVF is dependent on the number of embryos transferred and their implantation potential. The transfer of fewer embryos of high implantation potential maintains the probability of pregnancy and dramatically reduces the incidence of multiple pregnancy.[55]

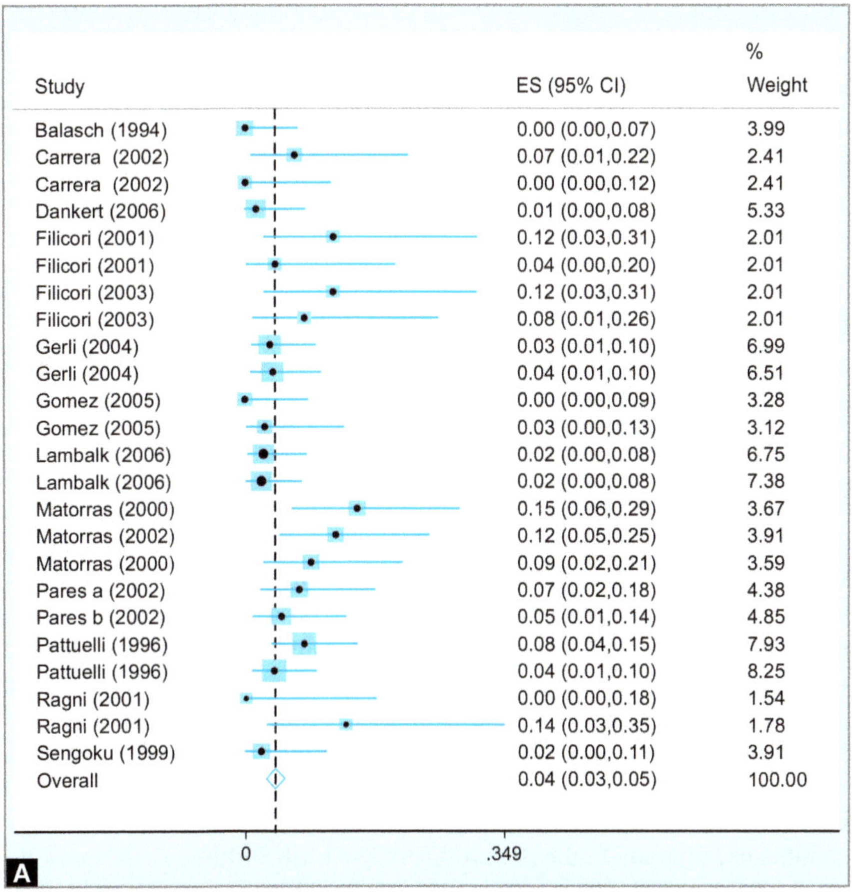

Fig. 15.14A: Incidence of multiple pregnancy per woman treated with the use of gonadotropins for the treatment of women with unexplained infertility.

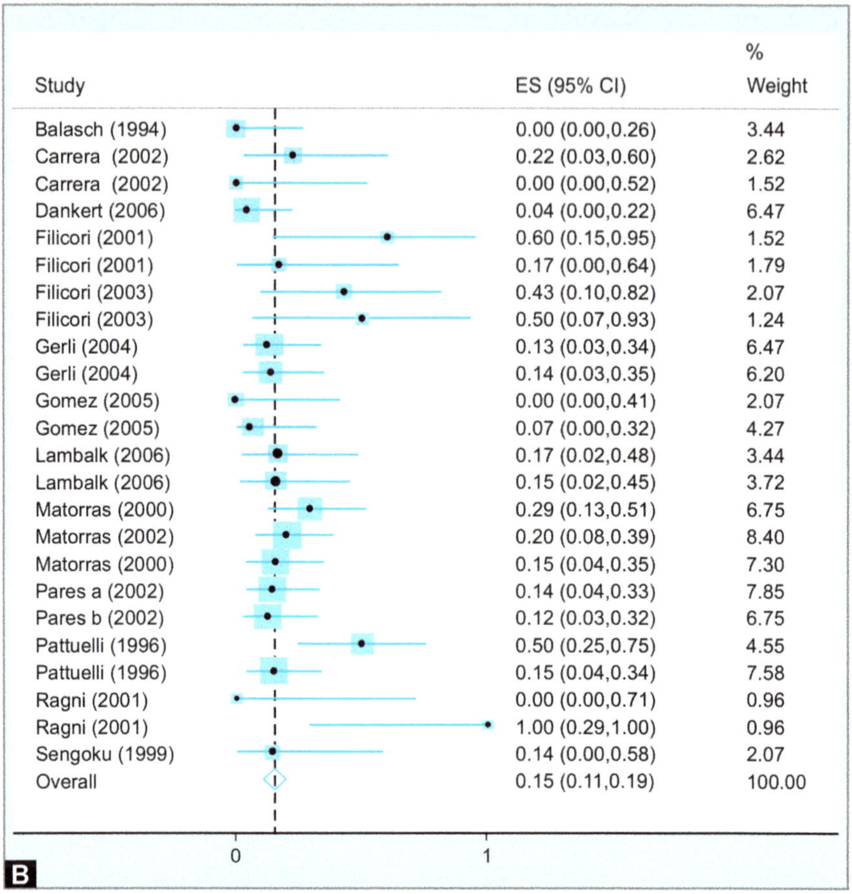

Fig. 15.14B: Incidence of multiple pregnancy per pregnancy achieved with the use of gonadotropins for the treatment of women with unexplained infertility.
(ES: Estimate; CI: Confidence interval).

Elective single embryo transfer has been widely accepted as a strategy eliminating the risk of twins particularly in young, good-prognosis women.[60,61] The principle of this policy is based on selecting a single embryo of the best morphological quality for transfer and freezing any additional embryos for replacement in subsequent cycles. Such a policy, however, appears to be associated with a decreased probability of pregnancy. In a systematic review and meta-analysis of studies performed in women less than 36 years old, it was shown that elective single embryo transfer compared with double embryo transfer was associated with a statistically significant reduction in the probability of live birth,[61] although the cumulative probability of live birth seems to be similar. This appears to be true even in women of advanced reproductive age.[62]

In Belgium, the application of a policy that restricts the number of embryos transferred, depending on the patient's age and treatment cycle resulted in reduction of multiple pregnancy rate from 29.1% to 9.5% in all patients and from 28.9% to 6.2% in women less than 36 years.[60] Despite the obvious advantages of single embryo transfer in eliminating multiple pregnancies, rates of single embryo transfer vary markedly across nations, with the highest reported in Sweden (69.4%) and the lowest in the USA (2.8%).[63]

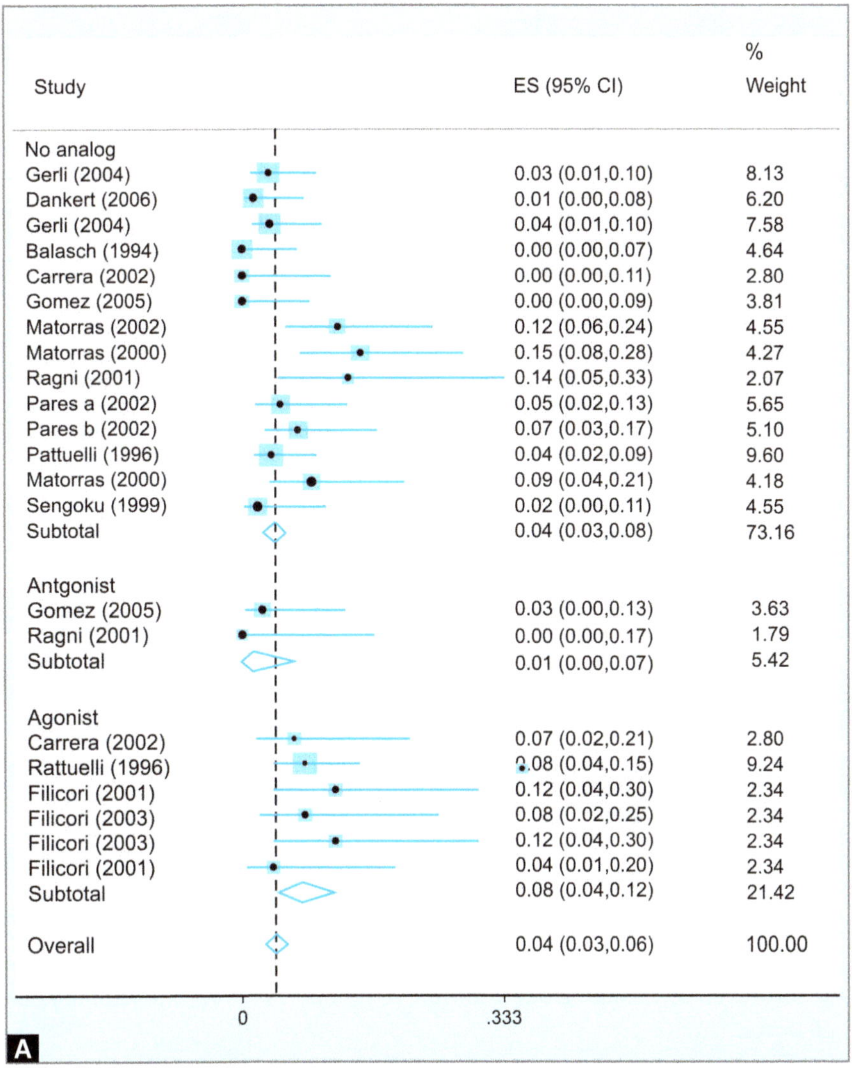

Fig. 15.15A: Incidence of multiple pregnancy per woman treated with follicle-stimulating hormone (FSH) without gonadotropin-releasing hormone (GnRH) analogs, with GnRH agonist or with GnRH antagonists.

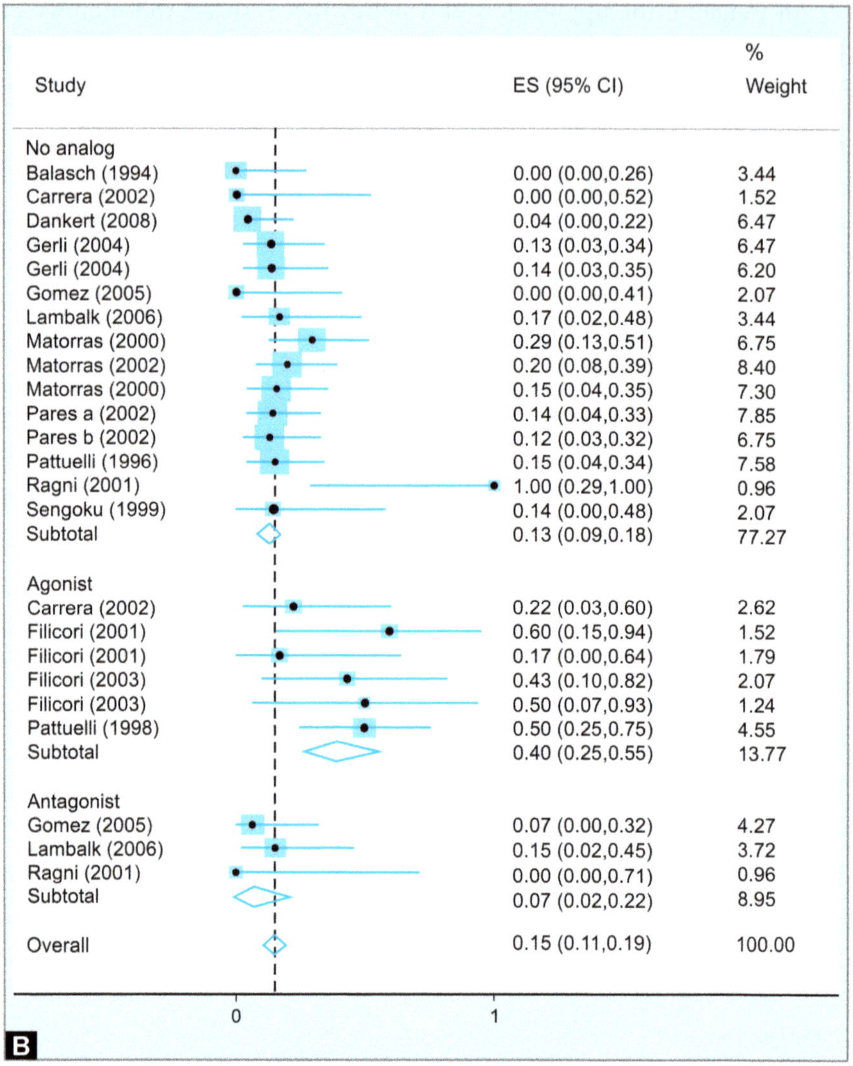

Fig. 15.15B: Incidence of multiple pregnancy per pregnancy achieved with the use of FSH without GnRH analogs, with GnRH agonist or with GnRH antagonists.
(ES: Estimate; CI: Confidence interval).

It should be noted that the transfer of multiple embryos is associated with an increase in the probability of pregnancy in women more than 40 years of age, however, in this age group multiple pregnancies (twins and triplets) can still occur.[64]

The use of preimplantation genetic screening (PGS) for selecting a single euploid blastocyst for transfer has been considered an important tool for eliminating multiple pregnancies and maintaining the probability of live birth particularly in patients of advanced reproductive age.[65,66] In a recent systematic review and meta-analysis, the use of comprehensive chromosome screening after blastocyst biopsy maintained similar ongoing pregnancy rates between PGS and control groups, while sharply decreasing multiple pregnancy rates.[67]

In the unfortunate case of triplets following embryo transfer, fetal reduction is considered as an appropriate management if ethical or religious issues are not present.[68-70] Fetal reduction was first described in the 1980s as a surgical procedure of selectively reducing the number of fetuses in an attempt to improve pregnancy outcomes by reducing the high adverse sequela of multiple pregnancies.[69] Although its benefits have been clearly shown for reduction of triplets to twins, it is still debatable whether the reduction of twins to singleton is justified.[69]

ADNEXAL TORSION

Acute abdominal pain, nausea, vomiting and ovarian enlargement at ultrasound are signs indicative of adnexal torsion. Following ovarian stimulation, cystic ovaries are predisposed to torsion,[5,71] the risk of which increases when ovarian stimulation is complicated with OHSS or leads to pregnancy.[71,72] In the first trimester of gestation following IVF, adnexal torsion should be suspected in all episodes of acute abdominal pain.[73,74]

The reported incidence of adnexal torsion in women who develop OHSS and do not achieve pregnancy is 2.3% (95% CI: 0.8–6.8), whereas in women who develop OHSS and achieve pregnancy the incidence increases to 16% (95% CI: 9.4–25.9).[75] In pregnant women who develop OHSS, ovarian cysts persist and this prolongs the period of increased risk for adnexal torsion.[72] In a series of 165 pregnant women who developed OHSS, the risk ratio for adnexal torsion was 3.7 (95% CI: 1.1–12.6) in twins as compared to singletons.[76]

It should be noted that history of adnexal torsion and the presence of multiple risk factors increase the probability of subsequent adnexal torsion.[77,78] The incidence of adnexal torsion recurrence is reported to be 19.5% (95% CI: 8.8–34.9) for pregnant and 9.1% (95% CI: 3.7–17.8) for nonpregnant women.[79]

Laparoscopy is a safe and effective first-line treatment for the management of adnexal torsion in both pregnant and nonpregnant women, minimizing postoperative discomfort and leading to shorter hospitalization.[80] However, special considerations should be present in pregnant women regarding the creation of pneumoperitoneum and the insertion of the Verres needle.[74]

Laparoscopic derotation of adnexal torsion is recommended even for ovaries which are already ischemic, since in 73% of cases it is sufficient to preserve ovarian function.[5] Unwinding of the affected adnexa is carried out by pushing the ovary contralaterally to the direction of the torsion using two blunt probes and if successful results in recoloration and disappearance of the congestion.[81] Complete absence of blood flow in the ovarian vessels has been suggested as an indication for adnexectomy.[74] Oophoropexy or shortening of utero-ovarian ligament have been advocated to avoid adnexal torsion recurrence.[5]

THROMBOEMBOLIC COMPLICATIONS

Thromboembolic complications both arterial and venous have been ascribed to the presence of OHSS, although they can also occur in its absence.[82] The exact mechanism by which OHSS creates a prothrombotic state is not clear.[83] However, high E2 concentrations, hemoconcentration after ovarian hyperstimulation as well as inherited thrombophilias are strongly hypothesized to be supportive of a hypercoagulable state, which induces the occurrence of thromboembolism.[6,84]

The development of thrombotic complications after ovarian stimulation is an infrequent event with an incidence for venous thrombosis ranging between 0.04% (95% CI: 0.01–0.11)[85] and 0.08% (95% CI: 0.01–0.29) per IVF cycle.[83] The incidence of arterial thrombosis is likely to be several times lower.[86] Women who develop arterial thrombosis are less often pregnant and have a lower rate of inherited thrombophilia, whereas those who develop venous thrombosis are more often pregnant and have underlying thrombophilic disorders.[86]

Prevention of thromboembolic complications involves administration of thromboprophylaxis in women at high risk, such as those who develop moderate-to-severe OHSS as well as in women with known thrombophilia, who undergo ovarian stimulation. For patients who develop moderate-to-severe OHSS, thromboprophylaxis should be initiated and be continued for a period of 4–8 weeks beyond resolution of OHSS.[86]

The management of thromboembolism requires appropriate therapy and adequate anticoagulation with close follow-up.[86] The use of aspirin, low molecular weight heparin (LMWH) and unfractionated heparin should be considered even when pregnancy is present and these patients would likely remain on therapeutic LMWH throughout pregnancy.[87]

REFERENCES

1. Kupka MS, D'Hooghe T, Ferraretti AP, et al. Assisted reproductive technology in Europe, 2011: results generated from European registers by ESHRE. Hum Reprod. 2016;31:233-48.
2. Birch Petersen K, Pedersen NG, Pedersen AT, et al. Mono-ovulation in women with polycystic ovary syndrome: a clinical review on ovulation induction. Reprod Biomed Online. 2016;32:563-83.
3. Abramov Y, Elchalal U, Schenker JG. Severe OHSS: An 'epidemic' of severe OHSS: a price we have to pay? Hum Reprod. 1999;14:2181-3.

4. Callahan TL, Hall JE, Ettner SL, et al. The economic impact of multiple-gestation pregnancies and the contribution of assisted-reproduction techniques to their incidence. N Engl J Med. 1994;331:244-9.
5. Spitzer D, Wirleitner B, Steiner H, et al. Adnexal torsion in pregnancy after assisted reproduction—case study and review of the literature. Geburtshilfe Frauenheilkd. 2012;72:716-20.
6. Stewart JA, Hamilton PJ, Murdoch AP. Thromboembolic disease associated with ovarian stimulation and assisted conception techniques. Hum Reprod. 1997;12:2167-73.
7. Mathur RS, Jenkins JM. Is ovarian hyperstimulation syndrome associated with a poor obstetric outcome? BJOG. 2000;107:943-6.
8. Fiedler K, Ezcurra D. Predicting and preventing ovarian hyperstimulation syndrome (OHSS): the need for individualized not standardized treatment. Reprod Biol Endocrinol. 2012;10:32.
9. Navot D, Bergh PA, Laufer N. Ovarian hyperstimulation syndrome in novel reproductive technologies: prevention and treatment. Fertil Steril. 1992;58: 249-61.
10. Mathur R, Jenkins J. Towards a clinically useful classification of OHSS. Reprod Biomed Online. 2009;19:434.
11. Randall JM, Templeton A. The effects of clomiphene citrate upon ovulation and endocrinology when administered to patients with unexplained infertility. Hum Reprod. 1991;6:659-64.
12. van Santbrink EJ, Eijkemans MJ, Laven JS, et al. Patient-tailored conventional ovulation induction algorithms in anovulatory infertility. Trends Endocrinol Metab. 2005;16:381-9.
13. Palomba S. Aromatase inhibitors for ovulation induction. J Clin Endocrinol Metab. 2015;100:1742-7.
14. Kar S. Clomiphene citrate or letrozole as first-line ovulation induction drug in infertile PCOS women: a prospective randomized trial. J Hum Reprod Sci. 2012;5:262-5.
15. Franik S, Kremer JA, Nelen WL, et al. Aromatase inhibitors for subfertile women with polycystic ovary syndrome. Cochrane Database Syst Rev. 2014;2: CD010287.
16. Melo AS, Ferriani RA, Navarro PA. Treatment of infertility in women with polycystic ovary syndrome: approach to clinical practice. Clinics (Sao Paulo). 2015;70:765-9.
17. Weiss NS, Nahuis M, Bayram N, et al. Gonadotrophins for ovulation induction in women with polycystic ovarian syndrome. Cochrane Database Syst Rev. 2015;9:CD010290.
18. Liu A, Zheng C, Lang J, et al. Letrozole versus clomiphene citrate for unexplained infertility: a systematic review and meta-analysis. J Obstet Gynaecol Res. 2014;40:1205-16.
19. Cantineau AE, Cohlen BJ, Heineman MJ. Ovarian stimulation protocols (anti-oestrogens, gonadotrophins with and without GnRH agonists/antagonists) for intrauterine insemination (IUI) in women with subfertility. Cochrane Database Syst Rev. 2011;2:CD005356.
20. Nisker J, Tummon I, Daniel S, et al. Conversion of cycles involving ovarian hyperstimulation with intra-uterine insemination to in-vitro fertilization. Hum Reprod. 1994;9:406-8.

21. Pasqualotto EB, Falcone T, Goldberg JM, et al. Risk factors for multiple gestation in women undergoing intrauterine insemination with ovarian stimulation. Fertil Steril. 1999;72:613-8.
22. Olufowobi O, Sharif K, Papaioannou S, et al. Role of rescue IVF-ET treatment in the management of high response in stimulated IUI cycles. J Obstet Gynaecol. 2005;25:166-8.
23. Antman AM, Politch JA, Ginsburg ES. Conversion of high-response gonadotropin intrauterine insemination cycles to in vitro fertilization results in excellent ongoing pregnancy rates. Fertil Steril. 2002;77:715-20.
24. Kawwass JF, Kissin DM, Kulkarni AD, et al. Safety of assisted reproductive technology in the United States, 2000-2011. JAMA. 2015;313:88-90.
25. Al-Inany HG, Youssef MA, Aboulghar M, et al. Gonadotrophin-releasing hormone antagonists for assisted reproductive technology. Cochrane Database Syst Rev. 2011;5:CD001750.
26. Tarlatzis BC, Griesinger G, Leader A, et al. Comparative incidence of ovarian hyperstimulation syndrome following ovarian stimulation with corifollitropin alfa or recombinant FSH. Reprod Biomed Online. 2012;24:410-9.
27. Griesinger G, Verweij PJ, Gates D, et al. Prediction of ovarian hyperstimulation syndrome in patients treated with corifollitropin alfa or rFSH in a GnRH antagonist protocol. PLoS One. 2016;11:e0149615.
28. Aboulghar MA, Mansour RT. Ovarian hyperstimulation syndrome: classifications and critical analysis of preventive measures. Hum Reprod Update. 2003;9:275-89.
29. Devroey P, Adriaensen P. OHSS Free Clinic. Facts Views Vis Obgyn. 2011;3:43-5.
30. Tarlatzis B, Bosdou J, Kolibianakis E. Elimination of OHSS by GnRH Agonist and Freezing Embryos. In: Rizk B, Gerris J (Eds). Complications and Outcomes of Assisted Reproduction. United Kingdom: Cambridge University Press; 2017. pp. 149-63. (In Press).
31. Humaidan P, Polyzos NP, Alsbjerg B, et al. GnRHa trigger and individualized luteal phase hCG support according to ovarian response to stimulation: two prospective randomized controlled multi-centre studies in IVF patients. Hum Reprod. 2013;28:2511-21.
32. Papanikolaou EG, Verpoest W, Fatemi H, et al. A novel method of luteal supplementation with recombinant luteinizing hormone when a gonadotropin-releasing hormone agonist is used instead of human chorionic gonadotropin for ovulation triggering: a randomized prospective proof of concept study. Fertil Steril. 2011;95:1174-7.
33. Decleer W, Osmanagaoglu K, Seynhave B, et al. Comparison of hCG triggering versus hCG in combination with a GnRH agonist: a prospective randomized controlled trial. Facts Views Vis Obgyn. 2014;6:203-9.
34. Pirard C, Donnez J, Loumaye E. GnRH agonist as luteal phase support in assisted reproduction technique cycles: results of a pilot study. Hum Reprod. 2006;21:1894-900.
35. Engmann L, DiLuigi A, Schmidt D, et al. The use of gonadotropin-releasing hormone (GnRH) agonist to induce oocyte maturation after cotreatment with GnRH antagonist in high-risk patients undergoing in vitro fertilization prevents the risk of ovarian hyperstimulation syndrome: a prospective randomized controlled study. Fertil Steril. 2008;89:84-91.
36. Lainas GT, Kolibianakis EM, Sfontouris IA, et al. Pregnancy and neonatal outcomes following luteal GnRH antagonist administration in patients with severe early OHSS. Hum Reprod. 2013;28:1929-42.

37. Lainas GT, Kolibianakis EM, Sfontouris IA, et al. Outpatient management of severe early OHSS by administration of GnRH antagonist in the luteal phase: an observational cohort study. Reprod Biol Endocrinol. 2012;10:69.
38. Griesinger G, Kolibianakis EM, Papanikolaou EG, et al. Triggering of final oocyte maturation with gonadotropin-releasing hormone agonist or human chorionic gonadotropin. Live birth after frozen-thawed embryo replacement cycles. Fertil Steril. 2007;88:616-21.
39. Bodri D, Guillen JJ, Galindo A, et al. Triggering with human chorionic gonadotropin or a gonadotropin-releasing hormone agonist in gonadotropin-releasing hormone antagonist-treated oocyte donor cycles: findings of a large retrospective cohort study. Fertil Steril. 2009;91:365-71.
40. Bodri D, Guillen JJ, Trullenque M, et al. Early ovarian hyperstimulation syndrome is completely prevented by gonadotropin releasing-hormone agonist triggering in high-risk oocyte donor cycles: a prospective, luteal-phase follow-up study. Fertil Steril. 2010;93:2418-20.
41. Castillo JC, Dolz M, Moreno J, et al. Triggering with GnRH agonist in oocyte-donation cycles: oestradiol monitoring is not necessary during ovarian stimulation. Reprod Biomed Online. 2012;24:247-50.
42. Hernandez ER, Gomez-Palomares JL, Ricciarelli E. No room for cancellation, coasting, or ovarian hyperstimulation syndrome in oocyte donation cycles. Fertil Steril. 2009;91:1358-61.
43. Acevedo B, Gomez-Palomares JL, Ricciarelli E, et al. Triggering ovulation with gonadotropin-releasing hormone agonists does not compromise embryo implantation rates. Fertil Steril. 2006;86:1682-7.
44. Galindo A, Bodri D, Guillen JJ, et al. Triggering with HCG or GnRH agonist in GnRH antagonist treated oocyte donation cycles: a randomised clinical trial. Gynecol Endocrinol. 2009;25:60-6.
45. Melo M, Busso CE, Bellver J, et al. GnRH agonist versus recombinant HCG in an oocyte donation programme: a randomized, prospective, controlled, assessor-blind study. Reprod Biomed Online. 2009;19:486-92.
46. Sismanoglu A, Tekin HI, Erden HF, et al. Ovulation triggering with GnRH agonist vs. hCG in the same egg donor population undergoing donor oocyte cycles with GnRH antagonist: a prospective randomized cross-over trial. J Assist Reprod Genet. 2009;26:251-6.
47. Griesinger G, Berndt H, Schultz L, et al. Intensified ovarian stimulation in a GnRH antagonist protocol with agonist triggering: a prospective, clinical feasibility study. Reprod Biomed Online. 2011;22:133-9.
48. Griesinger G, Schultz L, Bauer T, et al. Ovarian hyperstimulation syndrome prevention by gonadotropin-releasing hormone agonist triggering of final oocyte maturation in a gonadotropin-releasing hormone antagonist protocol in combination with a "freeze-all" strategy: a prospective multicentric study. Fertil Steril. 2011;95:2029-33, 33 e1.
49. Reddy J, Turan V, Bedoschi G, et al. Triggering final oocyte maturation with gonadotropin-releasing hormone agonist (GnRHa) versus human chorionic gonadotropin (hCG) in breast cancer patients undergoing fertility preservation: an extended experience. J Assist Reprod Genet. 2014;31:927-32.
50. Manzanares MA, Gomez-Palomares JL, Ricciarelli E, et al. Triggering ovulation with gonadotropin-releasing hormone agonist in in vitro fertilization patients with polycystic ovaries does not cause ovarian hyperstimulation syndrome despite very high estradiol levels. Fertil Steril. 2010;93:1215-9.

51. Practice Committee of the American Society for Reproductive Medicine. Electronic address: ASRM@asrm.org1; Practice Committee of the American Society for Reproductive Medicine. Prevention and treatment of moderate and severe ovarian hyperstimulation syndrome: a guideline. Fertil Steril. 2016;106: 1634-47.
52. RCOG. (2006). The Management of Ovarian Hyperstimulation Syndrome. Green-top Guideline No. 5. [online] Available from https://www.rcog.org.uk/globalassets/documents/guidelines/green-top-guidelines/gtg_5_ohss.pdf [accessed March, 2017].
53. Sebire NJ, Nicolaides KH. Screening for fetal abnormalities in multiple pregnancies. Baillieres Clin Obstet Gynaecol. 1998;12:19-36.
54. Scher AI, Petterson B, Blair E, et al. The risk of mortality or cerebral palsy in twins: a collaborative population-based study. Pediatr Res. 2002;52:671-81.
55. Fauser BC, Devroey P, Macklon NS. Multiple birth resulting from ovarian stimulation for subfertility treatment. Lancet. 2005;365:1807-16.
56. Farhi J, West C, Patel A, et al. Treatment of anovulatory infertility: the problem of multiple pregnancy. Hum Reprod. 1996;11:429-34.
57. Navot D, Goldstein N, Mor-Josef S, et al. Multiple pregnancies: risk factors and prognostic variables during induction of ovulation with human menopausal gonadotrophins. Hum Reprod. 1991;6:1152-5.
58. European Society of Human Reproduction and Embryology (ESHRE) Capri Workshop Group. Multiple gestation pregnancy. Hum Reprod. 2000;15: 1856-64.
59. Dickey RP. Strategies to reduce multiple pregnancies due to ovulation stimulation. Fertil Steril. 2009;91:1-17.
60. Van Landuyt L, Verheyen G, Tournaye H, et al. New Belgian embryo transfer policy leads to sharp decrease in multiple pregnancy rate. Reprod Biomed Online. 2006;13:765-71.
61. Gelbaya TA, Tsoumpou I, Nardo LG. The likelihood of live birth and multiple birth after single versus double embryo transfer at the cleavage stage: a systematic review and meta-analysis. Fertil Steril. 2010;94:936-45.
62. Fujimoto A, Morishima K, Harada M, et al. Elective single-embryo transfer improves cumulative pregnancy outcome in young patients but not in women of advanced reproductive age. J Assist Reprod Genet. 2015;32:1773-9.
63. Maheshwari A, Griffiths S, Bhattacharya S. Global variations in the uptake of single embryo transfer. Hum Reprod Update. 2011;17:107-20.
64. Klipstein S, Regan M, Ryley DA, et al. One last chance for pregnancy: a review of 2,705 in vitro fertilization cycles initiated in women age 40 years and above. Fertil Steril. 2005;84:435-45.
65. Yang Z, Liu J, Collins GS, et al. Selection of single blastocysts for fresh transfer via standard morphology assessment alone and with array CGH for good prognosis IVF patients: results from a randomized pilot study. Mol Cytogenet. 2012; 5:24.
66. Forman EJ, Hong KH, Ferry KM, et al. In vitro fertilization with single euploid blastocyst transfer: a randomized controlled trial. Fertil Steril. 2013;100:100-7 e1.
67. Dahdouh EM, Balayla J, Garcia-Velasco JA. Impact of blastocyst biopsy and comprehensive chromosome screening technology on preimplantation genetic screening: a systematic review of randomized controlled trials. Reprod Biomed Online. 2015;30:281-9.
68. Evans MI, Britt DW. Multifetal pregnancy reduction: evolution of the ethical arguments. Semin Reprod Med. 2010;28:295-302.

69. Evans MI, Andriole S, Britt DW. Fetal reduction: 25 years' experience. Fetal Diagn Ther. 2014;35:69-82.
70. Balasch J, Gratacos E. Delayed childbearing: effects on fertility and the outcome of pregnancy. Curr Opin Obstet Gynecol. 2012;24:187-93.
71. Rackow BW, Patrizio P. Successful pregnancy complicated by early and late adnexal torsion after in vitro fertilization. Fertil Steril. 2007;87:697 e9-12.
72. Gorkemli H, Camus M, Clasen K. Adnexal torsion after gonadotrophin ovulation induction for IVF or ICSI and its conservative treatment. Arch Gynecol Obstet. 2002;267:4-6.
73. Djakovic A, Honig A, Gross M, et al. Adnexal torsion in a patient with bichorial twin pregnancy in the 21st week of gestation treated by open laparoscopy: a case report. Arch Gynecol Obstet. 2006;274:248-9.
74. Arena S, Canonico S, Luzi G, et al. Ovarian torsion in in vitro fertilization-induced twin pregnancy: combination of Doppler ultrasound and laparoscopy in diagnosis and treatment can quickly solve the case. Fertil Steril. 2009;92: 1496 e9-13.
75. Mashiach S, Bider D, Moran O, et al. Adnexal torsion of hyperstimulated ovaries in pregnancies after gonadotropin therapy. Fertil Steril. 1990;53: 76-80.
76. Wiser A, Levron J, Kreizer D, et al. Outcome of pregnancies complicated by severe ovarian hyperstimulation syndrome (OHSS): a follow-up beyond the second trimester. Hum Reprod. 2005;20:910-4.
77. Weitzman VN, DiLuigi AJ, Maier DB, et al. Prevention of recurrent adnexal torsion. Fertil Steril. 2008;90:2018. e1-3.
78. Djavadian D, Braendle W, Jaenicke F. Laparoscopic oophoropexy for the treatment of recurrent torsion of the adnexa in pregnancy: case report and review. Fertil Steril. 2004;82:933-6.
79. Hasson J, Tsafrir Z, Azem F, et al. Comparison of adnexal torsion between pregnant and nonpregnant women. Am J Obstet Gynecol. 2010;202:536. e1-6.
80. Ko ML, Lai TH, Chen SC. Laparoscopic management of complicated adnexal masses in the first trimester of pregnancy. Fertil Steril. 2009;92:283-7.
81. Bassil S, Steinhart U, Donnez J. Successful laparoscopic management of adnexal torsion during week 25 of a twin pregnancy. Hum Reprod. 1999;14(3):855-7.
82. Whelan JG 3rd, Vlahos NF. The ovarian hyperstimulation syndrome. Fertil Steril. 2000;73:883-96.
83. Chan WS, Ginsberg JS. A review of upper extremity deep vein thrombosis in pregnancy: unmasking the 'ART' behind the clot. J Thromb Haemost. 2006;4:1673-7.
84. Ou YC, Kao YL, Lai SL, et al. Thromboembolism after ovarian stimulation: successful management of a woman with superior sagittal sinus thrombosis after IVF and embryo transfer: case report. Hum Reprod. 2003;18:2375-81.
85. Arya R, Shehata HA, Patel RK, et al. Internal jugular vein thrombosis after assisted conception therapy. Br J Haematol. 2001;115:153-5.
86. Chan WS. The 'ART' of thrombosis: a review of arterial and venous thrombosis in assisted reproductive technology. Curr Opin Obstet Gynecol. 2009;21: 207-18.
87. Bates SM, Greer IA, Hirsh J, et al. Use of antithrombotic agents during pregnancy: the Seventh ACCP Conference on Antithrombotic and Thrombolytic Therapy. Chest. 2004;126:627S-44S.

INDEX

Note: Page numbers followed by *f* refer to figure, *t* refer to table.

EU GSPR Authorised Reprsentative
Logos Europe, 9 rue Nicolas Poussin
1700, La Rochelle, France
Phone: +33 (0) 6 67 93 73 78
E-mail: contact@logoseurope.eu

www.ingramcontent.com/pod-product-compliance
Ingram Content Group UK Ltd.
Pitfield, Milton Keynes, MK11 3LW, UK
UKHW051917100926
8556IPUK00021B/1223
9789352700608